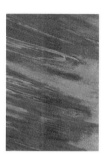

RESPIRATORY CARE EXAM REVIEW
Review for the Entry Level and Advanced Exams

Gary Persing, BS, RRT
Director of Clinical Education
Respiratory Therapy Program
Tulsa Community College
Tulsa, Oklahoma

W.B. SAUNDERS COMPANY
A Harcourt Health Sciences Company
Philadelphia   London   New York   St. Louis   Sydney   Toronto

W.B. SAUNDERS COMPANY
A Harcourt Health Sciences Company

The Curtis Center
Independence Square West
Philadelphia, Pennsylvania 19106

Acquistions Editor: Karen Fabiano
Developmental Editor: Mindy Copeland
Project Manager: Catherine Albright Jackson
Production Editor: Jodi Everding
Designer: Judi Lang
Cover Art: Judi Lang

NOTICE

Pharmacology is an ever-changing field. Standard safety precautions must be followed, but as new research and clinical experience broaden our knowledge, changes in treatment and drug therapy may become necessary or appropriate. Readers are advised to check the most current product information provided by the manufacturer of each drug to be administered to verify the recommended dose, the method and duration of administration, and contraindications. It is the responsibility of the treating physician, relying on experience and knowledge of the patient, to determine dosages and the best treatment for each individual patient. Neither the publisher nor the editor assumes any liability for any injury and/or damage to persons or property arising from this publication.

RESPIRATORY CARE EXAM REVIEW: ISBN 0-7216-8288-X
Review for the Entry Level and Advanced Exams

Printed in the United States of America

Last digit is the print number   9 8 7 6 5 4 3 2 1

This book is dedicated to Debbie, Lindsey, my mom and dad, Sundance, Greta, Abby, and most of all to Jesus Christ for His direction and wonderful "amazing grace."

Preface

One of the most satisfying accomplishments that may be achieved by respiratory care practitioners is the successful completion of the Entry Level Certification Exam and/or the Advanced Practitioner Written Registry/Clinical Simulation Exam offered by the National Board for Respiratory Care (NBRC). The credential of Certified Respiratory Therapist (CRT) is awarded to individuals with a score of 75% or higher on the 140-question CRT exam. Individuals attempting to obtain the credential of Registered Respiratory Therapist (RRT) must first be a CRT then score 70% or higher on the 100-question Written Registry exam, as well as successfully complete the Clinical Simulation exam, which consists of 10 simulations.

The purpose of this text is to prepare you to successfully complete both the CRT and RRT exams. The NBRC provides a test matrix that indicates the areas tested on these exams. This matrix was used as a guideline for the material in this text to better prepare you for these exams. Because the NBRC exams may exclude more current types of therapy or equipment, the clinical practices reflected in this book are not necessarily the most current in your region.

This textbook and CD-ROM contain more than 800 questions, both multiple-choice questions and open-ended questions. Each chapter begins with a pretest comprising several multiple-choice questions formatted like those found on the NBRC exams. After having completed the pretest, study the chapter and then answer the open-ended post-chapter study questions. If you have to return to the chapter to find the answers to some of the questions, don't be discouraged. By going back through the chapter and recording your answers on the post-chapter questions, you are reinforcing the information that will help you to retain the material. The answers to the pretest and post-chapter questions are on the last page of each chapter.

In each chapter, I have designated material that is exclusive to either the Entry Level exam or the Written Registry exam. This material is provided in boxes labeled "Exam Note." As you go through the book, you will notice that the majority of material will be found on both exams. Unless I have specifically stated that the material is exclusive to one exam, you should assume that the material may appear on both the CRT and RRT exams.

The major difference between the exams is that more "analysis" questions are asked on the RRT exam than on the CRT exam, while more "application" questions are asked on the CRT exam. There are also more "recall" questions on the CRT exam, which require less of an understanding of the material. (See the explanation for these three types of questions in the "Answer Key/Explanation" section.)

Over 70% of the Written Registry exam is composed of analysis questions, while only about 25% of the questions in the CRT exam fall into this category. Over half of the questions on the CRT exam are application questions.

You will also notice that some material has a star next to it or is typed in bold print. The star or bold print indicates especially important material that is commonly seen on the exams and should be reviewed thoroughly.

Following the chapters is a 140-question Entry Level Certification Practice Exam and a 100-question Advanced Practitioner Written Registry Practice Exam. I have tried to make these exams as close to the actual NBRC exams as possible so you will better know what to expect. At the end of each exam is the "Answer Key/Explanation" section that reveals the correct answer for each question and a detailed explanation for why the choice is correct. Also included is the complexity level of each question, which is described in more detail on the explanation page.

In addition to the Entry Level and Advanced Practitioner practice exams in the book, an example of each exam is also on the CD-ROM accompanying the text. The addition of these exams reflects the NBRC's move to computerized testing.

The CD-ROM also includes six clinical simulations. The simulations are written and developed in form and content to reflect those presented on the NBRC exam. Even if you are only preparing for the CRT exam the simulations are good practice and beneficial preparation.

When you take these practice exams, find a quiet place and give yourself the appropriate time allotted for each exam. Take the exam as if it were the actual exam. This will give you an idea of how to pace yourself when you take the "real thing." After taking the exam, pay close attention to your areas of strength and weakness. Return to the study guide chapters for further study, focusing more on your weak areas.

Proper preparation is essential to passing the NBRC exams. The NBRC provides excellent material to help you study for the credentialing exams. I highly recommend their self-assessment exams and practice clinical simulations and am sure you will find them very helpful. Over the course of your education in the field of respiratory care, you have surely accumulated many excellent textbooks and notes that are invaluable to your exam preparation. In this text, I have attempted to summarize, in a comprehensive and understandable way, the most important material necessary for you to understand in order to pass the NBRC registry exams. It is my sincere hope that whether you are preparing for the CRT or are already certified and working toward your RRT, this textbook will be beneficial to your preparation for the NBRC exams and you will be awarded the credential of Certified Respiratory Therapist or Registered Respiratory Therapist—whichever you are striving to achieve.

Gary Persing, BS, RRT

Acknowledgments

A special thanks goes to Andrew Allen for his ideas on the update of this book, Sue Hontscharik for her kindness and patience while answering all my questions, and Karen Fabiano and Mindy Copeland for their help during a time of transition. You have all made this a wonderful experience for me.

I especially want to thank Dennis Holland, Terry Krider, Robert Langenderfer, and Sharon McGenity-Hatfield for reviewing the material in this text. Your expertise and insight added greatly to the production of this book. I learned from each of you, and I am truly grateful.

Contents

ACRONYM LIST

2, 3–DPG	diphosphoglycerate
ABG	arterial blood gas
ADH	antidiuretic hormone
AGA	appropriate for gestational age
AIDS	acquired immunodeficiency syndrome
AMP	adenosine monophosphate
AP	anteroposterior
ARDS	acute respiratory distress syndrome
ASSS	American Standard Safety System
atm	atmosphere
AV	atrioventricular
BD	base deficit
BE	base excess
Bi-PAP	bilevel positive airway pressure
BPD	bronchopulmonary dysplasia
BSA	body surface area
BTPS	body temp and pressure saturation correction factor
$C(a-v)O_2$	arterial − venous oxygen content difference
CAD	coronary artery disease
CaO_2	total oxygen content of arterial
CCU	coronary care unit
CDC	Centers for Disease Control and Prevention
CGA	Compressed Gas Association
$CH_2=CH_2$	ethylene
CHF	congestive heart failure
CI	cardiac index
C_L	lung compliance
Cl	chloride continuous mechanical ventilation
CNS	central nervous system
CO	carbon monoxide
CO_2	carbon dioxide
COPD	chronic obstructive pulmonary disease
CPAP	continuous positive airway pressure
CPR	cardiopulmonary resuscitation
CPT	chest physical therapy
CVO_2	total oxygen content of mixed venous blood
CVP	central venous pressure
DIC	disseminated intravascular coagulation
DISS	Diameter Index Safety System
DKA	diabetic ketoacidosis
D_L	diffusion capacity of the lung
D_{LCO}	carbon monoxide diffusion capacity
ECF	Aeosinophilic chemotactic factor of anaphylaxis
ECG	electrocardiography, -phic, -gram
ECMO	extracorporeal membrane oxygenation
EEG	electroencephalogram, -phic, -phy
EMD	electromechanical dissociation
EOA	esophageal obturator airway
EPAP	expiratory positive airway pressure
ERV	expiratory reserve volume
ET	endotracheal
ETC	esophageal tracheal combitube
$FeCO_2$	fractional concentration of CO_2 in expired gas
$FEF_{200-1200}$	forced expiratory flow after first 200 mL
$FEF_{25\%-75\%}$	forced expiratory flow, mid-expiratory phase
FEO_2	fractional concentration of O_2 in expired gas
FET	forced expiratory technique
$FEV_{0.5}$	forced expiratory volume in 0.5 sec
FEV_1	forced expiratory volume in 1 sec
FEV_3	forced expiratory volume in 3 sec
FIO_2	fractional insired O_2 concentration
FRC	functional residual capacity
FVC	forced vital capacity
GI	gastrointestional
H_2CO_3	carbonic acid
Hb	hemoglobin
HbCO	carboxyhemoglobin
HBO	hyperbaric oxygen
HbO_2	oxyhemoglobin
HCO_3^-	bicarbonate
He	helium
HEPA	high-efficiency particulate air (filter)
HFJV	high-frequency jet ventilation
HFO	high-frequency oscillation
HFPPV	high-frequency positive pressure ventilation
HHN	handheld nebulizer
HMD	hyaline membrane disease
HME	heat moisture exchanger
Hz	hertz (cycles per second)
I/E	inspiratory to expiratory (ratio)
IC	inspiratory capacity
ICP	intracranial pressure
ICU	intensive care unit
ID	internal diameter
ILV	independent lung ventilation
IMV	intermittent mandatory ventilation
IPAP	inspiratory positive airway pressure
IPPB	intermittent positive pressure breathing
IRV	inspiratory reserve volume
IT	implantation tested
IV	intravenous
J	joules
K	potassium
L:S	lecithin-sphingomyelin (ratio)
LGA	large for gestational age
LMA	laryngeal mask airway
LVF	left ventricular failure
Mc	megacycle
MDI	metered-dose inhaler
MEP	maximum expiratory pressure
MI	myocardioal infarction
MIP	maximal inspiratory pressure
MPAP	mean pulmonary artery pressure
MSAP	mean systemic arterial pressure
MVV	maximum voluntary ventilation
Na	sodium
NaCl	sodium chloride
$NaHCO_3^-$	sodium bicarbonate
NG	nasogastric
NIF	negative inspiratory force
NO	nitrous oxide

O_2	oxygen
OD	outside diameter
P $(A-a)O_2$	alveolar-arterial oxygen pressure difference
PAC	premature atrial contraction
$PaCo_2$	partial pressure of carbon dioxide, arterial
Pao_2	partial pressure of oxygen, arterial
PAP	pulmonary artery pressure
Paw	mean airway pressure
PAWP	pulmonary artery wedge pressure
PB	barometric pressure
PCP	*Pneumocystis carinii* pneumonia
PCV	pressure-control ventilation
PCWP	pulmonary capillary wedge pressure
PDA	patent ductus arteriosus
PE	pulmonary embolism
PEEP	positive end-expiratory pressure
PEF	peak expiratory flow
PEP	positive expiratory pressure
$PETCo_2$	end-tidal carbon dioxide tension
PFC	persistent fetal circulation
PIP	peak inspiratory pressure
PISS	Pin Index Safety System
Pk	dissociation constant (6.1)
PPHN	persistent pulmonary hypertension of the neonate
PROM	premature rupture of membranes
psi	pounds per square inch
psig	pounds per square inch, gauge
PSV	pressure support ventilation
PT	prothrombin time
PTL	pharyngotracheal lumen (airway)
PTT	partial thromboplastin time
PVC	premature ventricular contractions
Pvo_2	partial pressure of oxygen, mixed venous blood
PVR	pulmonary vascular resistance
QS	shunted blood
QT	cardiac output (L/min)
Raw	airway resistance
RBC	red blood cell
RCP	respiratory care practitioner
RDS	respiratory distress syndrome
REE	resting energy expenditure (rate)
RLF	retrolental fibroplasia
RQ	respiratory quotient
RR	respiratory rate
RRT	registered respiratory therapist
RSV	respiratory syncytial virus
RV	residual volume
SA	sinoatrial
Sao_2	hemoglobin saturation with oxygen, arterial blood
SGA	small for gestational age
SIDS	sudden infant death syndrome
SIMV	synchronized intermittent mandatory ventilation
SPAG	small particle aerosol generator (nebulizer)
Spo_2	pulse oximetry
SRS	A slow-reacting substance of anaphylaxis
SV	stroke volume
Svo_2	hemoglobin saturation with oxygen mixed venous blood
SVR	systemic vascular resistance
TB	tuberculosis
$TcPo_2$	transcutaneous Po_2
TDP	therapist-driven protocol
TLC	total lung capacity
UAC	unbilical artery catheter
USN	ultrasonic nebulizer
V/Q	ventilation/perfusion (ratio)
VC	vital capacity
Vco_2	carbon dioxide production
V_{DS}	dead space volume
$\dot{V}_A$	alveolar minute volume
$\dot{V}_E$	minute volume
$\dot{V}o_2$	oxygen consumption per unit of time
V_T	tidal volume
VTG	thoracic gas volume
WBC	white blood cell
μm	micrometer (preferred over micron)

Chapter 1

Oxygen and Medical Gas Therapy

Answer the pre-test questions before studying the chapter. This will help you determine your strong and weak areas regarding the material covered.

1. A patient is receiving oxygen from an "E" cylinder at 4 L/min through a nasal cannula. The cylinder pressure is 1900 psig. How long will the cylinder run until it is empty?

   A. 47 minutes
   B. 1.7 hours
   C. 2.2 hours
   D. 3.6 hours

2. After setting up a partial rebreathing mask on a patient at a flow of 8 L/min, the reservoir bag collapses before the patient finishes inspiring. The respiratory care practitioner should do which of the following?

   A. Change to a 6 L/min nasal cannula.
   B. Decrease the flow.
   C. Change to a non-rebreathing mask.
   D. Increase the flow.

3. A patient with CO poisoning can best be treated with which of the following therapies?

   A. Nasal cannula at 6 L/min
   B. Hyperbaric O_2
   C. CPAP
   D. Non-rebreathing mask

4. The following blood gases have been obtained from a patient on a 60% aerosol mask.

pH	7.47
$PaCO_2$	31 mm Hg
PaO_2	58 mm Hg

   What should the respiratory care practitioner recommend at this time?

   A. Place the patient on CPAP.
   B. Place the patient on a 70% aerosol mask.
   C. Intubate and place the patient on mechanical ventilation.
   D. Place the patient on a non-rebreathing mask.

5. Given the following data, what is the patient's total arterial O_2 content?

pH	7.41
$PaCO_2$	37 mm Hg
PaO_2	88 mm Hg
HCO_3^-	26 mEq/L
SaO_2	95%
Hb	14 g/dL

   A. 12 vol%
   B. 14 vol%
   C. 16 vol%
   D. 18 vol%

6. A patient is on a 30% Venturi mask at an O_2 flow of 5 L/min. The total flow delivered by this device is which of the following?

   A. 36 L/min
   B. 45 L/min
   C. 54 L/min
   D. 60 L/min

Answers are at the end of the chapter.

★ I. STORAGE AND CONTROL OF MEDICAL GASES
   A. Storage of medical gases and cylinder characteristics
      1. Cylinders are constructed of chrome molybdenum steel.
      2. Gas cylinders are stored at high pressures; a full O_2 cylinder contains 2200 psig pressure.
      3. Cylinders are constructed in various sizes. The most common sizes for O_2 storage are the "H" cylinder and the "E" cylinder.
         a. The "H" cylinder holds 244 cu ft (6900 L) of O_2.

b. The "E" cylinder, used for transport, holds 22 cu ft (622 L) of O_2.

Note

There are 28.3 L in 1 cu ft.

---

4. Valves on the cylinder allow attachment of regulators that release the gas at various flow rates. The valves are constructed to allow the connection of only one type of gas regulator. For example, an O_2 regulator will not attach to a helium cylinder because of these cylinder and regulator safety systems.
   a. Large cylinders use the American Standard Safety System. Each type of gas cylinder valve has a different number of threads per inch and thread size, and the cylinder may require either a right or left hand turning motion for attachment to the regulator.
   b. Small cylinders use the Pin Index Safety System. Each cylinder valve has two holes drilled in unique positions that line up with corresponding pins on the appropriate regulator. There are six different hole placement positions.
5. Safety relief devices on cylinder valves allow escape of excess gas if the pressure in the cylinder increases. There are two types of safety relief devices.
   a. Frangible disk, which breaks at 3000 psig
   b. Fusible plug, which melts at 170°F
6. The CGA developed a color code system for gas cylinders that identifies the type of gas.

Type of Gas	Color of Cylinder
O_2	Green
O_2	White (international color code)
Helium	Brown
CO_2	Gray
NO	Light Blue
Cyclopropane	Orange
Ethylene	Red
Air	Yellow
CO_2/O_2	Gray shoulder and green body
Helium/O_2	Brown shoulder and green body

7. Cylinder markings
8. Cylinder testing
   a. Cylinders are visually tested by lowering a light bulb inside to look for corrosion.
   b. Cylinders are hydrostatically tested every 5 or 10 years, depending on the cylinder marking. A "star" next to the latest test date means the next test must be done 10 years

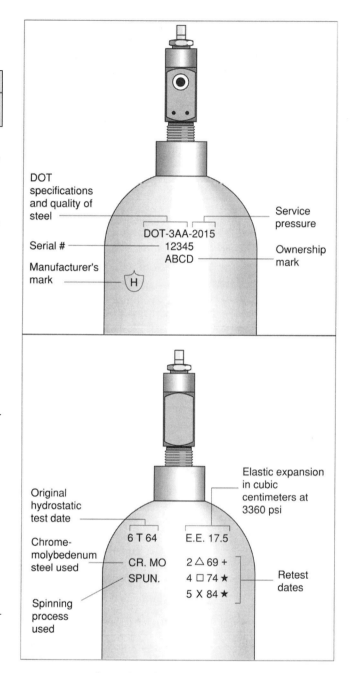

from that date. Hydrostatic testing determines the amount of:
   (1) Wall stress
   (2) Cylinder expansion
   (3) Leaks
9. Liquid gas systems
   a. One cubic foot of liquid O_2 expands to 860 cu ft as it changes to a gas. Liquid O_2 is much more economical than gas.
   b. The liquid O_2 is stored in Thermos containers at a pressure not to exceed 250 psig and a temperature below −297°F (the boiling point of O_2).
★ c. Liquid O_2 is most commonly produced by the process of fractional distillation.

★ B. Control of Medical Gases
   1. Regulators are devices attached to the cylinder valve to regulate flow and reduce cylinder pressure to working pressure (i.e., 50 psig).
   2. Types of reducing valves
      a. Single-stage, which reduces the cylinder pressure directly to 50 psig and has one safety relief device
      b. Double-stage, which reduces the cylinder pressure to approximately 150 psig, and then to 50 psig, and has two safety relief devices
      c. Triple-stage, which reduces the cylinder pressure to approximately 300 psig, then to 150 psig, and finally to 50 psig and has three safety relief devices

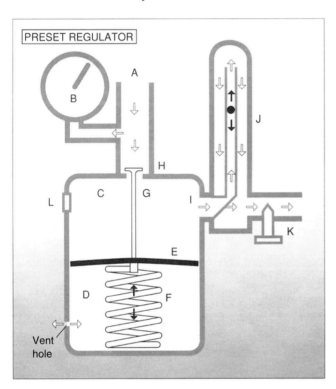

PRESET REGULATOR

pressure drops in the pressure chamber, the diaphragm assembly moves upward, allowing gas to enter the chamber again. In fact, the diaphragm assembly moves continually up and down, opening and closing the valve repeatedly, as gas passes through the chamber flowmeter (*J*) and needle valve (*K*). Excessive pressure in the pressure chamber is vented through a pressure relief valve (*L*). The spring tension on this regulator is preset at 50 psig.
      b. Adjustable regulator

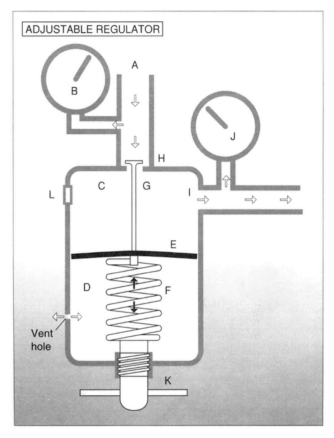

ADJUSTABLE REGULATOR

   3. Regulators may be preset or adjustable.
      a. Mechanics of a preset regulator
         Gas under high pressure from the cylinder enters the inlet (*A*) of the reducing valve where cylinder pressure is read on the Bourdon gauge (*B*). Gas then passes through the inlet valve (*H*) into the pressure chamber (*C*) and pushes down on the diaphragm (*E*), spring (*F*), and valve stem (*G*) assembly, closing the valve and cutting off gas flow into the pressure chamber. At the moment the valve closes, the gas pressure is equal to the spring pressure in the ambient chamber (*D*). Then, as gas exits the pressure chamber through the outlet (*I*),

This is an example of a Bourdon gauge regulator. It works just as a preset regulator does, except that the spring tension is adjustable by the user. The second gauge (*J*) indicates the pressure exerted by the spring. If a flowmeter or high pressure hose leading to a ventilator is attached to the outlet of the regulator, the spring should be adjusted to 50 psig. The gauge may also be calibrated in L/min to read flow. This is called a Bourdon gauge flowmeter.
   4. Technical problems associated with reducing valves and regulators
      a. Dust or debris entering the regulator from the cylinder valve may rupture the

diaphragm. Always "crack" the cylinder before attaching a regulator. This is accomplished by turning the cylinder on and back off quickly to blow out the debris from the cylinder outlet.

b. Constant pressure "trapped" in the pressure chamber after the cylinder is turned off may rupture the diaphragm. Always vent pressure in the regulator by turning the flowmeter back on after the cylinder is turned off.

c. A hole in the diaphragm will result in a continuous leak into the ambient chamber and out the vent hole (see diagram of regulator), causing failure of the regulator.

d. A weak spring can result in diaphragm vibration and inadequate flows that are caused by premature closing of the inlet valve.

★ e. When attaching a regulator to a small cylinder, make sure the plastic washer is in place or gas will audibly leak around the cylinder valve outlet and regulator inlet.

5. Calculating how long cylinder contents will last

$$\text{Minutes remaining in cylinder} = \frac{\text{cylinder pressure} \times \text{cylinder factor}}{\text{flowrate}}$$

Cylinder factors: H cylinder = 3.14 L/psig
                   E cylinder = .28 L/psig

EXAMPLE:

Calculate how long a full "H" cylinder will last running at 8 L/min.

$$\frac{2200 \text{ psig} \times 3.14 \text{ L/psig}}{8 \text{ L/min}} = \frac{6908}{8} = \frac{863.5 \text{ min}}{60} = 14.39 \text{ hr}$$

EXAMPLE:

An E cylinder of O_2 contains 1800 psig. If the respiratory care practitioner runs the cylinder at 4 L/min through a nasal cannula, how long will it take for the cylinder to reach a level of 200 psig?

$$\frac{(1800 \text{ psig-200 psig}) \times .28 \text{ L/psig}}{4 \text{ L/min}} = \frac{448}{4}$$

$$= \frac{112 \text{ min}}{60} = 1.9 \text{ hr}$$

---

6. Calculating the duration of flow for a liquid O_2 system

$$\text{Gas remaining} = \text{liquid wt (lbs)} \times 860 / 2.5 \text{ L/lb}$$
$$\text{Duration of contents (min)} = \text{Gas remaining (L)} / \text{Flow (L/min)}$$

EXAMPLE:

A liquid oxygen tank contains 5 lbs of liquid oxygen. The patient is receiving oxygen at 3 L/min through a nasal cannula. How long will the liquid oxygen last?

$$\begin{aligned}\text{Gas remaining} &= 5 \text{ lbs} \times 860 / 2.5 \text{ L/lb} \\ &= 4300 / 2.5 \\ &= 1720 \text{ L}\end{aligned}$$

$$\begin{aligned}\text{Duration of contents} &= 1720 \text{ L} / 3 \text{ L/min} \\ &= 573 \text{ minutes;} \\ 573 / 60 &= 9.6 \text{ hours or 9 hours, 36 minutes}\end{aligned}$$

---

7. Flowmeters
   a. Uncompensated flowmeter

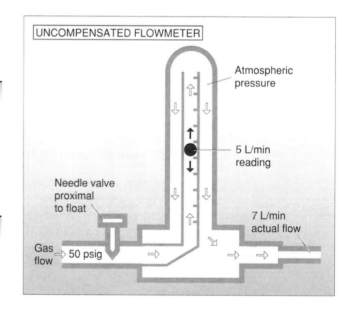

(1) The needle valve is located proximal to (before) the float, and therefore atmospheric pressure is in the Thorpe tube. Any back pressure in the tube affects the rise of the float.

(2) When a restriction, such as humidifier or nebulizer, is attached to the outlet, back pressure into the tube forces the float down and compresses the gas molecules closer together so that more molecules

go around the float than what the float indicates. Therefore, the flowmeter reading is lower than what the patient actually is receiving.

    (3) Uncompensated flowmeters should not be used clinically.

  b. Compensated flowmeter

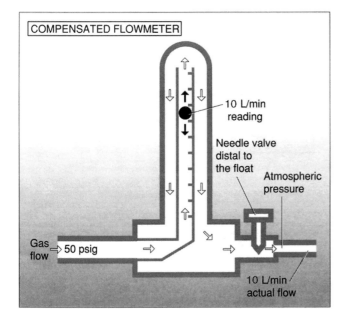

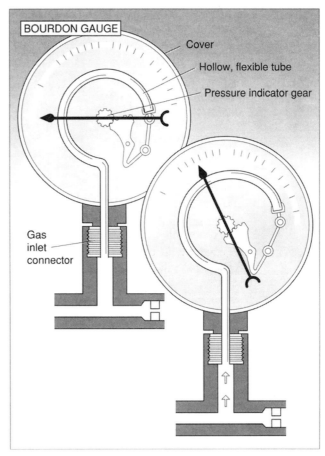

(1) The needle valve is located distal to (after) the float, and therefore 50 psig is in the tube. Only back pressure that exceeds 50 psig will affect the rise of the float.

(2) The flowmeter reads accurately with an attachment, such as a humidifier or nebulizer, on the outlet.

(3) There are three ways to determine if a flowmeter is compensated for pressure.

    (a) It is labeled as such on the flowmeter.

    (b) The needle valve is located after the float.

    (c) The float jumps when the flowmeter, while it is turned off, is plugged into a wall outlet.

(4) Flowmeter outlets use the Diameter Index Safety System, as does all gas-administering equipment that operates at less than 200 psig, to avoid attachment to the wrong gas source.

★ (5) If the flowmeter is turned completely off but gas is still bubbling through the humidifier or heard coming from the flowmeter, the valve seat is faulty and the flowmeter should be replaced.

  c. Bourdon gauge flowmeter

(1) The Bourdon gauge flowmeter is a pressure gauge that has been calibrated in liters per minute. It is uncompensated for back pressure.

(2) When a humidifier or nebulizer is attached to the Bourdon gauge's outlet, back pressure is generated into the gauge (which measures pressure) and the gauge reading is higher than what the patient is actually receiving.

(3) The gauge's mechanism operates by gas entering the hollow, flexible question mark-shaped tube, which tends to straighten as pressure fills it. A gear mechanism is attached to the tube, and as the tube straightens, it rotates a needle indicator that shows the pressure (flow).

(4) The advantage of the Bourdon gauge is that it, unlike Thorpe tube flowmeters, is not position-dependent. It reads just as accurately in a horizontal position as it does in a vertical position.

8. Air compressors are used to provide medical air through either portable compressors or large medical air piping systems. Two types of air compressors are generally used.

a. Piston air compressor

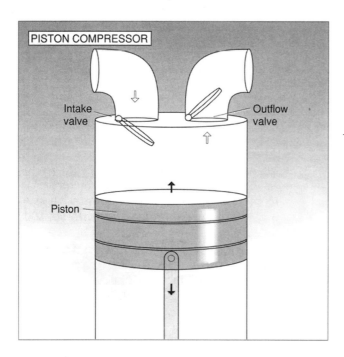

PISTON COMPRESSOR

Intake valve

Outflow valve

Piston

Air is drawn into the compressor, where it travels to a reservoir tank. From this tank, the air passes through a dryer to remove moisture and on to a pressure-reducing valve, which reduces the pressure to 50 psig to power a compressed-air wall outlet. As the piston drops, gas is drawn in through a one-way intake valve. On the upstroke, the intake valve closes and gas exits through a one-way outflow valve. Piston air compressors are seen most commonly on large medical air piping systems.

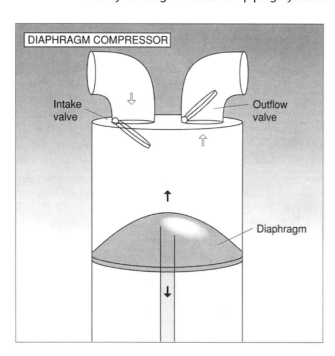

DIAPHRAGM COMPRESSOR

Intake valve

Outflow valve

Diaphragm

b. Diaphragm air compressor
   A diaphragm is used instead of a piston. On the downstroke, the flexible diaphragm bends downward, drawing air through a one-way intake valve. On the upstroke, air is forced out the one-way outflow valve. Diaphragm air compressors are commonly used on O_2 concentrators and portable air compressors.

★ II. OXYGEN THERAPY
   A. Indications for O_2 therapy
      1. Hypoxemia
      2. Labored breathing or dyspnea
      3. Increased myocardial work
   B. Signs and symptoms of hypoxemia
      1. Tachycardia
      2. Dyspnea
      3. Cyanosis
      4. Impairment of special senses
      5. Headache
      6. Mental disturbance
      7. Slight hyperventilation
   ★ C. Complications of O_2 therapy
      1. Respiratory depression: The patient with COPD who is breathing on the "hypoxic drive" mechanism is most affected. Maintain PaO_2 between 50 and 65 mm Hg on these patients.
      2. Atelectasis: High O_2 concentrations in the lung can wash out nitrogen in the lung and reduce the production of surfactant, which may lead to atelectasis. Maintain FiO_2 below 0.60.
      3. Oxygen toxicity: High O_2 concentrations result in increased O_2 free radicals and therefore lung tissue toxicity. This may lead to acute respiratory distress syndrome (ARDS). Maintain FiO_2 below 0.60.
      4. Reduced mucociliary activity: Maintain FiO_2 below 0.60.
      5. Retrolental fibroplasia (neonatal retinopathy): This is caused by high PaO_2 levels in infants and results in blindness. It is more common in premature infants. Maintain PaO_2 below 100 mm Hg. Normal level of PaO_2 in infants is 50 to 70 mm Hg.
   D. **Normal Pao₂ values by age**

Age (yr)	Normal Pao₂
< 60	80 mm Hg
70	70 mm Hg
80	60 mm Hg
90	50 mm Hg

   E. Four Types of Hypoxia
      1. Hypoxemic hypoxia
         a. Caused by lack of O_2 in the blood as a result of
            (1) Inadequate O_2 in the inspired air: administering O_2 is beneficial.

(2) Alveolar hypoventilation: administering O_2 alone may not be beneficial.

(3) Diffusion defects, i.e., pulmonary edema, atelectasis, pulmonary fibrosis: administering O_2 alone may not be beneficial

(4) A ventilation/perfusion mismatch: administering O_2 may be beneficial.

(5) An anatomic right to left shunt: administering O_2 is not beneficial.

★ b. If a normal PaO_2 cannot be maintained with a 60% O_2 mask, a large shunt is probable and should not be treated with higher O_2 concentrations. CPAP should be administered if the $PaCO_2$ is at normal or below normal levels. If the $PaCO_2$ level is elevated in a patient with hypoxemia, mechanical ventilation should be initiated.

2. Anemic hypoxia

   a. The blood's capacity to carry O_2 is reduced as a result of:

   (1) A decreased Hb level.

   (a) Normal Hb level is 12 to 16 g/dL of blood.

> **Note**
>
> g/dL = g/100 mL = g% = vol%

(b) **The PaO_2 level may be normal but because of the blood's reduced capacity to carry O_2, the tissues may be deprived of O_2. The Hb value must be determined to assess the patient's oxygenation status.**

(c) The Hb content may be increased by administering packed red blood cells.

(2) CO poisoning

(a) CO combines with Hb 200 to 250 times faster than O_2 does, and therefore occupies the iron-binding sites on Hb before O_2 can. This causes tissue hypoxia.

(b) Since Hb releases the CO more readily when levels of PaO_2 are high, the patient should immediately be placed on a non-rebreathing mask, which delivers high O_2 concentrations.

(c) Elevating the PaO_2 even higher to further increase the dissociation of Hb from CO may be achieved with hyperbaric O_2 therapy (discussed later in this chapter).

(d) Patients who have been involved in fires or have been breathing car

fumes must be treated immediately for CO poisoning.

★ (e) PaO_2 and Hb saturation (SaO_2) readings (discussed later in this chapter) may be within a normal range even though the patient is severely hypoxic.

★ (f) The level of CO bound to Hb (carboxyhemoglobin) may be determined with CO oximetry (discussed later in this chapter).

★ (g) The patient usually presents with a normal PaO_2 level and a low or normal $PaCO_2$ level. The pH level is usually low as a result of lactic acidosis (metabolic acidosis).

(3) Excessive blood loss: treated by administering blood.

(4) Methemoglobin: most commonly a result of nitrite poisoning, it is treated by administering ascorbic acid or methylene blue, which removes the chemical (nitrite) from the system.

(5) Iron deficiency, which is treated by increasing iron intake and administering blood.

b. The blood carries O_2 in two ways.

(1) Oxygen is bound to Hb: 1.34 mL of O_2 combines with 1 g of Hb (1.34 × Hb × SaO_2).

(2) Oxygen is dissolved in plasma: .003 mL of O_2 dissolves in plasma for every 1 mm Hg of O_2 tension (PaO_2), or (.003 × PaO_2)

> **Note**
>
> The sum of these two mechanisms equals the total arterial O_2 content in mL/dL of blood, which is the most effective method for determining the O_2-carrying capacity of a patient's blood.

EXAMPLE:

Given the following information, calculate the patient's total arterial O_2 content.

ABG study results	
pH	7.42
PCO_2	41 mm Hg
PO_2	90 mm Hg
SaO_2	98%
Hb	15 g/dL

O_2 bound to Hb = 1.34 × 15 × .98 = 19.7 mL/dL
O_2 dissolved in plasma = .003 × 90 = .27 mL/dL
Total arterial O_2 content = 19.7 mL + .27 mL = 19.97 mL/dL

3. Stagnant (circulatory) hypoxia
   a. The O_2 content and carrying capacity is normal but capillary perfusion is diminished as a result of
      (1) Decreased heart rate
      (2) Decreased cardiac output
      (3) Shock
      (4) Embolism
   b. May be seen as a localized problem, such as peripheral cyanosis resulting from exposure to cold weather.
4. Histotoxic hypoxia
   a. The oxidative enzyme mechanism of the cell is impaired as a result of
      (1) Cyanide poisoning
      (2) Alcohol poisoning
   b. Rarely accompanied by hypoxemia but is accompanied by increased venous Po_2 levels.

F. **Oxygen Delivery Devices**
1. Low flow O_2 systems: an O_2 delivery device that does not meet the patient's inspiratory flow demands; therefore, room air must make up the remainder of the patient's V_T. The normal inspiratory flow rate is 25 to 30 L/min. The following devices are connected to humidifiers; however, in some institutions, humidifiers are not used if less than 5 L/min is being delivered.
   a. Nasal catheter
      (1) Delivers 24% to 44% O_2 at flow rates of 1 to 6 L/min (at about a 4% increase for every liter per minute increase).
      (2) Catheter should be lubricated with water-soluble gel and inserted nasally to just above the uvula. Catheter may be measured against patient's nose-to-ear length to help insert it the appropriate distance.
      (3) If catheter is inserted too far, air swallowing and gastric distention may result.
      (4) Change catheter to alternate nostril every 8 hours.
   b. Transtracheal O_2 catheter
      (1) A catheter inserted directly into the trachea to deliver low flow rates (1 to 3 L/min) of O_2.
      (2) Conserves O_2 for home patients by bypassing of anatomic dead space, which results in a reduction in the work of breathing.
      (3) Possible complications include accidental removal of the catheter and irritation or infection at the insertion site and in the trachea.

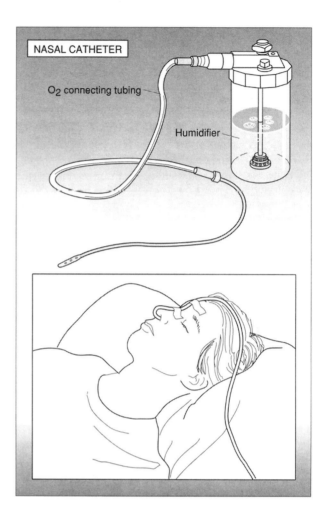

NASAL CATHETER

O_2 connecting tubing

Humidifier

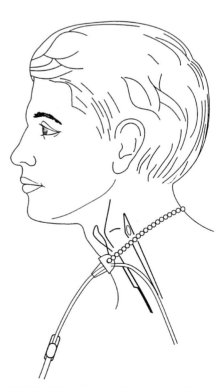

From Scanlan C, Wilkins R, Stoller J: Egan's Fundamentals of Respiratory Care, ed 7, St. Louis, 1999, Mosby.

c. Nasal cannula

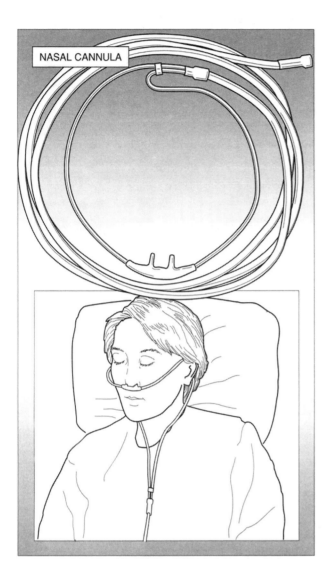

(1) **Delivers 24% to 44% O$_2$ at flow rates of 1 to 6 L/min** (at about a 4% increase for every liter per minute increase).

(2) Much better tolerated by the patient than a nasal catheter.

Note

Two types of O$_2$-conserving cannulas, called reservoir cannulas, have become popular.

1. Nasal reservoir cannula
   a. The reservoir, which is positioned just below the nose, stores approximately 20 mL of O$_2$ that the patient inhales during the early part of inspiration.

b. Since the patient receives more O$_2$ with each breath, the flow needed for a prescribed level of O$_2$ may be decreased, thus conserving O$_2$.

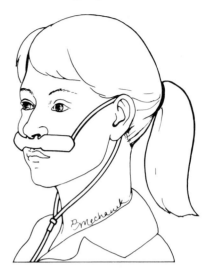

From Scanlan C, Wilkins R, Stoller J: Egan's Fundamentals of Respiratory Care, ed 7, 1999, St. Louis, Mosby.

2. Pendant reservoir cannula
   a. The pendant reservoir cannula uses a pendant-shaped inflatable reservoir that expands as the patient exhales, forcing the stored O$_2$ out of the pendant and up the cannula tubing to the patient.

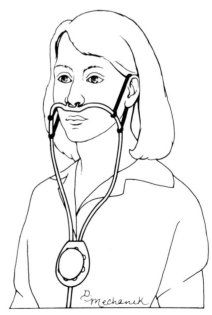

From Scanlan C, Wilkins R, Stoller J: Egan's Fundamentals of Respiratory Care, ed 7, 1999, St. Louis, Mosby.

b. For this device to function properly, the patient must exhale through the nose, so the exhaled air passes through the cannula tubing to inflate the reservoir.

c. Since the pendant may be hidden beneath clothing and the nasal reservoir is much larger than typical cannulas, the patient may prefer the pendant cannula.

Note

In place of O_2 flowmeters, pulse-dose O_2 delivery systems may be employed in conjunction with the nasal cannula, transtracheal catheter, and reservoir cannulas. Pulse-dose systems supply gas to the cannula only during inspiration. The device, plugged into a 50-psig O_2 wall outlet, senses patient effort, and a solenoid valve opens, delivering a "pulse" of O_2 at the set flow rate. This system also results in equivalent O_2 at a lower flow rate, thus conserving O_2.

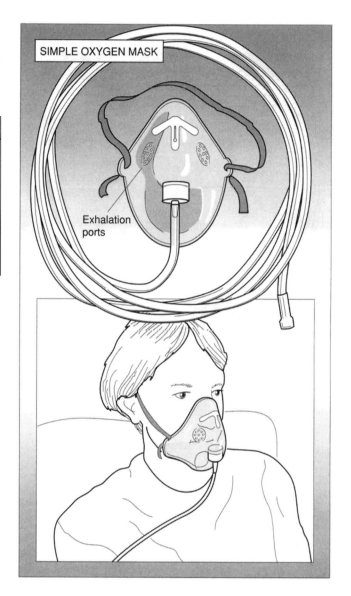

SIMPLE OXYGEN MASK

Exhalation ports

d. Simple O_2 mask
  (1) **Delivers 35% to 55% O_2 at flow rates of 5 to 12 L/min**
  ★ (2) Minimum flow rate of 5 L/min is required to prevent build up of exhaled CO_2 in the mask.
e. Partial rebreathing mask
  (1) Delivers 35% to 60% O_2 at flow rates of 8 to 15 L/min.
  ★ (2) Flowrate must be sufficient to keep the reservoir bag at least one-third to one-half full at all times.
  (3) Must ensure that the patient is not positioned so that the reservoir bag gets kinked or cuts off flow, because this results in a lower F_{IO_2}.
  (4) Only the first part of the patient's exhaled gas enters the reservoir bag. This is gas that was left in the upper airway from the previous inspiration and is therefore high in O_2 and low in CO_2. It is gas that did not participate in gas exchange at the alveolar-capillary level.
f. Non-rebreathing mask
  (1) **Delivers 60% to 80% O_2 at flow rates of 8 to 15 L/min.**
  ★ (2) Flow rate must be sufficient to keep the reservoir bag at least one-third to one-half full at all times.
  (3) The non-rebreathing mask is equipped with a one-way flutter valve between the mask and the reservoir bag, which will not allow exhaled gases into the reservoir bag.
  (4) One-way flutter valves are located on both exhalation ports of the mask to prevent room air entrainment. If one

valve is used, F_{IO_2} decreases and the mask is considered a low-flow mask, but if both valves are used, no air entrainment can occur, F_{IO_2} increases, and the mask is considered a high-flow device.
  (5) Must ensure that the reservoir bag doesn't kink or cut flow off especially if both exhalation ports have one-way valves, because no room air would be available to the patient. (For this reason one valve is often left off.)
★ g. Low-flow O_2 devices are adequate O_2 delivery systems only if the patient meets the following criteria.
1. Regular and consistent ventilatory pattern
2. Respiratory rate of less than 25/min
3. Consistent V_T of 300 to 700 mL

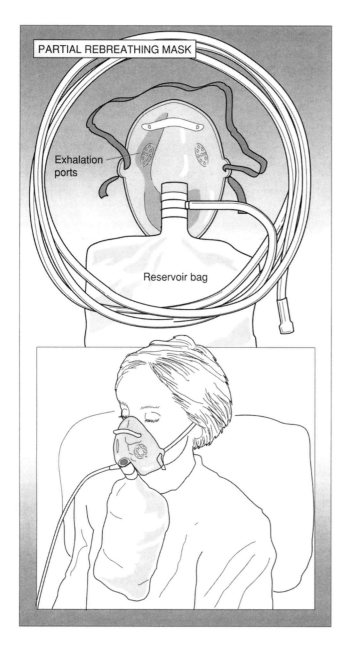

PARTIAL REBREATHING MASK

Exhalation ports

Reservoir bag

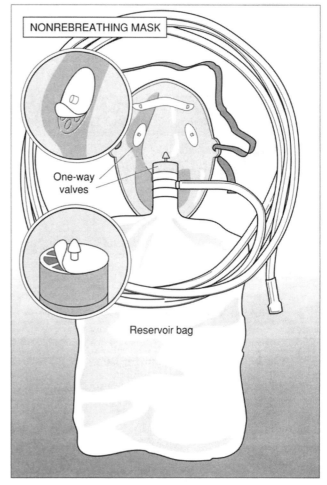

NONREBREATHING MASK

One-way valves

Reservoir bag

Note

★ Any patient requiring supplemental O_2 who does not meet these criteria should be placed on a high-flow O_2 delivery device (discussed later).
★ The percentage of O_2 delivered by a low-flow device is variable, depending on the patient's V_T, respiratory rate, inspiratory time, and ventilatory pattern.

2. High-flow O_2 delivery devices provide all of the inspiratory flow required by the patient at relatively accurate and consistent O_2 percentages. With the exception of the Venturi mask, these devices are attached to nebulizers.
   a. **Venturi mask (air entrainment mask) provides 24% to 50% O_2.**

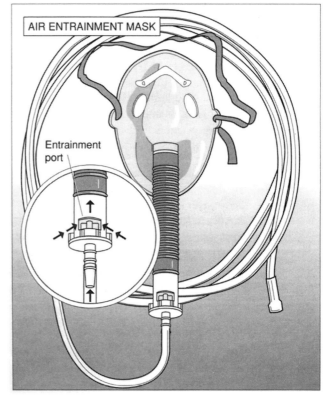

AIR ENTRAINMENT MASK

Entrainment port

(1) Increasing the flow rate on the device will not alter F_{IO_2}. The jet size and entrainment port alter F_{IO_2}.

    (a) The larger the entrainment port, the more air entrained and the lower the F_{IO_2}.

    (b) Likewise, the smaller the entrainment port, the less air entrained and the higher the F_{IO_2}.

    (c) The larger the jet size, the less air entrained and the higher the F_{IO_2}.

    (d) The smaller the jet size, the more air entrained and the lower the F_{IO_2}.

Note

The entrainment port must be prevented from becoming occluded (e.g., by the patient's hand, bedsheet), because this decreases the amount of air entrainment and thus increases the delivered O_2 percentage.

---

(2) Air/O_2 entrainment ratios

O_2 Percentage	Air/O_2 Entrainment Ratio
24%	25 : 1
28%	10 : 1
30%	8 : 1
35%	5 : 1
40%	3 : 1
50%	1.7 : 1
60%	1 : 1

These ratios may be calculated by the following formula:

$$\frac{100 - x}{x - 20\star} = \frac{\text{parts of air entrained}}{1 \text{ part } O_2}$$

use 21 on percentages of less than 40%

EXAMPLE:

Calculate the air/O_2 ratio for 40% O_2.

$$\frac{100 - 40}{40 - 20} = \frac{60}{20} = \frac{3}{1} = 3 : 1$$

This means that for every liter of O_2 (source gas) delivered from the flowmeter, 3 L of air are entrained into the device. Another method to calculate air/O_2 ratios is the "magic box" method. It's not really magic, but most people like it better than the above equation.

20	60
	40
100	20

---

1. Draw a tic-tac-toe box and place 20 or 21 (depending on percentage you are calculating) in the upper left corner.
2. Place 100 in the lower left corner.
3. Place the percentage you are calculating in the middle box of the middle row (in this example, use 40).
4. Subtract 20 from 40 and place the answer in the lower right corner, and subtract 40 from 100 and place the answer in the upper right corner.
5. After subtracting, you should have 60 in the upper right corner (representing air) and 20 in the lower right corner (representing O_2). Now divide 60 by 20, and you get 3, or a 3 : 1 air-O_2 ratio.

    (3) Calculating total flow

Note

If a venturi mask is set on 40% oxygen and a flow rate of 12 L/min, the total flow delivered would be:

$$
\begin{array}{r}
12 \text{ L/min of } O_2 \\
+\ 36 \text{ L/min of air } (12 \times 3) \\
\hline
48 \text{ L/min of total flow}
\end{array}
$$

FASTER METHOD: Add the ratio parts together and multiply by the flow.

40% (3 : 1 air/O_2 ratio)
$3 + 1 = 4$ and $4 \times 12 = 48$ L/min

EXAMPLE:

A venturi mask is set on 24% O_2 and a flow of 4 L/min. Calculate the total flow.

$$\frac{100 - 24}{24 - 21} = \frac{76}{3} = \text{approx.} \frac{25}{1} = 25 : 1 \text{ air/} O_2 \text{ ratio}$$

$$
\begin{array}{r}
4 \text{ L/min of } O_2 \\
+\ 100 \text{ L/min of air} \\
\hline
104 \text{ L/min of total flow}
\end{array}
$$

OR

Sum of the ratio of parts multiplied by flow:

$$[(25 + 1) = 26] \times 4 = 104 \text{ L/min}$$

EXAMPLE:

The physician has ordered a 40% aerosol mask to be placed on a patient who has a total inspiratory flow of 44 L/min. What is the minimum flow rate setting on the flowmeter that will meet this patient's inspiratory flow demands?

Since the air/O_2 ratio for 40% O_2 is 3:1, add the ratio parts together:

$$3 + 1 = 4$$

We now must set the flowmeter on the lowest L/min flow that multiplied by 4 delivers a total flow of at least 44 L/min, or 4 × ? = 44. Therefore, the flowmeter must be set at a minimum of 11 L/min.

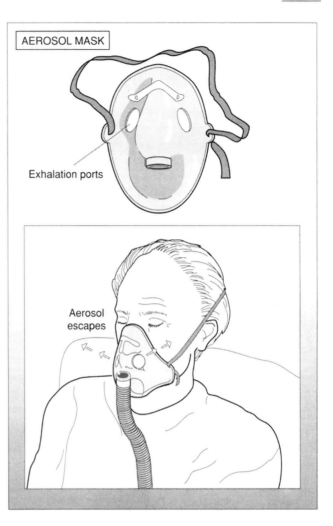

AEROSOL MASK

Exhalation ports

Aerosol escapes

Note

To determine a patient's inspiratory flow, use the following equation:

$$\text{Inspiratory flow} = \frac{V_T \ (L)}{\text{inspiratory time (sec)}}$$

The flow will be in L/sec, so multiply by 60 to change to L/min.

EXAMPLE:

The physician has ordered O_2 for a patient with a spontaneous V_T of 550 mL and an inspiratory time of 1 sec. The O_2 device must deliver what flow rate to meet the patient's inspiratory demands?

$$\text{Inspiratory flow} = \frac{.55 \ L}{1.0 \ sec} = .55 \ L/sec \times 60 = 33 \ L/min$$

In other words, the O_2 delivery device used must be able to deliver a total flow of at least 33 L/min to meet the patient's inspiratory flow demands. Which of the following would produce the necessary flow?

A. *40% air entrainment mask at 8 L/min*
B. *50% air entrainment mask at 12 L/min*
C. *35% air entrainment mask at 6 L/min*
D. *50% air entrainment mask at 10 L/min*

Flow rates are A, 32 L/min; B, 32 L/min; C, 36 L/min; and D, 27 L/min. Choice "C" exceeds the patient's inspiratory flow demands, and therefore is the correct choice.

    b. Aerosol mask
      (1) **This mask delivers 21% to 100% O_2 (depending on nebulizer setting) at flow rates of 8 to 5 L/min.**
      (2) If the nebulizer is set on 100%, the device probably would not meet the patient's inspiratory flow demands. Room air would enter the mask through the exhalation ports during inspiration, decreasing FIO_2.

      (3) **Mist should be visible at all times to ensure adequate flow rates.**
    c. Face tent
      (1) **Delivers 21% to 40% O_2 (depending on nebulizer setting) at flow rates of 8 to 15 L/min.**

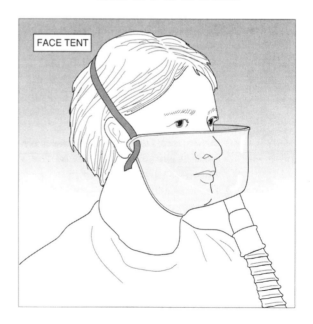

FACE TENT

(2) Used primarily for patients with facial trauma or burns or for those who cannot tolerate a mask.

d. T-tube flow-by or Briggs adaptor

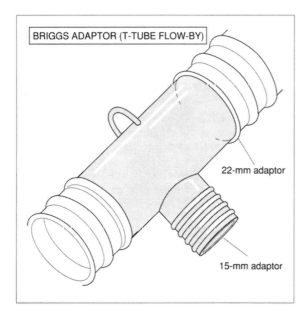

BRIGGS ADAPTOR (T-TUBE FLOW-BY)

22-mm adaptor

15-mm adaptor

(1) **Delivers 21% to 100% O_2 (depending on nebulizer setting) at flow rates of 8 to 15 L/min**

(2) Used on the intubated or tracheostomy patient

(3) A 50-mL piece of reservoir tubing should be attached to the end of the T-piece (opposite from where the aerosol tubing from the nebulizer is attached). This prevents air from entering the T-piece during inspiration and if the reservoir falls off, FIO_2 may decrease.

(4) **Adequate flows are ensured by visible mist flowing out of the 50-mL reservoir at all times.**

e. Tracheostomy mask (collar)

(1) **Delivers 35% to 60% O_2 (depending on nebulizer setting) at flow rates of 10 to 15 L/min**

(2) **Adequate flows are ensured by visible mist flowing out of the exhalation port at all times.**

(3) Mask should fit directly over the tracheostomy tube.

f. Oxygen Tent

(1) **Delivers 21% to 50% O_2 at flow rates of 10 to 15 L/min**

(2) Used primarily on children with croup or pneumonia.

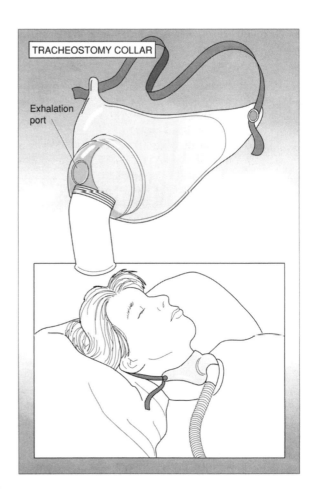

TRACHEOSTOMY COLLAR

Exhalation port

(3) Not an ideal O_2 delivery device because of the leakage and reduced O_2 delivery when the tent is opened for patient care.

(4) A fire hazard exists if electrical devices or friction toys, which may spark, are left in the tent.

G. **Important Points Concerning High-Flow Devices**

★ 1. High-flow O_2 devices set on 60% or higher may deliver a total flow rate of less than 25 to 30 L/min, thereby not meeting the patient's

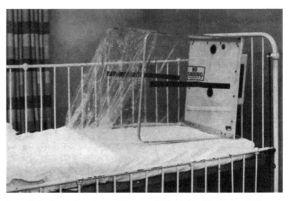

From Safar P, ed: Respiratory Therapy. Philadelphia: FA Davis. 1965.

inspiratory flow demands and essentially acting as a low-flow device with the patient breathing in room air to make up the difference. When this happens, it means the O_2 percentage setting on the nebulizer is no longer accurate, and the patient is receiving less delivered O_2 than the setting suggests.

2. To ensure adequate flow rates on a device set on 60% or higher, use two flowmeters connected in line together.
3. To ensure adequate flow rates, set the flowmeter to a rate that delivers a total flow of at least 40 L/min.
4. **A restriction, such as kinked aerosol tubing or water in the tubing, causes back pressure into the nebulizer, decreasing the amount of air entrainment and therefore increasing the percentage of O_2.**
5. Increasing the flow on a high-flow device does not increase the delivered F_{IO_2}. It will only increase the total flow.

H. **Calculating F_{IO_2}**

$$F_{IO_2} = \frac{O_2\ flow + (air\ flow \times .2)}{total\ flow}$$

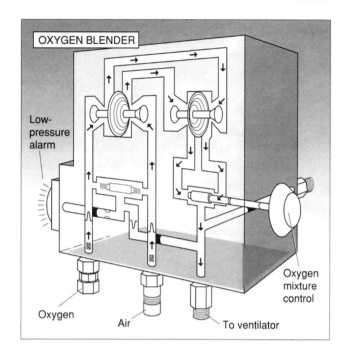

OXYGEN BLENDER

Low-pressure alarm

Oxygen mixture control

Oxygen   Air   To ventilator

3. Blenders provide a stable F_{IO_2} as long as the outlet flow exceeds the patient's inspiratory flow demands.

III. MIXED GAS THERAPY

EXAMPLE:

A nebulizer set on 40% dilution mode and connected to an O_2 flowmeter running at 10 L/min has an air bleed-in rate of 6 L/min downstream. Calculate the F_{IO_2}.

O_2 flow	= 10 L/min
Air flow	= 30 L/min (entrained through nebulizer)
Air flow	= 6 L/min (bleed-in)
Total flow	= 46 L/min

$$F_{IO_2} = \frac{10 + (36 \times .2)}{46} = \frac{10 + 7.2}{46} = \frac{17.2}{46} = .37$$

I. **Oxygen blender**
   1. These devices use 50-psig gas sources to mix or blend O_2 and compressed air proportionately to deliver 21% to 100% O_2 at flow rates of 2 to 100 L/min.
   2. A blender consists of pressure-regulating valves that regulate O_2 and air inlet pressure, a mixture control (precision metering device), and an audible alarm system, which sounds if there is a drop in inlet pressure.

> *Exam Note*
>
> Helium/O_2 and CO_2/O_2 therapy appears on the *RRT examination only.*

A. **Helium/O_2 therapy**
   1. Helium is the second lightest gas, and therefore when combined with O_2, decreases the total density of the gas. This allows the gas to pass through obstructions more easily.
   2. Helium/O_2 mixtures (heliox) are stored in brown-and-green cylinders.
   3. Helium does not support life and therefore must be mixed with O_2. Two common mixtures are
      a. 80% Helium and 20% O_2
      b. 70% Helium and 30% O_2
   4. Running these gas mixtures through an O_2 flowmeter will give inaccurate readings, since the gas is lighter than pure O_2. A correction factor may be used to make the reading accurate.
      a. For an 80:20 mixture of helium and O_2, multiply the flowmeter reading by 1.8 to determine the correct flow rate. Divide the flow rate by 1.8, if you want to deliver a specific flow.

An 80:20 mixture of helium and O_2 is running through an O_2 flowmeter at 10 L/min. What is the actual flow rate?

$$10 \times 1.8 = 18 \text{ L/min}$$

You want to deliver 12 L/min of an 80:20 mixture of helium and O_2 to the patient. What must you set the O_2 flowmeter on to deliver this flow rate?

$$\frac{12}{1.8} = 6.6 \text{ L/min}$$

   ★ b. For a 70:30 mixture of Helium and O_2, multiply the flowmeter reading by 1.6. Divide by 1.6 to obtain a specific flow rate. (See example above and substitute 1.6 for 1.8.)
   ★ 5. Helium and O_2 mixtures must be delivered in a tightly closed system, such as a non-rebreathing mask, ET tube, or tracheostomy tube, to prevent this lighter gas from leaking out.
   6. The only side effect of Helium/O_2 therapy is distortion of the voice.
   7. Extreme caution must be used when mixing heliox from a helium cylinder and an O_2 cylinder. Inaccurate flow readings may result in the patient receiving less than 21% O_2. A pre-mixed Helium/O_2 cylinder is recommended.
   8. Helium/O_2 mixtures are safe and may be of benefit in the treatment of
      a. Obstruction from secretions
      b. Asthma (during episodes of bronchospasm)
B. **CO_2 and O_2 therapy**

> **Note**
>
> In the past, respiratory therapists have used CO_2/O_2 gas mixtures for a variety of reasons. Although at present they are used only sparingly, the concepts behind their use are important for the practitioner to understand.

   1. Physiologic actions of CO_2
      a. The gas mixture is a respiratory stimulant in concentrations of up to 10%, resulting in increased respiratory rate and V_T.
      b. The gas mixture is a respiratory depressant in concentrations of more than 10%, resulting in decreased respiratory rate and V_T.
      c. Increased blood pressure results from systemic vasoconstriction.

d. Increased heart rate
e. Increased cerebral blood flow results from cerebral vasodilation
f. Vasodilation of capillary beds
g. CO_2 is a CNS depressant in low concentrations (5% to 10%) resulting in mental depression or unconsciousness
h. CO_2 is a CNS stimulant in high concentrations (more than 30%), resulting in seizures
   2. Indications for CO_2 therapy

> **Note**
>
> The CO_2/O_2 mixture most commonly used consists of 95% O_2 and 5% CO_2. This is commonly referred to as a 95/5 treatment.

      a. To improve cerebral blood flow
         (1) After stroke
         (2) In persons who have fainting spells
         (3) In acute hearing loss
      b. To stimulate deep breathing
         (1) To prevent or treat atelectasis
         (2) Since respiratory rate is usually increased and not V_T, this is not effective in treating atelectasis.
      c. To treat hiccoughs
         May interfere with the spasm of the phrenic nerve and thereby stop the hiccoughs
      d. To stop seizure activity
         Low concentrations (5%) cause CNS depression
      e. To treat CO poisoning
         Low concentrations (3% to 7%) enhance the release of the CO from Hb
   3. Side effects of CO_2 therapy
      a. Dyspnea
      b. Dizziness
      c. Muscle tremors
      d. Nasal irritation
      e. Paresthesia
      f. Headache
      g. Nausea (CO_2 toxicity)
      h. Vomiting (CO_2 toxicity)
      i. Disorientation (CO_2 toxicity)
      j. Severe elevation in blood pressure (CO_2 toxicity)
   4. Important points concerning CO_2 therapy
      a. No more than 5% CO_2 should be used.
      b. The treatment should not exceed 10 min.
      c. The treatment should be given with a non-rebreathing mask that is held over the face and not strapped on, so that it can be easily removed if necessary.

d. The treatment is contraindicated in patients who have compromised central respiratory centers, such as those with severe COPD.

e. CO_2/O_2 therapy is not the treatment of choice for deep breathing. Other methods are much more effective and much safer.

IV. HBO THERAPY

A. Hyperbaric chambers

1. Fixed multiplace chamber

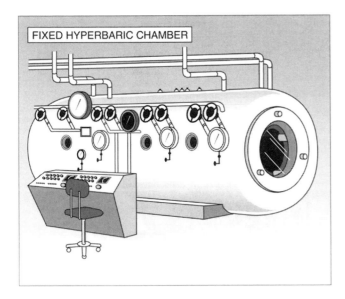

FIXED HYPERBARIC CHAMBER

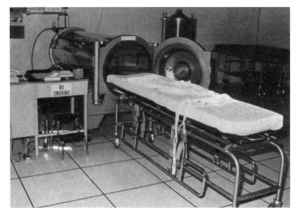

From Davis JC, Hunt TK. *Hyperboric Oxygen Therapy.* Bethesda MD: Undersea Medical Society, 1977.

2. Portable monoplace chamber

B. Hyperbaric O_2 therapy is the delivery of O_2 at greater than atmospheric pressure and is accomplished by placing the patient in a hyperbaric chamber.

C. The multiplace chamber is a walk-in unit, which will accommodate several people.

D. The monoplace unit will accommodate only one person at a time.

E. The chambers are usually pressurized to 3 atm, or three times atmospheric pressure, as the patient breathes 100% O_2.

F. This increased pressure likewise increases the amount of O_2 in the blood and body tissues. While breathing room air at 1 atm, the PaO_2 is about 100 mm Hg with about 0.3 vol% O_2 dissolved in the plasma; however, while breathing 100% O_2 at 3 atm, the PaO_2 is about 1800 mm Hg with 6.2 vol% O_2 dissolved in the plasma.

G. Physiologic effects of hyperbaric O_2

1. Elevated PaO_2 levels
2. Vasoconstriction
3. New capillary bed formation
4. Metabolic alteration of aerobic and anaerobic organisms
5. Reduction of nitrogen bubbles in the blood

H. Indications for hyperbaric O_2 therapy

1. CO poisoning
2. Cyanide poisoning
3. Decompression sickness ("the bends")
4. Gas gangrene
5. Gas embolism
6. Osteonecrosis

I. HBO treatments, or "dives" (as they are often called), usually require 90 min at 2 to 3 atm, two to four times a day.

V. OXYGEN ANALYZERS

A. **Galvanic cell O_2 analyzers**

1. Electrolyte gel is used to chemically reduce O_2 to electron flow.
2. A Clark electrode is used to measure O_2 concentration.
3. *The analyzer* reading is affected by water, positive pressure, high altitude, torn membrane, or lack of electrolyte gel.

B. **Polarographic O_2 analyzers**

1. A battery polarizes the electrodes to allow O_2 reduction to occur, giving off electron flow.
2. The Clark electrode is used to measure O_2 concentration.
3. *The analyzer* reading is affected by water, positive pressure, high altitude, torn membrane, or lack of electrolyte gel.
4. Electrodes last longer on the galvanic cell analyzer, but the polarographic analyzer has a quicker response time.

> ### Note
>
> Other specialty gas analyzers may be used in the hospital setting. Helium analyzers are seen in pulmonary function laboratories. Although much could be said on how these analyzers function, the most important aspect to remember for the examination is that these analyzers read zero when calibrated to room air.

VI. OXYGEN SATURATION MONITORING (PULSE OXIMETRY)

A. Use of the pulse oximeter
1. Pulse oximeters are devices that measure SaO_2 by the principle of spectrophotometry. This is also referred to as SpO_2.
2. Light from the probe is directed through a capillary bed to be absorbed in different amounts, depending on the amount of O_2 bound to Hb. The result is displayed on the monitor as a percentage of saturation.
3. The probe is noninvasive and may be attached to the finger, toe, or ear of adults and the ankle or foot of infants.
4. Pulse oximeters seem to be quite accurate, although some studies show they may be less accurate when used for "spot checks" rather than continuous monitoring.

B. Causes of inaccurate readings
1. Low blood perfusion.
2. CO poisoning.
3. Severe anemia.
4. Hypotension.
5. Hypothermia.
6. Cardiac arrest.
7. Nail polish, especially blue, green, brown and black colors, may cause lower oximetry readings. Polish should be removed or the oximeter placed on the ear lobe instead of the fingers.
8. Ambient light sources, such as direct sunlight, phototherapy, and fluorescent lights, affect the accuracy of the pulse reading. Wrapping the sensor site with a towel or gauze to block the light can eliminate this problem.
9. Dark skin pigmentation.

VII. CO-OXIMETRY

A. This procedure requires arterial blood to be obtained. The oximeter, part of the blood gas analyzer, is able to measure the amount of Hb, HbO_2, and HbCO in blood.

B. This procedure uses the principle of spectrophotometry to measure the blood level of CO bound to Hb (HbCO).
1. HbCO is usually expressed as a percentage of total Hb.
2. HbCO as high as 10% may be seen in heavy smokers, but higher levels are measured in patients who have inhaled large amounts of car fumes or smoke.
3. Patients with HbCO levels of less than 20% are usually asymptomatic.
4. HbCO levels of more than 20% result in nausea and vomiting. Fatal levels are 60% to 80%.

POST-CHAPTER STUDY QUESTIONS

1. List the air/O_2 ratios for 60% O_2, 40% O_2, 35% O_2, 30% O_2, and 24% O_2.
2. Give four examples of high-flow O_2 delivery devices.
3. What is the primary benefit of using a reservoir cannula?
4. Calculate total O_2 content, given the following ABG test results.

pH	7.36
$PaCO_2$	40 mm Hg
PaO_2	82 mm Hg
SaO_2	96%
Hb	13 g/dL

5. What is the total flow delivered by an aerosol mask on 60% O_2, running at 12 L/min?
6. List the three ventilatory criteria that should be met by patients receiving O_2 from a low-flow device.
7. An 80:20 mixture of Helium/O_2 running through an O_2 flowmeter at 6 L/min is delivering how much flow to the patient?
8. Calculate how long an "E" cylinder with 1900 psig will run at 5 L/min.
9. Give examples of three low-flow O_2 delivery devices.
10. List five conditions that affect the accuracy of pulse oximeters.
11. List five indications for the use of hyperbaric O_2 therapy.
12. How does water in the aerosol tubing of a mask affect the delivered FIO_2?
13. The physician orders O_2 therapy for a patient with a V_T of 400 mL and an inspiratory time of 0.5 sec. What flow must the mask deliver to meet this patient's inspiratory flow demands?

Answers are at the end of the chapter.

REFERENCES

Eubanks O and Bone R: Comprehensive Respiratory Care, ed 2, St. Louis, 1990, The CV Mosby Co.

Fink J and Hunt G: Clinical practice in respiratory care, Philadelphia, 1999, JB Lippincott Co. Malley W: Clinical blood gases: application and noninvasive alternatives, Philadelphia, 1990, WB Saunders Co.

McPherson SP: Respiratory therapy equipment, ed 5, St. Louis, 1995, The CV Mosby Co.

Scanlan C, Wilkins R, and Stoller J: Egan's fundamentals of respiratory care, ed 7, St. Louis, 1999, The CV Mosby Co.

PRE-TEST ANSWERS

1. C
2. D
3. B
4. A
5. D
6. B

ANSWERS TO POST-CHAPTER STUDY QUESTIONS

1. 60%, 1:1; 40%, 3:1; 35%, 5:1; 30%, 8:1; and 24%, 25:1
2. Venturi mask, aerosol mask, T-piece (Briggs adaptor), face tent, tracheostomy collar
3. Conserves O_2 by storing it in the reservoir.
4. 17 vol%,

$$1.34 \times 13 \times .96 = \ 16.7$$
$$.003 \times 82 \quad = +\ \ .25$$
$$\overline{16.95 \quad \text{or} \quad 17 \text{ vol\%}}$$

5. 24 L/min,

60% (1:1 air/O_2 ratio)
1 + 1 = 2, 2 × 12 L/min = 24 L/min

6. Consistent ventilatory pattern, V_T 300 mL to 700 mL, respiratory rate of less than 25/min
7. 10.8 L/min,

$$1.8 \times 6 = 10.8 \text{ L/min}$$

8. 1 hour, 46 minutes,

$$\frac{1900 \times .28}{5} = \frac{532}{5} = 106 \text{ min} = 1 \text{ hr } 46 \text{ min}$$

9. Nasal cannula, simple O_2 mask, partial rebreathing mask
10. Poor perfusion, severe anemia, hypotension, elevated HbCO level, direct light, phototherapy and fluorescent light sources, nail polish, dark skin pigmentation
11. CO poisoning, cyanide poisoning, decompression sickness, gas gangrene, gas embolism
12. Increases FIO_2
13. 48 L/min,

$$\text{Insp. flowrate} = \frac{V_T}{\text{Insp. time}} = \frac{.4L}{.5 \text{ sec}}$$
$$= .8 \text{ L/sec} \times 60 = 48 \text{ L/min}$$

Chapter 2

Humidity and Aerosol

PRE-TEST QUESTIONS

Answer the pre-test questions before studying the chapter. This will help you determine your strong and weak areas regarding the material covered.

1. Secretions tend to become thicker if the inspired air has which of the following characteristics?

    A. *A relative humidity of 100% at body temperature*
    B. *32 mg H_2O per liter of gas*
    C. *A water vapor pressure of 47 mm Hg*
    D. *48 mg H_2O per liter of gas*

2. A patient receiving 38 mg H_2O per liter of gas from a nebulizer has a humidity deficit of which of the following?

    A. *6 mg/L*
    B. *9 mg/L*
    C. *12 mg/L*
    D. *18 mg/L*

3. After connecting a nasal cannula to the humidifier outlet, you kink the tubing and hear a whistling noise coming from the humidifier. Which of the following most likely has caused this?

    A. *The humidifier jar is cracked.*
    B. *The capillary tube in the humidifier is disconnected.*
    C. *The humidifier has no leaks.*
    D. *The top of the humidifier is not screwed on tightly.*

4. You notice that the patient's secretions have become thicker and more difficult to suction since replacing the ventilator humidifier with a heat moisture exchanger. The respiratory therapist should recommend which of the following?

    A. *Increase inspiratory flow.*
    B. *Increase the temperature to the heat moisture exchanger.*
    C. *Replace with a new heat moisture exchanger.*
    D. *Replace the heat moisture exchanger with a conventional heated humidifier.*

5. Which of the following are indications for bland aerosol therapy?

    I. Cough must be induced for sputum collection.
    II. Mobilization of secretions must be improved.
    III. Post-extubation inflammation of the upper airway must be treated.

    A. *I only*
    B. *I and II only*
    C. *II and III only*
    D. *I, II and III*

6. You notice that very little mist is being produced by a nebulizer attached to an aerosol mask. Which of the following could be responsible for this?

    I. The liter flow is too high.
    II. The nebulizer jet is clogged with soap residue.
    III. The filter on the capillary tube is obstructed.

    A. *I only*
    B. *II only*
    C. *I and III only*
    D. *II and III only*

Answers are at the end of the chapter.

REVIEW

I. **HUMIDITY THERAPY**
   A. **Humidity** is the quality of wetness in air or a gas caused by the addition of water in a gaseous state or vapor. Also called "molecular water" or "invisible moisture."

> **Note**
>
> The objective of humidity therapy is to make up for water loss that occurs when dry gas is delivered or when the upper airway is bypassed. Adding "liquid" water or mist to the airway to thin secretions is accomplished by **aerosol therapy** (discussed later).

B. **Clinical Uses of Humidity**
   1. To humidify dry therapeutic gases.
   2. To provide 100% body humidity of the inspired gas for patients with ET tubes or tracheostomy tubes.
C. **Normal Airway Humidification**
   1. The nose warms, humidifies, and filters inspired air.
   2. The pharynx, trachea, and bronchial tree also warm, humidify, and filter inspired air.
   3. By the time inspired air reaches the oropharynx, it has been warmed to approximately 34°C and is 80% to 90% saturated with H_2O.
   4. By the time the inspired air reaches the carina, it has been warmed to body temperature (37°C) and is 100% saturated.
   5. When the inspired air is fully saturated (100%) it holds **44 mg H_2O per liter of gas and exerts a water vapor pressure of 47 mm Hg.**
D. **Absolute and Relative Humidity**
   1. **Absolute humidity** is the amount of water in a given volume of gas and its measurement is expressed in mg/L.
   2. **Relative humidity** is a ratio between the amount of water in a given volume of gas and the maximum amount it is capable of holding at that temperature (capacity). Its measurement is **expressed as a percentage and obtained with a hygrometer.**
   3. **Relative humidity = $\dfrac{\text{absolute humidity}}{\text{capacity}} \times 100$**

EXAMPLE:

The amount of moisture in a given volume of gas at 31°C is 24 mg H_2O per liter of gas. Calculate the relative humidity. (Note: At 31°C, air can hold 32.01 mg H_2O per liter.)

Relative humidity $= \dfrac{24 \text{ mg/L}}{32.01 \text{ mg/L}} = .75 \times 100 = $ **75%**

EXAMPLE:

A gas at 22°C has a relative humidity of 54%. Calculate the absolute humidity. (Note: At 22°C, air can hold 19.42 mg H_2O per liter.)

Absolute humidity = relative humidity × capacity

Absolute humidity $= .54 \times 19.42 \text{ mg/L} = $ **10.5 mg/L**

E. **Body Humidity**
   1. Body humidity is the relative humidity at body temperature and is expressed as a percentage.

2. Body humidity $= \dfrac{\text{absolute humidity}}{44 \text{ mg/L}} \times 100$

Note

44 mg/L is the capacity of water at body temperature.

EXAMPLE:

If the gas that the patient is inspiring contains 21 mg of H_2O per liter of gas, what is the body humidity?

Body humidity $= \dfrac{21 \text{ mg/L}}{44 \text{ mg/L}} = .48 \times 100 = $ **48%**

   3. A 48% body humidity indicates the inspired air is holding only 48% of the water it takes to fully saturate the gas in the airway at body temperature. The body's humidification system adds the other 52% by the time the air reaches the carina.
F. **Humidity Deficit**
   1. Inspired air that is not fully saturated at body temperature creates a humidity deficit. This deficit is corrected by the body's own humidification system.
   2. Humidity deficit may be expressed in mg/L or as a percentage.
   3. **Humidity deficit = 44 mg/L − absolute humidity** or when expressed as a percent:

$$\dfrac{\textbf{Humidity deficit (mg/L)}}{\textbf{44 mg/L}} \times \textbf{100}$$

EXAMPLE:

A patient on T-tube flow-by is inspiring air from an Ohio nebulizer that contains 18 mg H_2O per liter of air. What is this patient's humidity deficit?

44 mg/L − 18 mg/L = **26 mg/L**

As a percentage:

$\dfrac{26}{44} \text{ mg/L} \times 100 = $ **59%**

   4. This is why it is important to deliver humidified gas at body temperature to patients with artificial airways that bypass the patient's upper airway.
   ★5. If adequate humidity is not provided, the patient's airway can dry out, leading to thickening of secretions and resulting in increased airway resistance.

6. Gas being delivered to a patient with an ET tube or tracheostomy tube that contains **less than 44 mg H₂O per liter of gas or a water vapor pressure of less than 47 mm Hg tends to dry secretions, making them thicker and more difficult to mobilize.**

G. **Efficiency of Humidifiers**

Depends on three important factors.

   a. Duration of contact between the gas and water (longer duration results in increased humidity)
   b. Surface area of gas and water contact (greater surface area results in increased humidity)
   c. Temperature of the gas and water (higher temperature results in increased humidity)

H. **Types of Humidifiers**

1. **Pass-over humidifier** (nonheated humidifier)

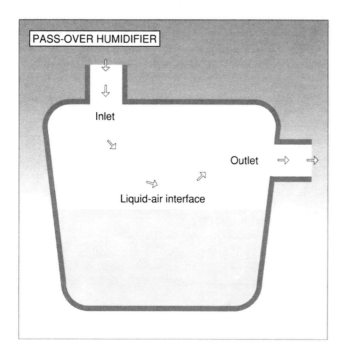

PASS-OVER HUMIDIFIER

Inlet

Outlet

Liquid-air interface

   a. Gas simply passes over the surface of the water, picking up moisture and delivering it to the patient.
   b. Produces low humidification because of the limited time of gas and water contact and the small surface area involved.
   c. Provides a body humidity of approximately 25%.

2. **Bubble humidifier** (nonheated humidifier)

   a. The most common type of humidifier used with oxygen delivery devices.
   b. O₂ entering the humidifier travels through a tube under the surface of the water and exits through a diffuser at the lower end of the tube.

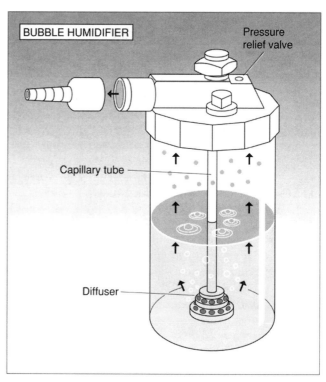

BUBBLE HUMIDIFIER

Pressure relief valve

Capillary tube

Diffuser

   c. **Provides a body humidity of 35% to 40%.**

3. **Wick humidifier** (heated humidifier)

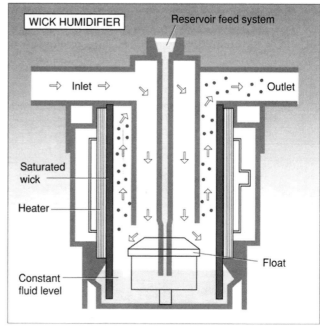

WICK HUMIDIFIER

Reservoir feed system

Inlet

Outlet

Saturated wick

Heater

Constant fluid level

Float

   a. Gas from the flowmeter or ventilator enters the humidifier and is exposed to the wick (made of cloth, sponge, or paper), which is partially under the surface of the water.

b. As gas passes the wick, it absorbs water that is delivered to the patient.

c. Because the water bath or the gas is heated, a body humidity approaching 100% is delivered to the patient. This method is ideal for patients with artificial airways and those who are on mechanical ventilators.

4. **Cascade humidifier** (heated humidifier)

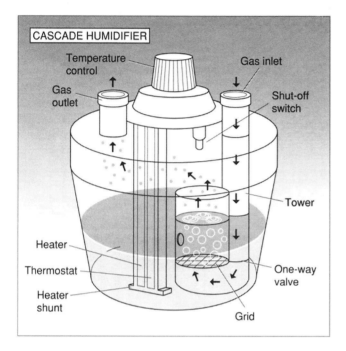

a. Gas travels down the tower and hits the bottom of the jar, which displaces the water upward over a grid, forming a liquid film. The gas travels back up through the grid (from underneath), picking up moisture and delivering it to the patient.

b. Since the humidifier is heated, this method is capable of delivering gas at **100% body humidity.**

★ c. Should the humidifier be allowed to run dry, the thermostat automatically turns the heater off, preventing the reservoir from being damaged or allowing hot dry gas to be delivered to the patient.

I. **Important Points Concerning Humidifiers**

1. Most nonheated humidifiers have a pressure pop-off valve set at **2 psi.** After the device is set up, the tubing of the oxygen delivery device (e.g., cannula, mask) should be kinked to obstruct flow. If the pop-off sounds, there are no leaks. If no sound is heard, all connections, as well as the humidifier top, should be tightened.

2. Water levels of all humidifiers should be maintained at the levels marked on the humidifier jar to ensure maximum humidity output.

3. Condensation occurs in the tubing of heated humidifiers. This water should be discarded in a trash container or basin and should **never** be put back into the humidifier.

4. The temperature of inspired gas should be monitored continuously with an in-line thermometer when using heated humidifiers. The thermometer should be as close to the patient wye as possible.

5. Warm moist areas, such as heated humidifiers, are a breeding ground for microorganisms (especially *Pseudomonas* species). The humidifier should be replaced **every 24 hours.**

> **Note**
>
> Bacteria that is growing in a heated humidifier probably will not be delivered to the patient (and cause a nosocomial infection) because the humidified particles are too small to carry the bacterial particles. Nebulizers are a more likely source of nosocomial infections because of the larger water particles produced, which are able to carry the bacteria to the patient.

J. **Heat Moisture Exchanger** (artificial nose)

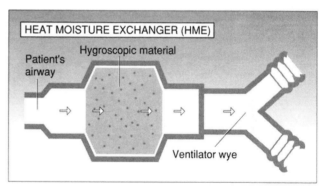

1. This device is placed in-line between the patient and the patient wye of the ventilator circuit.

2. As the patient exhales, gas at body humidity and body temperature enters the heat moisture exchanger (HME), heating the hygroscopic filter (made of felt, plastic foam, or cellulose sponge) and condensing water into it. During the next inspiration, gas passes through the HME and is warmed and humidified.

3. Under ideal conditions the HME can produce 70% to 90% body humidity.

> **Note**
>
> If the patient's secretions begin to thicken while using a heat moisture exchanger, the HME should be replaced with a conventional heated humidifier.

4. The HME may be used for temporary humidification during patient transport or for long-term humidification for ventilator-dependent patients. If ventilatory pressure begins to increase, check for water or secretions in the HME and, if there are obstructions, change to a new HME. If secretions are causing obstruction, a conventional heated humidifier should be used.

II. **AEROSOL THERAPY**

A. Aerosol is defined as a suspension of water in particulate form (or a mist) in gas. Nebulizers produce aerosolized gas.

B. **Clinical Uses For Aerosol Therapy**
1. To improve the mobilization of pulmonary secretions
2. To administer medications (via HHN or USN)
3. To prevent dehydration
4. After extubation to prevent or relieve bronchospasm or inflammatory reactions
5. To hydrate the airway of a tracheostomy patient
6. To induce cough for sputum collection

C. **Hazards of Aerosol Therapy**
1. Bronchospasm: administration of a bronchodilator may decrease the potential of this hazard.
2. Overhydration
3. Overheating of inspired gas
4. Tubing condensation draining into the airway
5. Delivery of contaminated aerosol to the patient

D. **Characteristics of Aerosol Particles**
1. The ideal particle size for therapeutic use in respiratory care is 0.5 to 3.0 μm.
2. Numerous factors affect the penetration and deposition of aerosol particles.
   a. **Gravitational sedimentation:** The larger a particle is, the more effect gravity has on it and the sooner it will deposit.
   b. **Brownian movement:** Affects particles of 0.1 μm or smaller in size, which will deposit too soon (possibly in the aerosol tubing).
   c. **Inertial impaction:** Larger particles have greater inertia, which keeps them moving in a straight line. They cannot make directional changes in the airway, therefore they deposit sooner.
   d. **Hygroscopic properties:** Aerosol particles are hygroscopic (retain moisture). As they travel down the airway, they may increase in size as they retain moisture, altering the time at which they deposit.
   e. **Ventilatory pattern:** To obtain optimal particle penetration, the patient should be instructed to take **slow, moderately deep breaths** with a 2-3 second breath hold at end inspiration.

E. **Types of Nebulizers (Pneumatic)**
1. **Mechanical nebulizer** (entrainment nebulizer)

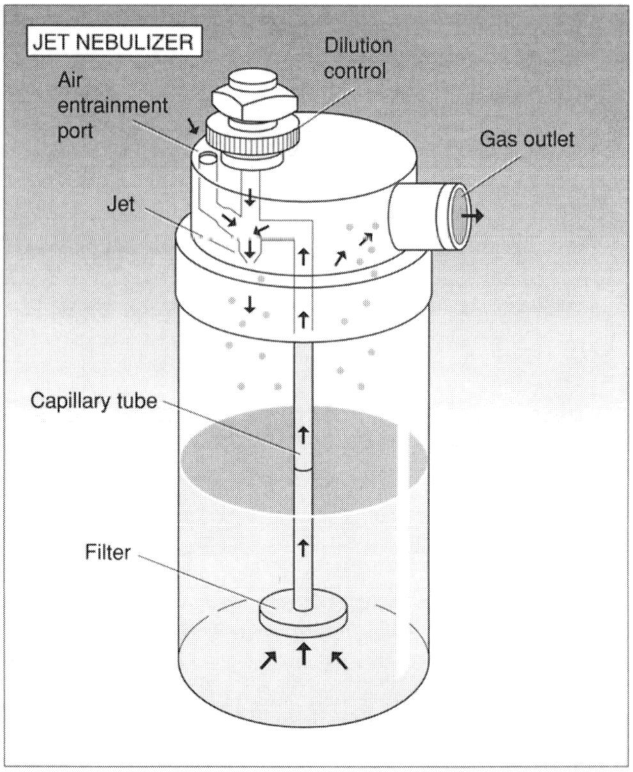

   a. Uses viscous shear forces (see later note) to draw water up the capillary tube into the gas stream to produce aerosol (mist).
   b. Uses either a **Venturi** or **Pitot tube** for the entrainment of air to obtain various oxygen percentages.
      (1) **Venturi tube:** The objective is to allow air entrainment, increase flow, and restore postrestriction pressure toward prerestriction pressure.
      (2) **Pitot tube:** The objective is to maintain high forward velocity of the gas after air entrainment occurs, which results in a high forward pressure that is better able to counteract back pressure into the device and to maintain more stable oxygen percentages of the gas. (Postrestriction lateral pressure is not restored to prerestriction levels.)

Note

Current theories in the literature suggest that the negative pressure created to entrain air is the result of viscous shear forces that occur as gas *passes through a restriction*. As the gas travels through a narrowed orifice, the flow becomes turbulent and the swirling of the gas causes a drop in pressure, allowing air to be entrained in the area of lower pressure.

c. Mechanical nebulizers produce about **50%** of their particles in the **0.5- to 3.0-μg** size range.

2. **Hydrosphere (Babington nebulizer)**

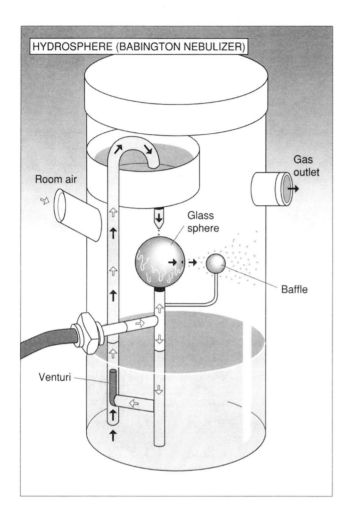

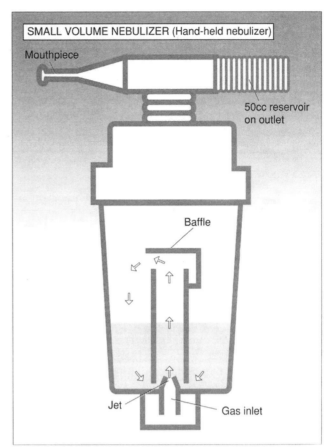

a. Water is pumped up into a reservoir above a glass sphere and drops out of the reservoir onto the sphere. The sphere has a small hole with high-velocity gas coming through it that decreases the pressure pulling the water over the sphere. Water is hit by high-velocity gas, producing an aerosol, and the particles hit a baffle, further reducing particle size.

b. About 97% of the aerosol particles produced fall within the 1- to 10-μg size range, with 50% measuring less than 5 μg.

c. The hydrosphere is commonly used to deliver aerosol to an oxygen tent.

3. **Small-volume nebulizer**

a. Used as a handheld nebulizer or as a nebulizer on a ventilator or IPPB circuit to deliver medications.

b. Usually holds 3 to 6 mL of liquid medications.

4. **Metered-dose inhaler (MDI)**

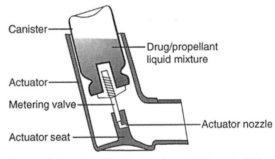

From Rau JL: Respiratory Care Pharmacology. ed 5, St. Louis, 1998, Mosby.

a. This device delivers medication in aerosol form by squeezing the vial (in which the medication is stored) upward into the delivery port. This activates a small valve that allows the pressurized gas to nebulize the medication and deliver it to the patient.

b. MDIs have become a very popular method for delivering aerosolized drugs to the respiratory tract.

c. The particle size produced varies from 2 to 40 μg. Only about 10% of the dose actually reaches the lower respiratory tract.

d. The patient **must be instructed thoroughly and correctly** on proper use of the MDI to assure optimal aerosol particle penetration.

e. These points should be emphasized in teaching the patient proper use of the MDI.
   (1) Do not place your lips around the delivery port, but keep your mouth opened wide so that the teeth and lips will not obstruct the flow of aerosol.
   (2) Hold the MDI about 1 in from the mouth, with the delivery port opening directed inside the mouth.
   (3) Inhale as slowly and as deeply as possible. **The MDI should be activated just after you start inhaling.**
   (4) Depending on the prescription, take two or three aerosol doses (puffs) in one breath.
   (5) Hold your breath at peak inspiration for **5 to 10 sec** for optimal aerosol penetration.

f. MDIs are also used on ventilator-dependent patients by placement of the device directly into the inspiratory limb of the circuit and activated by the respiratory care practitioner. Ideally, the aerosol should be delivered during a sigh breath with an inspiratory hold.

g. Spacers and holding chambers, which are extensions placed on the outlet of the MDI, have proved to be effective in minimizing aerosol loss and increasing the evaporation of the propellant. This increases the stability of

the aerosol and and results in deeper penetration of the particles.

5. **Small particle aerosol generator (SPAG nebulizer)**

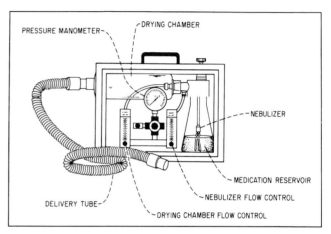

From Scanlon C, Spearman C, Sheldon R. Egan's Fundamentals of Respiratory Care. ed 5, St. Louis, 1990, CV Mosby.

★ a. This device is used to deliver the antiviral drug Ribavirin (Virazole) to infant and pediatric patients with respiratory syncytial virus (RSV) or bronchiolitis (see chapter on neonatal and pediatric respiratory care).

b. The drug exits the nebulizer through a jet and passes through a drying gas chamber that contains anhydrous (dry) gas. This further reduces the size of the particles, **the majority of which are less than 5 μg in size.**

F. **Types of Nebulizers (Electric)**
   1. **Impeller nebulizer** (spinning disk or room humidifier)

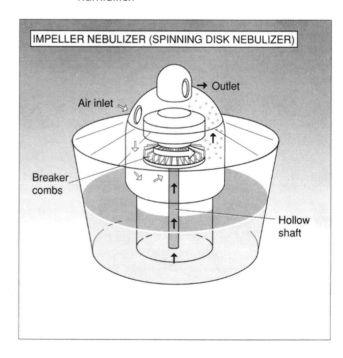

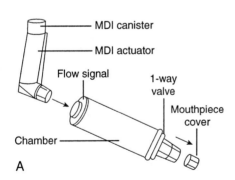

A

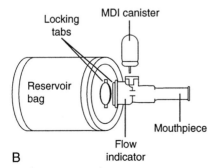

B

Types of spacers and holding chambers
From Rau JL: Respiratory Care Pharmacology. ed 5, St. Louis, 1998, Mosby.

a. The disk rotates rapidly, drawing water up from the reservoir and throwing it through a slotted baffle, which reduces the size of the particles.
b. These devices are popular for home use but, clinically, do not produce adequate aerosol output.
c. These devices are difficult to keep clean.

2. **Ultrasonic nebulizer**

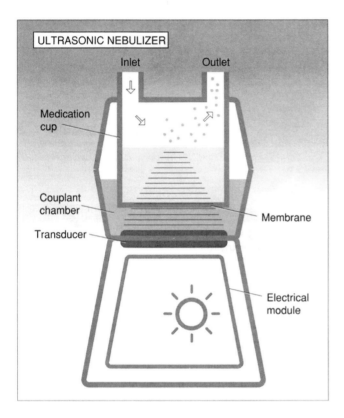

ULTRASONIC NEBULIZER

Inlet   Outlet

Medication cup

Couplant chamber

Transducer

Membrane

Electrical module

a. A piezoelectric transducer located in the bottom of the couplant chamber of the unit is electrically charged and produces high-frequency vibrations. These vibrations are focused on the bottom of the medication cup that sits in the couplant chamber. The vibrations break the medications in the cup into small particles, which are delivered to the patient.
b. **The frequency (which determines the particle size)** of the electric energy supplied to the transducer is approximately 1.35 Mc (Mc = 1 million Hz).
c. The couplant chamber contains **tap water** to help absorb mechanical heat and to act as a transfer medium for the sound waves to the medication cup.
d. The amplitude control determines the volume of the aerosol output. Volume may be as high as 6 mL/min, which is twice the

output of pneumatic nebulizers, **making the ultrasonic nebulizer the best choice for patients with thick, retained sputum.**
e. A built-in blower delivers 20 to 30 L/min of air to the medication cup to aid in aerosol delivery and help evacuate heat.
★ f. 90% of the aerosol particles produced fall within the 0.5- to 3.0-μg range.
g. The temperature of the delivered aerosol is between 3°C and 10°C above room temperature during normal operation.
h. **Hazards of ultrasonic therapy**
 (1) Overhydration
 (2) Bronchospasm
 (3) Sudden mobilization of secretions
 (4) Electrical hazard
 (5) Water collection in the tubing
 (6) Swelling of secretions from the absorption of saline, which may obstruct the airway
 (7) Changes in drug dosage, caused by the drug reconcentrating because of the solvent in the medication cup, leading to an increasingly stronger dose as the treatment continues

G. **Important Points Concerning Nebulizers**
★ 1. Of all respiratory equipment, heated nebulizers are the greatest source of delivery of contaminated moisture to the patient; *Pseudomonas* species are the most common contaminate. These nebulizers should be replaced every 12 to 24 hr.
★ 2. Make sure that jets and capillary tubes are clear of debris or buildup of minerals by cleaning after each use. If the nebulizer isn't producing adequate mist, a clogged capillary tube or jet may be the cause.
3. All nebulizers have pressure pop-off valves that should be checked after the nebulizer is set up (valves are usually set at 2 psi). The pop-off valve will be effective only if the nebulizer is set on 100% since an open entrainment port would constitute a leak in the nebulizer.
4. Keep water drained out of the aerosol tubing because this will **increase** the percentage of oxygen delivered to the patient.
5. Keep the water level at the appropriate markings on the nebulizer to ensure optimal aerosol output.
6. Soap should not be used to clean the couplant chamber or medication cup of the ultrasonic nebulizer, because residue interferes with the ultrasonic activity. Should this occur, a small amount of isopropyl alcohol in the couplant chamber or medication cup will help.

7. Make sure the filter at the end of the capillary tubes of pneumatic nebulizers are decontaminated properly. A dirty or clogged filter does not allow the fluid to be drawn up the tube adequately, reducing aerosol output.

POST-CHAPTER STUDY QUESTIONS

1. List five hazards of aerosol therapy.
2. What medication is delivered through the SPAG nebulizer?
3. If the inspired air can hold 32 mg of H_2O per liter and is holding 8 mg/L, what is the relative humidity?
4. How much of a humidity deficit exists when a patient inspires air holding 30 mg of H_2O per liter?
5. Give an example of a humidifier that can deliver gas at 100% body humidity.
6. List four hazards of ultrasonic nebulizer therapy.
7. A clogged filter or capillary tube on a jet nebulizer has what affect on the operation of the device?
8. List six clinical indications for aerosol therapy.
9. List one reason why an HME should be changed to a conventional heated humidifier.
10. How should a patient be instructed to breathe while a bronchodilating agent is being administered via a small-volume nebulizer?
11. An HME can produce a body humidity in what range?

Answers are at the end of the chapter.

REFERENCES

Eubanks D and Bone R: Comprehensive Respiratory Care, ed 2, St. Louis, 1990, The CV Mosby Company.

McPherson SP: Respiratory therapy equipment, ed 5, St. Louis, 1995, The CV Mosby Co.

McPherson SP: Respiratory home care equipment, Dubuque IA, 1988, Kendall/Hunt Publishing Co.

Scanlan C, Wilkins R, and Stoller J: Egan's fundamentals of respiratory care, ed 7, St. Louis, 1999, Mosby, Inc.

PRE-TEST ANSWERS

1. B
2. A
3. C
4. D
5. D
6. D

ANSWERS TO POST-CHAPTER STUDY QUESTIONS

1. Bronchospasm; overhydration; overheating of inspired gases; tubing condensation affecting F_{IO_2} or draining into patient's airway, delivering contaminated water to the patient
2. Ribavirin
3. 25%
4. 14 mg/L
5. Heated cascade or wick humidifier
6. Overhydration, bronchospasm, sudden mobilization of secretions, electrical hazard, condensation in tubing, swelling of secretions resulting in airway obstruction, drug reconcentration
7. Decreased water output
8. Improve secretion mobilization, delivery of aerosolized medications, prevent dehydration, induce cough, relieve upper airway inflammation, hydration of airways
9. If secretions thicken and become difficult to mobilize
10. Slow, moderately deep breaths, with a 2- to 3-sec breath hold at end of inspiration
11. 70% to 90%

Chapter 3

Assessment of the Cardiopulmonary Patient

PRE-TEST QUESTIONS

Answer the pre-test questions before studying the chapter. This will help you determine your strong and weak areas regarding the material covered.

1. A patient coughs up yellow sputum after an IPPB treatment. Which one of the following statements is TRUE in regard to this sputum production?

   A. It is old and contains little water.
   B. It is termed hemoptysis.
   C. It contains WBCs.
   D. It is a normal color for sputum.

2. The term used to describe a condition in which a patient has difficulty breathing while in a supine position is which of the following?

   A. Orthopnea
   B. Hypoventilation
   C. Paroxysmal nocturnal dyspnea
   D. Kussmaul's respirations

3. A patient enters the emergency department, and on initial examination, the respiratory care practitioner observes paradoxical respirations. Which of the following should the practitioner suspect?

   A. Pulmonary edema
   B. Pneumonia
   C. Flail chest
   D. Pleural effusion

4. Perfusion in the extremities may best be determined by which of the following methods?

   A. Obtaining ABG studies and determining the Pa_{O_2} level.
   B. Assessing the Sa_{O_2} level with a pulse oximeter.
   C. Assessing capillary refill.
   D. Palpating a brachial pulse.

5. While palpating the chest, the respiratory care practitioner determines that there are decreased vibrations over the right lower lobe. This may be the result of which of the following?

   I. Pneumothorax
   II. Pleural effusion
   III. Pneumonia

   A. I only
   B. II only
   C. I and II only
   D. II and III only

6. A chest x-ray film taken after ET intubation shows the tip of the ET tube is resting at the fourth rib. Which of the following actions should be taken?

   A. The tube should be advanced 2 cm.
   B. The tube should be advanced until equal breath sounds are heard.
   C. The tube should remain at this level.
   D. The tube should be withdrawn 3 cm.

Answers are at the end of the chapter.

REVIEW

I. **PATIENT HISTORY**
   A. Patient interview: obtain the following information
      1. Chief complaint
      2. Symptoms that the patient has and when they started
      3. Past medical problems
      4. Occupation
      5. Medications currently prescribed
      6. Allergies
      7. Exercise tolerance and daily activities
      8. Living environment
      9. Nutritional status
      10. Social support systems available
   B. Techniques for an effective patient interview
      1. Introduce yourself and establish a rapport with the patient so that the patient feels comfortable and open to discussion.

2. Try to avoid leading questions, such as "Are you still short of breath?" These questions may illicit a different response than asking "How is your breathing at this time?"
3. Always show respect for the patient's attitudes and beliefs.
4. Promote a relaxed atmosphere and avoid difficult medical terms that the patient may not understand.

EXAMPLE:

When describing the use of hyperinflation therapy, do not say, "This therapy will help you reach your inspiratory capacity and help prevent atelectasis." Do say, for example, "This therapy will help encourage you to breathe deeper to help prevent your lungs from collapsing."

---

5. To promote better understanding of the information discussed, the RCP must be able to modify terminology to fit the age or education level of the patient. Use simpler terms than the medical terms, which may be difficult for the patient.

II. **ASSESSMENT OF SYMPTOMS**
   A. **Common Symptoms in Patients with Pulmonary Disease**
      1. **Cough:** Aids in clearing the airway of secretions
         a. Nonproductive cough is caused by
            (1) Irritation of the airway
            (2) Acute inflammation of the respiratory mucosal membrane
            (3) Presence of a growth
            (4) Irritation of the pleura
            (5) Irritation of the tympanic membrane
         b. Productive cough: sputum color must be monitored
            (1) White and translucent: contains normal mucus
            (2) Yellow: indicates infection and contains WBCs; called **purulent sputum**
            (3) Green: contains old, retained secretions
          ★ (4) Green and foul-smelling: indicates *Pseudomonas* species infection
            (5) Brown: contains old blood
            (6) Red: contains fresh blood

> **Note**
>
> Foul-smelling sputum that often settles into several layers is characteristic of bronchiectasis. (See chapter 12 on disorders of the airway.)

c. When cough is productive, it is important to record the amount, consistency, odor, and color of sputum, because changes in these qualities over 24 hr are important in diagnosis of pulmonary disease.
d. Sputum collection and laboratory analysis are important parts of the pulmonary assessment. Steps in sputum collection:
   (1) Explain to patient the intent to collect a sample.
   (2) Good oral hygiene prevents the collection from being contaminated by oral secretions.
   (3) Sputum sample must be from a deep cough.

> **Note**
>
> If patient cannot cough adequately, nasotracheal suctioning for the sample may be necessary. To collect the sputum, a sputum trap or a Lukens tube catheter is necessary.

e. Characteristics of a cough
   (1) Bark-like cough usually indicates croup.
   (2) Harsh, dry cough with inspiratory stridor usually indicates upper airway problems.
   (3) Wheezing type of coughs usually indicate lower airway pathology.
   (4) Chronic productive coughs are indicative of chronic bronchitis.
   (5) Frequent hacking cough and throat clearing may be the result of smoking or sinus or viral infection.
2. **Dyspnea** is difficult or labored breathing.
   a. A subjective symptom that is influenced by the patient's reactions and emotional state.
   b. Causes of dyspnea
      (1) Increased airway resistance
      (2) Upper airway obstruction
      (3) Asthma and other chronic lung diseases
      (4) Decreased lung compliance
      (5) Pulmonary fibrosis
      (6) Pneumothorax
      (7) Pleural effusion
      (8) Abnormal chest wall
      (9) Anxiety state, when there is no physiologic explanation
   c. Types of dyspnea
      (1) **Orthopnea** is dyspnea while lying down. The condition is usually seen in patients with heart failure and is caused by increased congestion of the lungs while lying down. It is often observed in patients with emphysema

because of their inadequate diaphragmatic movement during ventilation.

(2) **Paroxysmal nocturnal dyspnea** is sudden onset of shortness of breath after being in bed for several hours. It is seen in cardiac patients and results in acute pulmonary edema, which usually subsides quickly after the patient is positioned upright.

(3) **Exertional dyspnea** is often seen in patients with cardiopulmonary disease. The severity is determined by the amount of exertion. It is important to determine at what point the patient experiences dyspnea: Does it begin after walking up a light of stairs or just walking across the room?

3. **Hemoptysis** is coughing up blood from the respiratory tract.
   a. Blood-tinged or blood-streaked sputum is not hemoptysis.
   b. Hemoptysis is determined by the coughing up of a certain volume of blood; the amount indicates the severity of the symptom.
   c. Causes of hemoptysis
      (1) Pneumonia
      (2) Tuberculosis
      (3) Bronchiectasis
      (4) Lung abscess
      (5) Fungal lung infection: histoplasmosis
      (6) Neoplasms: bronchogenic carcinoma
      (7) Pulmonary embolism
      (8) Valvular heart diseases
      (9) Mitral valve stenosis
   d. Patients may think they are "coughing up blood" from the lungs when the blood is from the gastrointestinal tract. The origin of the blood must be determined.

4. **Chest pain**
   a. The thoracic wall is the most common source of chest pain.
   b. The pain may be from nerves, muscles, or the skin or bones of the thoracic wall.
   c. The lung parenchyma is not sensitive to pain.
   d. The parietal pleura (layer lining the chest wall) is very sensitive to pain and is usually the source of pain associated with pneumonias, pleurisy, and other inflammatory processes.
   e. Chest pain may be associated with **pulmonary hypertension** caused by the increased tension on the walls of the vessels and increased workload on the right side of the heart.

   f. Chest pain may originate from the heart as a result of inadequate blood supply. This pain is called **angina pectoris.**
   g. Chest pain is also associated with a ruptured aorta, myocardial infarction, and esophageal problems.

III. **OTHER PHYSICAL ASSESSMENTS**
   A. **Breathing Patterns**
      1. **Eupnea:** the normal rate and depth of respirations, which is 10 to 20 breaths per min.
      2. **Bradypnea:** less than the normal respiratory rate. May be seen with respiratory center depression caused by head trauma or drug overdose.
      3. **Apnea:** absence of breathing for a specific period of time (usually at least 10 sec). Seen in patients with respiratory arrest caused by asphyxia, severe drug overdose, central and obstructive sleep apnea, and other central respiratory center disorders.
      4. **Tachypnea:** faster than the normal respiratory rate but with the normal depth of breathing. May indicate decreased lung compliance and is associated with restrictive diseases, pneumonia, and pulmonary edema.
      5. **Hypopnea:** shallow respirations (about half of normal depth) with slower than normal respiratory rate. Hypopnea is normal in well-conditioned athletes and is accompanied by a slow pulse rate. May be seen in patients with damage to the brain stem and is accompanied by a weak, rapid pulse.
      6. **Hyperpnea:** deep, rapid, and labored breathing. Associated with conditions in which there is an inadequate oxygen supply, such as cardiac and respiratory diseases. Usually refers to hyperventilation.
      7. **Kussmaul's respiration:** increased rate and depth of breathing. Usually seen in patients with severe metabolic acidosis (diabetic ketoacidosis).
      8. **Biot's respiration:** irregular depth of breathing with periods of apnea. Breathing may be slow and deep or rapid and shallow. Associated with elevated ICP or meningitis.
      9. **Cheyne-Stokes respiration:** deep, rapid breathing followed by apnea. The breaths begin slow and shallow and gradually increase to above normal volume and rate, then gradually diminish in volume and rate to apnea. Apnea may last 10 to 20 sec before the cycle is repeated. Seen with respiratory center depression caused by stroke or head injury, pneumonia in the elderly, or drug overdose.

B. **Chest Inspection:** This should be performed with the patient seated and clothing removed above the waist. If patient is not able to sit in a chair, he or she should be placed in bed in Fowler's position (i.e., head of bed elevated 45°). **Inspection should include:**

1. The rate, depth, and regularity of breathing compared with the norms for the patient's age and activity level.
2. Skin color, temperature, and condition, such as bruises or scars. Is patient diaphoretic (perspiring)?
3. Chest symmetry: make a comparison of one side of the chest to the other.
   a. Observe chest excursion while standing in front of the patient to determine if both sides are expanding equally.
   ★ b. Unequal expansion may indicate:
      ★ (1) Atelectasis
      ★ (2) Pneumothorax
      (3) Chest deformities
      (4) Flail chest: **"Paradoxical"** respirations may be observed, in which chest moves in on inspiration and out on expiration.
4. Shape and size of chest: in comparison to norms
   a. Observe the AP diameter.
   b. An increased AP diameter is called a **"barrel chest" and is indicative of chronic lung disease.**
5. Work of breathing
   a. Should be evaluated to determine the level of breathing difficulty.
   b. While observing the patient's breathing process, determine the following factors:
      (1) Is the chest movement symmetric?
      (2) Are the accessory muscles being used?

Note

The intercostal muscles and diaphragm are the major muscles for normal ventilation. The accessory muscles are the scalene and the sternomastoid muscles in the neck and the pectoralis major muscle in the anterior chest. When accessory muscles are used during ventilation, it is a sign of respiratory distress.

---

(3) What is the shape of the chest?
(4) What is the respiratory rate?
(5) Is the breathing pattern regular or irregular?
(6) Are there any bony deformities of the ribs, spine, or chest?

(7) Is the patient's VT normal in relation to size and age?
(8) Is expiration prolonged, shorter than inspiration, or equal to inspiration?
(9) Are substernal, suprasternal, or intercostal retractions or nasal flaring observed? **These are all signs of respiratory distress.**

C. **Inspection of the Extremities**
   1. **Digital clubbing**

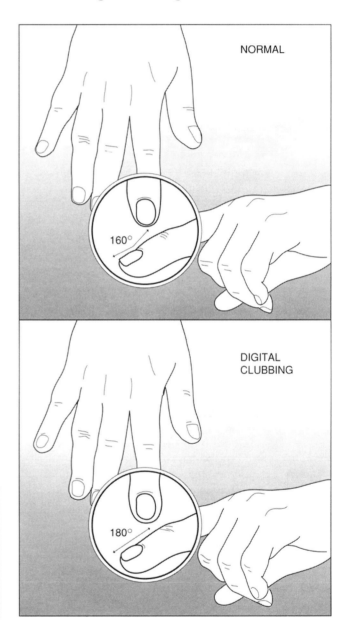

a. Digital clubbing is indicative of longstanding pulmonary disease: 75% to 85% of all clubbing is the result of pulmonary disease.
b. Consists of enlargement of the distal phalanges of the fingers and, less commonly,

the toes. There is a loss of the angle between the nail and dorsum of the terminal phalanx.

c. It is the result of **chronic hypoxemia.**

2. **Pedal edema**

a. This refers to an accumulation of fluid in the subcutaneous tissues of the ankles.

b. This symptom is commonly observed in patients with chronic pulmonary disease, in which their chronic hypoxemic state results in pulmonary vasoconstriction.

c. This results in an increased workload on the right heart, right ventricular hypertrophy, and eventually, right heart failure (cor pulmonale).

d. Venous blood flow returning to the heart is diminished, and the peripheral blood vessels become engorged. The ankles are most affected as a result of gravity.

3. **Cyanosis**

a. Refers to the bluish discoloration of the skin and nailbeds resulting from a **5 g/dL decrease in oxygenated hemoglobin.**

b. Cyanosis may indicate decreased oxygenation or reduced peripheral circulation.

c. Patients with decreased hemoglobin levels (anemia) may not exhibit cyanosis even if tissue hypoxia is present. An anemic patient has a low oxygen-carrying capacity, which may result in tissue hypoxia but does not cause cyanosis unless 5 g/dL of unsaturated hemoglobin is present. If there is not enough hemoglobin in the blood to manifest it, cyanosis will not occur.

d. Conversely, a patient with an increased level of hemoglobin (polycythemia) has an increased capacity for carrying oxygen. This patient may have a level of 5 g/dL of unsaturated hemoglobin, and therefore be cyanotic, yet have enough saturated hemoglobin to adequately oxygenate the tissues.

4. **Capillary refill**

a. Perfusion to the extremities may be determined by assessing capillary refill.

b. This is performed by compressing the patient's fingernail for a short time, then releasing it, and observing the time it takes for blood flow to return to the nailbed.

c. Normal refill time is less than 3 sec.

d. Patients with decreased cardiac output and poor digital perfusion have a longer refill time.

D. **Chest Deformities**

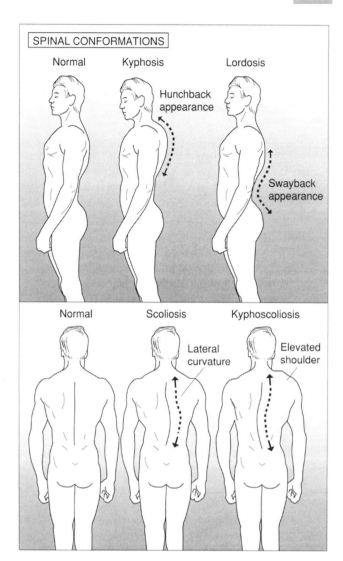

1. **Kyphosis**

a. Backward curvature of the spine, resulting in "hunchback" appearance.

b. Caused by degenerative bone disease or age or may be seen with COPD.

2. **Lordosis**

a. Backward curvature of the lumbar spine, resulting in a "swayback" appearance.

b. Usually not a cause of respiratory difficulties.

3. **Scoliosis**

a. Lateral curvature of the thoracic spine, resulting in chest protrusion posteriorly and the anterior ribs flattening out. Chest protrudes on right or left side.

b. Depending on severity, it may result in impaired lung movement.

4 **Kyphoscoliosis**

a. Combination of kyphosis and scoliosis

b. May be most adequately observed by noticing different heights of the shoulders.

c. Cardiopulmonary problems don't normally present until patients reach their 40s or 50s.

d. Pulmonary signs and symptoms of kyphoscoliosis
★ (1) Dyspnea
   (2) Hypoxemia
   (3) Hypercapnia
   (4) Progressive respiratory insufficiency
   (5) Cardiac failure
   (6) Decreased lung capacity evidenced by results of pulmonary function tests **(restrictive disease)**
   (7) Frequent pulmonary infections
   (8) Uneven ventilation/perfusion ratio

5. **Pectus carinatum**

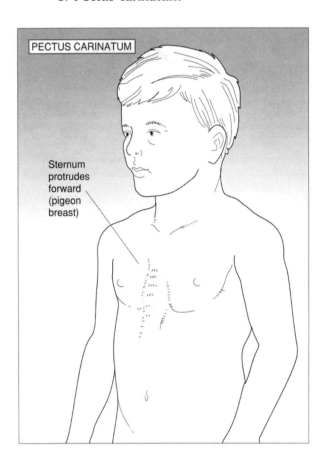

a. Also called "pigeon breast"; results in the forward projection of the xiphoid process and lower sternum.
b. Usually a congenital condition.
c. May cause dyspnea on exercise and more frequent respiratory infections as a result of interference with heart and lung movement.
d. In severe cases, surgical correction may be indicated.

6. **Pectus excavatum**
   a. Also called "funnel chest"; results in a funnel-shaped depression over the lower sternum.
   b. Usually a congenital condition.

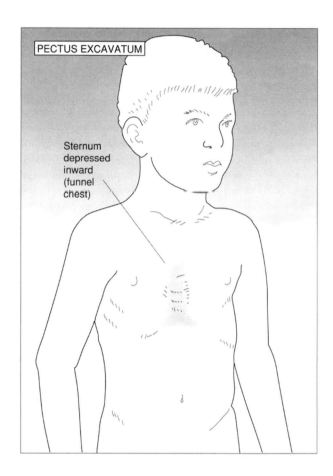

c. May lead to dyspnea on exertion and more frequent respiratory infections.

7. **Barrel chest**
★ a. Results from the premature closure of the airways that causes trapping of air and hyperinflated lungs, giving the chest a "barrel" appearance.

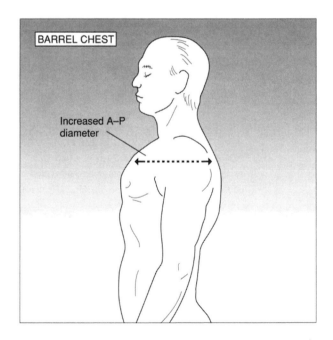

b. The increased tone and development of the accessory muscles, which are used during breathing by patients with COPD, also contributes to the barrel appearance.

★ c. Seen almost exclusively on patients with chronic lung disease.

★ d. This hyperinflated state of the lungs pushes down on the diaphragm, restricting its movement. The diaphragm is a dome-shaped muscle that is innervated by the phrenic nerve. Contraction of the muscle causes a drop in pressure within the lungs below atmospheric levels, and air enters the airway. Hyperinflated lungs tend to flatten the diaphragm, diminishing its contracting ability. This decreases alveolar ventilation and chest excursion, resulting in labored breathing.

e. Muscles normally used for ventilation are the **diaphragm and external intercostals,** but since the diaphragms of COPD patients are flattened, they use their accessory muscles during normal ventilation.

E. **Palpation of the Chest**
1. Using the sense of touch on the chest wall to assess physical signs.
2. Hands are placed on the chest to assess chest movement and vibration.
3. Vibrations felt on the chest wall as the patient speaks are called "tactile fremitus." The vibrations originate at the vocal cords and are transmitted down the tracheobronchial tree, through the alveoli to the chest wall.
   a. With the practitioner's hands on the patient's chest, the patient is asked to say certain words, such as "ninety-nine," as the practitioner palpates over different areas of the chest.
   b. Vibrations are decreased over pleural effusions, fluid, and pneumothorax.
   c. Vibrations are increased over atelectasis, pneumonia, and lung masses.
4. Position of the trachea
   a. Assessed by placing both thumbs on each side of the suprasternal notch and gently pressing inward. Only soft tissue should be palpable. If the trachea is felt, it indicates that the trachea has shifted and is no longer positioned midline, as it should be.

★ b. A shift of the trachea's position may be the result of a tension pneumothorax or massive atelectasis.
   (1) Tension pneumothorax: **trachea shifts to the unaffected side (opposite side of pneumothorax)**

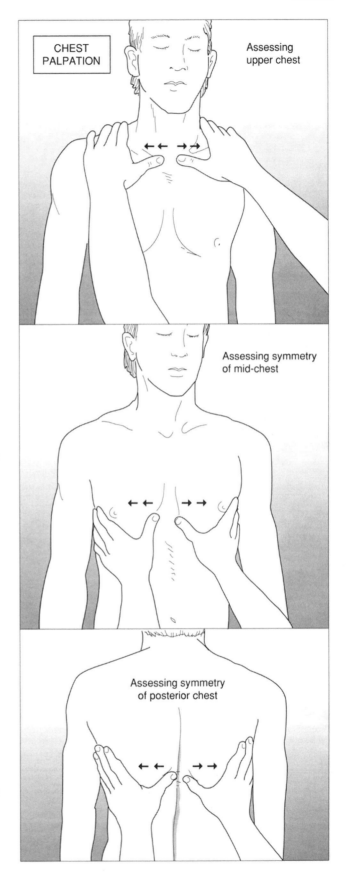

CHEST PALPATION

Assessing upper chest

Assessing symmetry of mid-chest

Assessing symmetry of posterior chest

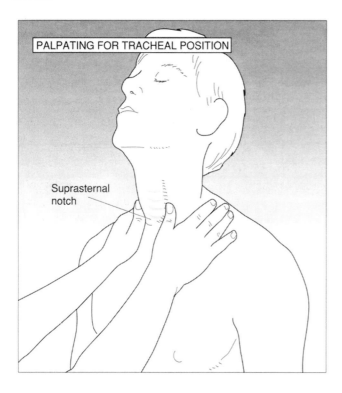

PALPATING FOR TRACHEAL POSITION

Suprasternal notch

(2) Atelectasis: **trachea shifts toward the affected side (same side as atelectasis)**

F. **Percussion of the Chest Wall**
1. This involves tapping on the chest directly with one finger or indirectly by placing one finger on chest area and tapping on that finger over different areas of the chest.
2. There are five different sounds heard during percussion.
   a. **Hyperresonance**
      (1) A loud, low-pitched sound of long duration that is produced over areas that contain a greater proportion of air than tissue.
      (2) Examples: air-filled stomach, emphysema (air trapping), pneumothorax
   b. **Resonance**
      (1) A low-pitched sound of long duration that is produced over areas with equal distribution of air and tissue.
      (2) Example: normal lung tissue
   c. **Dullness**
      (1) A sound of medium intensity and pitch of short duration that is produced over areas that contain a higher proportion of tissue or fluid than air.
      (2) Examples: atelectasis, consolidation, pleural effusion, pleural thickening, pulmonary edema
   d. **Flatness**

      (1) A sound of low amplitude and pitch that is produced over areas that contain a higher proportion of tissue than air.
      (2) Examples: massive pleural effusion, massive atelectasis, pneumonectomy
   e. **Tympany**
      (1) A drum-like sound
      (2) Example: tension pneumothorax
G. **Auscultation of Breath Sounds**
   1. **Normal breath sounds**
      a. **Vesicular**
         (1) Gentle rustling sound heard over the entire chest wall, except the right supraclavicular area.
         (2) Inspiration is longer than expiration, with no pause between.
      b. **Bronchial**
         (1) Loud and generally high-pitched sound heard over the upper portion of the sternum, trachea, and both mainstem bronchi.
         (2) Expiration is longer than inspiration, with a short pause between.
         (3) If heard in other lung areas, indicates atelectasis or consolidation
      c. **Bronchovesicular**
         (1) A combination of bronchial and vesicular breath sounds, normally heard over the sternum, between the scapulae, and over the right apex of the lung
         (2) Inspiration and expiration are of equal duration, with no pause between.
      d. **Tracheal**
         (1) Harsh and high-pitched sound heard over the trachea.
         (2) Expiration is slightly longer than inspiration.
   2. **Adventitious breath sounds**
      a. **Crackles**
         (1) Bubbling or crackling sound heard primarily on inspiration, produced by air flowing through fluid in the alveoli or small airways.
         (2) Crackles are commonly heard in patients with pulmonary edema, pneumonia, emphysema, atelectasis, or fibrosis. Crackles are also heard at the end of inspiration resulting from alveoli popping open.
      b. **Rhonchi**
         (1) Sounds that are produced in airways filled with secretions or fluids. Typically, a rumbling sound is heard on expiration, primarily in larger airways.

(3) Caused by asthma, emphysema, mucus plugs, or stenosis.

> **Note**
>
> A distinguishing feature between crackles and rhonchi is that rhonchi generally clear after coughing, while crackles usually do not.

c. **Wheezes**
   (1) Often considered a rhonchi with a musical quality, produced by air flow through constricted airways
   (2) May be heard on both inspiration and expiration
   ★ (3) Wheezes are heard characteristically with asthma and are a result of bronchoconstriction.
d. **Pleural friction rub**
   (1) Clicking or grating sound caused by friction that is produced as the parietal and visceral pleura rub against each other during the breathing process
   (2) Most commonly associated with pleurisy and is very painful

H. **Auscultation of heart sounds**
   1. **Normal heart sounds:** Heart sounds are thought to be produced as a result of sudden changes in blood flow through the heart that cause a vibration of the valves and chambers inside the heart. The normal heart sound is a "lubb-dub" sound.
      a. The first heart sound ("lubb") represents the closing of the AV valves.
         (1) The AV valves are the mitral valve (between the left atrium and left ventricle) and the tricuspid valve (between the right atrium and right ventricle).
         (2) The first heart sound is designated **S1.**
      b. The second heart sound ("dub") represents the closing of the semilunar valves.
         (1) The semilunar valves consist of the pulmonic valve (between the right ventricle and the pulmonary artery) and the aortic valve (between the left ventricle and aorta).
         (2) The second heart sound is designated **S2.**
      c. A third and fourth heart sound (**S3 and S4**) may be heard, but they are more difficult to hear than **S1 and S2** and are more easily heard in children.
         (1) **S3** is thought to result from blood rushing into the ventricles during early ventricular diastole.
         (2) **S4** is thought to result from atrial contraction.
   2. **Abnormal heart sounds (murmurs)**
      a. Murmurs usually occur when blood flows in a turbulent fashion through heart structures that have a decreased cross-sectional area.
      b. Murmurs are described by the location of the sound, the part of the cardiac cycle in which they occur, and the intensity of the sound.
      c. **Conditions resulting in heart murmurs**
         (1) Aortic valve disease (stenosis, regurgitation, etc.)
         (2) Mitral valve disease (stenosis, regurgitation, etc.)
         (3) Pulmonic valve stenosis
         (4) Tricuspid valve insufficiency

> **Note**
>
> An abnormal sound heard over the heart or arteries or veins that is caused by turbulent blood flow or an obstruction is referred to as a bruit.

I. **Chest X-ray Film Interpretation**
   1. Useful terms when interpreting chest films
      a. **AP view:** chest film taken from front to back
      b. **Consolidation:** well-defined, solid-appearing lung that appears light on the film and is **caused by pneumonia.**
      c. **Radiodensity** describes white areas on the film that indicate fluids and solids; radiodensity is **caused by pneumonia and pleural effusion, for example.**
      d. **Infiltrates** are **scattered or patchy white areas on the film** that are caused by inflammatory processes that indicate **atelectasis or disease.**
      e. **Radiolucency appears dark on x-ray film and indicates air; hyperlucency is characteristic of emphysema, asthma, or subcutaneous emphysema.**
   2. RCPs most commonly examine chest x-ray film for the following
      a. **Atelectasis**
         (1) Appears lighter than normal lung tissue
         (2) May be indicated by elevated diaphragm, mediastinal shift (toward

area of atelectasis), or increased density and decreased volume of a lung area

b. **Pneumonia**
   (1) Appears white on x-ray film
   (2) Consolidation of entire lobe or more may cause **mediastinal shift toward the consolidation.**

c. **Pneumothorax**
   (1) Air found in the pleural cavity appears dark with no vascular markings in the involved areas.
   (2) **Tension pneumothorax** may result in mediastinal shift and a tracheal **shift away from the side of the pneumothorax.**

d. **ET tube placement**
   ★ (1) Tube should rest about 2 to 7 cm above the carina, which is located on x-ray film at the level of the fourth rib or fourth thoracic vertebra.
   (2) If ET tube is inserted too far, it has a greater tendency to enter the **right mainstem bronchus.**
   (3) If right mainstem is inadvertently intubated, diminished breath sounds would be heard on the left and asymmetrical chest movement may be observed.

e. **Heart shadow**
   (1) Should appear white in the middle of the chest, with the left heart border easily determined
   (2) A normal heart should be less than half the width of the chest. Increased heart size may indicate CHF.

f. **Diaphragm**
   (1) Should be rounded or dome-shaped
   (2) Appears white on x-ray film at the level of the sixth rib
   ★ (3) Patients with hyperinflated lungs (i.e., who have COPD) have flattened diaphragms.
   (4) Both hemidiaphragms should be assessed for height and angle to the chest wall.
   (5) The dome of the right hemidiaphragm is normally 1 to 2 cm higher than the left because of space needed for the liver.
   (6) Elevation of one hemidiaphragm may be the result of gas in the stomach or of atelectasis.

J. **Pulse**
1. Pulse is a direct indicator of the heart's action.
2. Normal heart rate in adult: 60 to 90 beats/min

3. Normal heart rate in child: 90 to 120 beats/min
4. An abnormally low heart rate is called **bradycardia;** caused by infection, hypothermia, or heart abnormalities.
5. An abnormally high heart rate is called **tachycardia;** caused by hypoxemia, fever, loss of blood volume, heart abnormalities, and anxiety.
6. **Peripheral edema and venous engorgement** indicate inadequate pumping action of the heart, resulting from right heart failure (cor pulmonale) or left heart failure (CHF).
7. **Paradoxical pulse** (pulsus paradoxus) is a pulse that becomes weaker on inspiration; it may be defined as a decrease in systolic pressure of more than 10 mm Hg during inspiration and may be seen in patients with severe COPD, including asthma, pericarditis, pulmonary embolism, CHF, and pericardial effusion. If paradoxical pulse is observed after chest trauma or cardiothoracic surgery, cardiac tamponade should be suspected. Cardiac tamponade is a life-threatening condition in which blood collects in the pericardial sac and causes pressure that prevents the heart from pumping adequately.
8. **Pulsus alternans** is an alternating pattern of strong and weak pulses. The ventricle ejects more than the normal amount of blood with a contraction and then less than the normal amount of blood with the next contraction. This is commonly observed in patients with LVF and usually indicates bigeminal PVCs (see chapter on cardiac monitoring).

K. **Blood pressure**
1. Blood pressure is measurement of the pressure within the arterial system.
2. Normal range for adults: 100/60 mm Hg to 140/90 mm Hg
3. Normal range for children: 95/60 mm Hg to 110/65 mm Hg
4. Normal range for neonates: 60/30 mm Hg to 90/60 mm Hg
5. Systolic pressure (first or top number) is the pressure measured during ventricular contraction.
6. Diastolic pressure (last or bottom number) is the pressure measured while the ventricles are at rest.
7. The diastolic pressure is the most critical measurement because it is the lowest pressure that the heart and arterial system experience.

8. An abnormally low blood pressure is called **hypotension;** usually caused by shock, high-volume blood loss, positioning, and CNS depressant drugs.
9. An abnormally high blood pressure is called **hypertension;** usually caused by cardiovascular imbalances, stimulant drugs, stress, and fluid retention resulting from renal failure.
10. Many factors affect blood pressure.
    a. Blood volume
    b. Blood viscosity
    c. Heart's pumping action
    d. Elasticity of the blood vessels
    e. Resistance to blood flow through the vessels
11. Blood pressure is measured with a sphygmomanometer (blood pressure cuff).

L. **Body temperature**
1. Normal body temperature is 98.6°F (37°C).
2. Slightly higher temperature in children is normal as a result of a higher metabolic rate.
3. An abnormally low body temperature is called **hypothermia** and is caused by sweating (diaphoresis), blood loss, exposure to cold temperatures, and abnormally high heat loss.
4. An abnormally high body temperature is called **hyperthermia** and is caused by decreased heat loss, infection, or increased environmental temperature.

> **Note**
>
> A fever results in increased oxygen consumption, leading to an increased work of breathing to meet the increased oxygen demands of the body.

5. The term used to describe a person with normal body temperature is **afebrile;** the term used to describe a person with a fever is **febrile.**

M. **Assessing Mental Status**
1. **Level of consciousness**
    a. Alert: patient is awake and responds to stimuli
    b. Obtunded and confused: patient is awake but responds slowly to commands and may be disoriented
    c. Lethargic: patient seems unconscious but, when stimulated, will awaken
    d. Coma: patient is unconscious and, when stimulated, will not awaken
2. **Orientation to time and place**
    a. Ask patient the date
    b. Ask if patient knows where he or she is
3. **Ability to cooperate**
    a. Ask patient to follow simple commands

b. Patient cooperation is necessary for effective therapy, such as incentive spirometry or IPPB
4. **Emotional state**
    a. Ask patient to describe his or her feelings
    b. Note patient's emotional response while you are asking questions

IV. **ASSESSMENT OF LABORATORY TEST RESULTS**

> **Exam Note**
>
> Reviewing the patient chart for laboratory values appears on the CRT examination. Reviewing the laboratory values, recommending procedures to obtain more data, and evaluating and monitoring lab data appears on the RRT examination only.

A. **Serum Electrolytes**
1. **Sodium** (Na^+)
    ★ a. Normal level: 135 to 145 mEq/L
    b. Sodium is the major cation in the extracellular fluid, and its concentration is controlled by the kidneys by means of regulating the amount of water in the body.
    c. **Hyponatremia** is an Na^+ level < 135 mEq/L; causes include:
       (1) Renal failure
       (2) CHF
       (3) Excessive fever or sweating
       (4) Long-term diuretic administration
       (5) Inadequate sodium intake
       (6) Excessive water ingestion
       (7) Severe burns
       (8) GI fluid losses (vomiting, diarrhea)
    d. **Clinical symptoms of hyponatremia**
       (1) Muscle weakness, **making ventilator weaning difficult**
       (2) Confusion
       (3) Muscle twitching progressing to convulsions
       (4) Anxiety
       (5) Alterations in level of consciousness
    e. **Hypernatremia** is an Na^+ level > 145 mEq/L; causes include
       (1) Excessive water loss (sweating, diarrhea)
       (2) Renal failure
       (3) Inadequate water intake
       (4) Mannitol diuresis
       (5) Corticosteroid administration
    f. **Clinical symptoms of hypernatremia**
       (1) Confusion
       (2) CNS dysfunction
       (3) Seizure activity

(4) Coma
2. **Potassium** (K^+)
  ★ a. Normal value: 3.5 to 5.0 mEq/L
  b. Potassium is the major intracellular cation.
  c. **Hypokalemia** is a K^+ level < 3.5 mEq/L; causes include:
    (1) Diuretic therapy
    (2) Adrenocorticosteroid administration
    (3) Vomiting, diarrhea
    (4) Burns
    (5) Severe trauma
  d. **Clinical symptoms of hypokalemia**
  ★ (1) Muscle weakness leading to paralysis, respiratory failure, and hypotension
  ★ (2) Cardiac arrhythmias
    (a) Premature atrial contractions and PVCs
    (b) Atrial and ventricular tachycardia
    (c) Asystole
    (3) ST segment depression on ECG
    (4) Decreased GI tract motility resulting in abdominal distention
  e. **Hyperkalemia** is a K^+ level > 5.0 mEq/L; causes include:
    (1) Acidosis
    (2) Renal insufficiency
    (3) Tissue necrosis
    (4) Hemorrhage
  f. **Clinical symptoms of hyperkalemia**
    (1) Paralysis
  ★ (2) ECG abnormalities
    (a) Shortened QT interval
    (b) Widened QRS complex
    (c) Prolonged PR interval
    (d) Absence of P wave
  ★ (3) Cardiac arrhythmias
    (a) Ventricular arrhythmias
    (b) Nodal arrhythmias
3. **Chloride** (Cl^-)
  ★ a. Normal value: 95 to 105 mEq/L
  b. Chloride is the major anion in the body; two-thirds of chloride in the body is found in extracellular compartments. Since chloride is generally excreted with potassium as potassium chloride by the kidney, decreased levels of one results in decreased levels of the other.
  c. **Hypochloremia** is a Cl^- level < 95 mEq/L; causes include:
    (1) Vomiting, diarrhea
    (2) Furosemide (Lasix) diuresis

Note

Hypochloremia may result in metabolic alkalosis.

---

d. **Clinical symptoms of hypochloremia**
    (1) Muscle spasm
    (2) Coma (in severe hypochloremia)
  e. **Hyperchloremia** is a Cl^- level > 105 mEq/L; causes include:
    (1) Respiratory alkalosis
    (2) Metabolic acidosis
    (3) Dehydration
    (4) Administration of excessive amounts of $NaCl^-$ and K^+
  f. **Clinical symptoms of hyperchloremia**
    (1) Headache
    (2) Malaise
    (3) Weakness
    (4) Unconsciousness
    (5) Coma
4. **Calcium** (Ca)
  ★ a. Normal value: 4.25 to 5.25 mEq/L
  b. Most of the body's calcium is contained in the bones; it plays a major role in neuromuscular function and cellular enzyme reactions.
  c. **Hypocalcemia** is a Ca level < 4.25 mEq/L; causes include:
    (1) Severe trauma
    (2) Renal failure
    (3) Severe pancreatitis
    (4) Vitamin D deficiency
    (5) Parathyroid hormone deficiency
  d. **Clinical symptoms of hypocalcemia**
    (1) Muscle spasm
    (2) abdominal cramping
    (3) convulsions (rare)
    (4) Prolonged QT interval on ECG
  e. **Hypercalcemia** is a Ca level > 5.25 mEq/L; causes include:
    (1) Hyperthyroidism
    (2) Vitamin A or D intoxication
    (3) Hyperparathyroidism
    (4) Sarcoidosis
    (5) Cancer metastasis to the bone
  f. **Clinical symptoms of hypercalcemia**
    (1) Muscle weakness, **making ventilator weaning difficult**
    (2) Fatigue
    (3) Mental depression
    (4) Anorexia
    (5) Nausea, vomiting
    (6) Coma (in severe cases)
5. **Bicarbonate** (HCO_3^-) (see chapter on ABG interpretation)
B. **Blood Urea Nitrogen** (BUN)
  1. Urea is a substance produced in the liver; it is carried in the blood to the kidneys, where it is excreted in the urine.

2. If the kidneys fail to remove urea from the blood adequately, the blood urea concentration increases.

★3. The normal BUN level is 7 to 20 mg/dL.

   4. **An elevated BUN level is indicative of renal failure.**

C. **Glucose**

★ 1. Normal serum level: 70 to 105 mg/dL

★2. Elevated levels observed in diabetic ketoacidosis; patient compensates with alveolar hyperventilation (Kussmaul's respirations, as mentioned earlier in this chapter).

D. **Hematology Tests**

   1. **Red blood cells** (RBC)

      a. The number of red blood cells, also referred to as **erythrocytes,** determine the adequacy of oxygen transport.

      b. Normal level: 4 to 6 million/mm^3 of blood.

   ★ c. A decreased RBC count (or anemia) indicates an inadequate oxygen-carrying capacity of the blood. Treatment is a blood transfusion.

   2. **Hemoglobin** (Hb)

      a. Hemoglobin is the portion of the red blood cell that carries oxygen, so it is an indicator of the oxygen-carrying capacity of the blood.

   ★ b. Normal level: 13.5 to 18.0 g/dL in males; 12 to 16 g/dL in females

      c. A subnormal hemoglobin level indicates inadequate oxygen-carrying capacity in the blood. Treatment is a blood transfusion.

   3. **Hematocrit** (Hct)

      a. The hematocrit is the percentage of the total blood volume that is RBCs.

      b. Normal levels: 43% to 50% in males; 37% to 43% in females. Average levels: 35% to 45%.

      c. A decreased hematocrit level indicates inadequate oxygen-carrying capacity in the blood. Treatment is a blood transfusion.

   4. **White blood cells** (WBCs)

      a. The WBC count determines the presence or absence of infection. WBCs are also referred to as **leukocytes.**

   ★ b. Normal Level: 5,000 to 10,000/mm^3 of blood

   ★ c. An elevated WBC count indicates the presence of infection. The RCP should recommend a chest x-ray film and sputum culture to determine lung involvement.

E. **Coagulation Studies**

   1. Platelet count

      a. Normal level: 150,000 to 400,000/mm^3 of blood

      b. Platelets are the smallest cells in the blood and are essential for coagulation (clotting).

      c. Decreased platelet count may be the result of bone marrow diseases or DIC.

   2. Prothrombin time (PT)

      a. A test used to determine the clotting ability of the blood.

      b. Normal PT: 11.0 to 12.5 sec

   3. Partial thromboplastin time (PTT)

      a. Another test to determine the clotting ability of the blood.

      b. Normal PTT: 60 to 85 sec

Note

It is important for the RCP to assess these coagulation studies. Patients with decreased platelet counts or increased PT or PTT are at increased risk of hemorrhaging. This means great care must be taken during nasotracheal suctioning or arterial puncture. Nasotracheal suctioning should be minimized, and puncture sites should be compressed longer after an arterial stick than for other patients.

F. **Urinalysis** is a routine analysis that includes chemical analysis to detect protein (proteinuria), sugar (glucosuria), and ketones (ketonuria) and microscopic analysis to detect WBCs and RBCs.

   1. Proteinuria is usually a sign of kidney disease.

   2. Glucosuria is commonly found in diabetics or patients with kidney disorders.

   3. Ketonuria is observed in patients affected by starvation, diabetes, and alcohol intoxication. Ketones are formed as the body breaks down fat.

   4. Hematuria is defined as blood in the urine and is observed in patients with renal and genitourinary disorders.

G. **Fluid Balance:** Important in all patients, but especially so for mechanical ventilator-dependent patients. Recording fluid input and output volumes is mandatory.

Exam Note

Questions relating to fluid balance (intake and output) appear on the RRT examination only.

---

   1. Signs of **dehydration**

      a. Hypotension

      b. Decreased cardiac output

      c. Thick pulmonary secretions

      d. Decreased urine output

   2. Causes of **dehydration**

      a. Vomiting and diarrhea

b. Inadequate humidification of inspired gases
c. Excessive ventilation
d. Inadequate IV fluids
e. Excessive urination

3. Treatment for **dehydration**
   a. Increase IV fluids.
   b. Ensure adequate humidification of the airway by using conventional heated humidifiers in place of HMEs.
   c. Direct instillation of saline down the ET tube to help thin secretions.
   d. Provide water via USN therapy.

4. Signs of **overhydration**
   a. Increased $P(A-a)O_2$
   b. Evidence of CHF on chest x-ray
   c. Decreasing lung compliance
   d. Increased PCWP
   e. Pulmonary edema
   f. Crackles (rales) on auscultation

5. Causes of **overhydration**
   a. Excessive fluid intake (near-drowning, excessive IV fluids, water intoxication)
   b. Inadequate excretion (renal insufficiency)
   c. Increased levels of ADH
   d. Prolonged USN therapy

6. Treatment for **overhydration**
   a. Reduction in IV fluid volume
   b. Restrict oral intake
   c. Diuretic therapy

Note

Normal urine output is 700 to 2000 mL/day.

V. REVIEWING THE PATIENT CHART

A. Once the patient has been admitted and requires respiratory care, the chart should be reviewed for the following information.

1. Patient history
2. Physical examination on admission
3. Current vital signs
   a. Heart rate
   b. Respiratory rate: If the rate remains elevated or there is little or no change in the patient's respiratory distress, the RCP should recommend modifications in the prescribed oxygen therapy (such as increasing the FIO_2, placement on CPAP, or institution of mechanical ventilation) (see chapter on ventilator management).
   c. Blood pressure: A decrease in blood pressure may indicate excessive PEEP levels, requiring a decrease in the prescribed

level of PEEP (see chapter on ventilator management).

4. Current respiratory care orders
   a. Oxygen delivery device
   b. Percentage or flow rate of oxygen
   c. Type of ventilator and prescribed parameters
   d. Frequency and duration of prescribed treatments
   e. Medications ordered with the treatment

5. Patient progress notes

6. **ABG levels:** Abnormal values in PaO_2 and/or $PaCO_2$ indicate that changes in oxygen therapy or ventilatory parameters are necessary (see chapters on ABG interpretation and ventilator management).

7. Pulmonary function test results
   a. Determine severity of lung dysfunction
   b. Determine obstructive or restrictive abnormalities
   c. Recommendation for before and after bronchodilator studies to determine responsiveness to therapy

VI. CLINICAL APPLICATION OF COMPUTERS

A. **Computerized Charting**

1. Practitioners are now using handheld computers to chart information, rather than recording in the patient chart manually.

2. Patient orders, progress notes, treatment times, and ventilator settings are often charted through the computer. This information can be downloaded into a central workstation or may be printed for all practitioners to use. This can be very helpful when giving reports to the oncoming shift.

B. **Computerized Monitoring**

1. The most common types of computer monitoring of the patient are hemodynamic monitoring, ventilator monitoring, and ECG monitoring. Data collected can be stored so that an interpretation may be done at any time.

2. Interpretations of ABG levels may be accomplished through computer software specifically designed for this purpose.

3. Computer software provides for the calculation and interpretation of ventilation parameters, such as static lung compliance, $P(A-a)O_2$, shunt calculations, and many other pulmonary and hemodynamic parameters.

4. Computerized technology has been used for pulmonary function testing for several years. Interpretation of results is accomplished with program algorithms.

VII. DEVELOPING RESPIRATORY CARE PLANS AND PROTOCOLS

Many institutions around the country have adopted Therapist Driven Protocols (TDPs).

1. TDPs are guidelines that are used to determine the appropriateness of respiratory care treatments; they include the correct delivery method, indications, and discontinuation protocols.
2. TDPs are written in either algorithm or outline form.
3. Advantages of TDPs
   a. The practitioner is more actively involved with determining therapy modifications as the patient's clinical status changes.
   b. Improved treatment allocation
   c. Improved cost management

POST-CHAPTER STUDY QUESTIONS

1. What is yellow sputum indicative of?
2. What bacterial organism should be suspected if the patient's sputum is green and foul-smelling?
3. List nine causes of dyspnea.
4. What does the term orthopnea mean and in which patients is it most commonly found?
5. Describe Kussmaul's respirations and in which patients this breathing pattern is most often seen.
6. List three conditions in which asymmetrical chest movement may be observed.
7. Describe paradoxical respiration and name a condition in which it is most commonly observed.
8. Define pedal edema and what causes it.
9. Name a condition that results in the trachea shifting toward the side of the body that condition is affecting.
10. Name a condition that results in the trachea shifting away from the affected side.
11. Which muscles are used for normal ventilation?
12. What causes the "barrel chest" appearance in patients with COPD?
13. Name two conditions in which a hyperresonant percussion note would be heard.
14. Name two conditions in which a dull percussion note would be heard.
15. List four conditions that result in heart murmurs.
16. List the normal values for the following electrolytes: sodium, potassium, and chloride.
17. Why would decreased sodium and potassium levels make weaning a patient from the ventilator more difficult?
18. What does an elevated BUN level indicate?
19. How does the respiratory system compensate when glucose levels increase in a diabetic patient?

20. List the normal levels for each of the following: RBC count, Hb level, Hct, and WBC count.
21. What do decreases in Hb level, Hct, and RBC count indicate?
22. Name two conditions that cause a decreased platelet count.
23. Patients with a decreased platelet count and increased PT are at a greater risk for what occurrence?
24. List four signs of dehydration.
25. List six causes of dehydration.
26. List six signs of overhydration.

Answers are at the end of the chapter.

REFERENCES

Eubanks DH and Bone RC: Comprehensive respiratory care, ed 2, St. Louis, 1990, The CV Mosby Co.

Farzan S: A concise handbook of respiratory diseases, ed 4, Stamford, CT, 1997, Appleton & Lange.

Levitzky M, Introduction to respiratory care, Philadelphia, 1990, WB Saunders Co.

Scanlan CL, Wilkins RL, and Stoller JK: Egan's fundamentals of respiratory care, ed 7, St. Louis, 1999, Mosby, Inc.

Clinical assessment in respiratory care, ed 3, St. Louis, 1995, Mosby-Yearbook, Inc.

PRE-TEST ANSWERS

1. C
2. A
3. C
4. C
5. C
6. D

ANSWERS TO POST-CHAPTER QUESTIONS

1. Infection (increased WBC count)
2. *Pseudomonas* species
3. Increased airway resistance, COPD, upper airway obstruction, decreased lung compliance, pulmonary fibrosis, pneumothorax, pleural effusion, abnormal chest wall, anxiety
4. Difficulty sleeping while lying down (supine), COPD, chronic cardiac disease, obese patients
5. Deep, rapid breathing pattern (hyperventilation), diabetic ketoacidosis (DKA)

6. Atelectasis, pneumothorax, chest deformities, flail chest
7. Chest moves in during inspiration and out during expiration; flail chest or other chest trauma
8. Fluid around the ankles that results from right-sided or left-sided heart failure
9. Massive atelectasis
10. Tension pneumothorax
11. Diaphragm, external intercostal muscles
12. Air-trapping, enlarged accessory muscles of the chest
13. Pneumothorax, emphysema
14. Atelectasis, consolidation, pleural effusion, pleural thickening, pulmonary edema
15. Aortic valve disease, mitral valve disease, pulmonic valve stenosis, tricuspid valve insufficiency
16. Na^+, 135 to 145 mEq/L; K^+, 3.5 to 5.0 mEq/L; Cl^-, 95 to 105 mEq/L

17. Both result in muscle weakness
18. Renal failure
19. Alveolar hyperventilation
20. RBCs, 4 to 6 million/mm^3; Hb, males 13 to 18 g/dL, females 12 to 16 g/dL; Hct, 35% to 45%; WBC 5000 to 10,000/mm^3
21. Inadequate oxygen-carrying capacity
22. Bone marrow diseases, DIC
23. Hemorrhaging
24. Hypotension, decreased cardiac output, thick pulmonary secretions, decreased urine output
25. Vomiting, diarrhea, inadequate humidification of inspired air, excessive ventilation, excessive urine output, inadequate IV fluids
26. Increased $P(A-a)O_2$, CHF findings on x-ray studies, decreased lung compliance, increased PCWP, pulmonary edema, crackles on auscultation

Chapter 4

Management of the Airway

PRE-TEST QUESTIONS

Answer the pre-test questions before studying the chapter. This will help you determine your strong and weak areas regarding the material covered.

1. Which of the following are hazards of an EOA?

    I. Tracheal intubation
    II. Rupture of esophagus
    III. Vomiting on removal of the EOA

    A. I only
    B. I and II only
    C. II and III only
    D. I, II and III

2. Opening the patient's airway using an oropharyngeal airway is most beneficial when the obstruction is caused by which of the following?

    A. Secretions
    B. Foreign body
    C. Edema
    D. Tongue

3. McGill forceps are used during which of the following procedures?

    A. Nasotracheal intubation
    B. Oral intubation
    C. Tracheotomy
    D. Insertion of an EOA

4. The physician wants to begin weaning a patient from a tracheostomy tube. How may this best be accomplished?

    A. Deflate the cuff every 2 hours.
    B. Change to a fenestrated tracheostomy tube.
    C. Keep the cuff inflated and remove the inner cannula.
    D. Change to a tracheostomy tube with a foam cuff.

5. You are called to a patient's room because a ventilator alarm is sounding. You hear an audible leak around the patient's ET tube during a ventilator breath and notice the exhaled volume reading is 150 mL less than the set V_T. You check the cuff pressure and find that it is 12 mm Hg. The appropriate action is which of the following?

    A. Maintain the current cuff pressure and increase the patient's V_T to compensate for the leak.
    B. Instill enough air to maintain a cuff pressure of 30 mm Hg.
    C. While listening with a stethoscope at the larynx, instill air into the cuff until a slight leak is heard on inspiration.
    D. Instill enough air until only a slight audible leak is heard.

6. You want to attempt to pass a suction catheter into the patient's left lung to obtain a sputum specimen. What would be the most appropriate method to achieve this?

    A. Have the patient turn the head to the left.
    B. Have the patient turn the head to the right.
    C. Use a coudé suction catheter.
    D. Use a catheter that is one-half the internal diameter of the patient's airway.

Answers are at the end of the chapter.

REVIEW

I. **UPPER AIRWAY OBSTRUCTION**
   A. **Main Causes of Upper Airway Obstruction**
      1. Tongue falling back against the posterior wall of the pharynx, resulting from unconsciousness or CNS abnormality.
      2. Edema, or postextubation inflammation and swelling, of the glottic area.
      3. Bleeding
      4. Secretions
      5. Foreign substances
         a. Foreign bodies

b. False teeth

c. Vomitus

6. Laryngospasm

B. **Signs of Partial Upper Airway Obstruction**

1. Crowing, gasping sounds on inspiration

2. Not able to cough (with a slight obstruction, the patient may be able to cough)

3. Increasing respiratory difficulty

4. Good to poor air exchange (depending on severity of obstruction)

5. Exaggerated chest and abdominal movement without comparable air movement

6. Cyanosis (depending on severity of obstruction)

C. **Signs of Complete Upper Airway Obstruction**

1. Inability to talk

2. Increased respiratory difficulty with no air movement

3. Cyanosis

4. Sternal, intercostal, and epigastric retractions

5. Use of accessory muscles of the neck and chest

6. Extreme panic

7. Unconsciousness and respiratory arrest, if obstruction is not removed

D. **Treatment of Airway Obstruction**

1. If the patient is conscious and has a partial airway obstruction, patient should be left alone and allowed to try to relieve the obstruction on his or her own.

2. If the patient is conscious and has a complete airway obstruction caused by food or a foreign object, abdominal thrusts must be performed until the object is dislodged (see chapter on CPR).

3. If the patient is unconscious and has a partial or complete airway obstruction that is most likely caused by the tongue, the head tilt and chin lift maneuver will help relieve the obstruction by moving the tongue forward.

II. **ARTIFICIAL AIRWAYS**

A. **Oropharyngeal Airway**

1. Maintains a patent airway by lying between the base of the tongue and the posterior wall of the pharynx, preventing the tongue from falling back and occluding the airway.

2. **Must only be used on the unconscious patient,** because a conscious patient would gag on the airway, potentially leading to aspiration.

3. This airway should **never** be taped in place, because if the patient becomes conscious, the airway must be easily removable to prevent vomiting and aspiration.

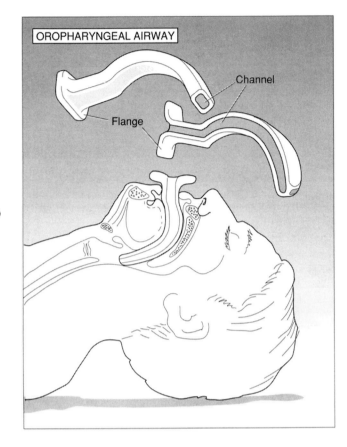

OROPHARYNGEAL AIRWAY

Channel

Flange

4. Proper insertion of the oropharyngeal airway

a. Measure the airway from the corner of the lip to the angle of the jaw to ensure proper length.

b. Remove foreign substances from the mouth.

c. Hyperextend the neck.

d. Using the cross-finger technique, open the patient's mouth and insert the airway with the tip pointing toward the roof of the mouth.

e. Observe the airway passing the uvula and rotate the airway 180°.

5. **Hazards of oropharyngeal airways**

a. Gagging or fighting the airway; if this occurs, remove the airway immediately

b. Base of tongue pushed into the back of the throat and obstructing the airway if inserted improperly

c. Pushing the epiglottis into the laryngeal area with an airway that is too large

d. Aspiration of the airway or ineffectiveness in relieving obstruction because airway is too small

6. **Important points concerning oropharyngeal airways**

★ a. Oropharyngeal airways may be used in the unconscious, orally intubated patient to prevent the patient from biting the ET tube.

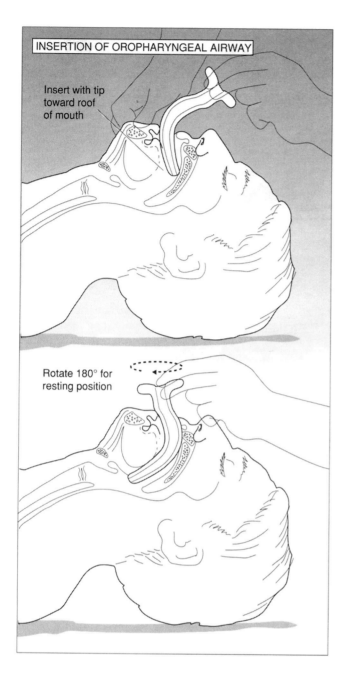

INSERTION OF OROPHARYNGEAL AIRWAY

Insert with tip toward roof of mouth

Rotate 180° for resting position

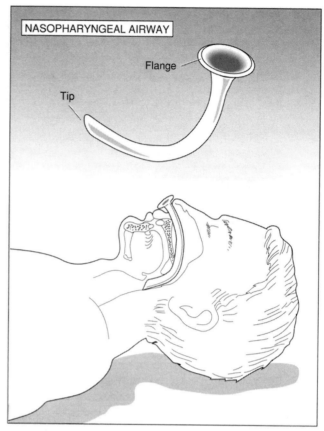

NASOPHARYNGEAL AIRWAY

Flange

Tip

tragus of the ear. The outside diameter of the airway should be equal to the inside diameter of the patient's internal nares.
b. Lubricate the airway with a water-soluble gel and insert into patient's nostril.
c. The flanged end should rest against the nose and the distal tip should rest behind the uvula.
d. Place tape around the flanged end to secure in place. (Safety pin may be inserted through the flange and the pin taped to the face.)
3. This airway is tolerated by the conscious patient.
4. This airway is most commonly used to facilitate nasotracheal suctioning.
5. **Hazards of nasopharyngeal airways**
   a. Aspiration of an airway that is too small
   b. Nasal irritation; to prevent this, alternate nostrils daily
C. **Esophageal Obturator Airway** (EOA)

b. Berman airways are made of hard plastic and have a groove down either side to guide a suction catheter to the glottic area.
c. Guedel airways are made of a soft, pliable material, which has an opening through the middle to allow the passing of a suction catheter into the glottic area.
B. **Nasopharyngeal Airway**
1. Maintains a patent airway by lying between the base of the tongue and the posterior wall of the pharynx.
2. Constructed of soft pliable rubber; it is inserted as follows:
   a. Select the proper size by measuring the airway from the tip of the nose to the

Exam Note

The EOA appears on the RRT examination only, but will likely be replaced with the LMA and/or ETC (see below).

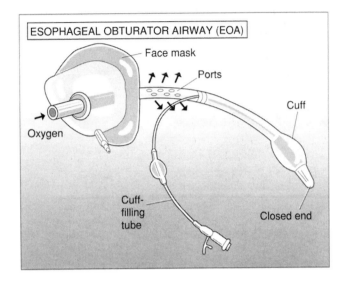

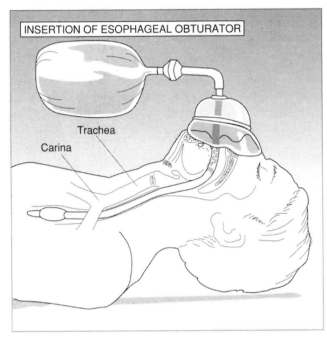

1. Developed in 1973 as an alternative to tracheal intubation, especially for those not skilled in tracheal intubation.
2. The tube is placed in the esophagus to prevent air from entering the stomach during manual ventilation. A resuscitator bag is attached to the proximal end of the tube, and gas exits small holes in the tube in the laryngeal area. Since the stomach is sealed off with a cuff, gas enters the lungs only.
3. Used in emergency situations for **unconscious, apneic patients.**
4. The tube is 30 to 37 cm long with a closed distal end and a 30-mL cuff just above the end of the tube.
5. Steps for proper insertion of the EOA
   a. Check the cuff and lubricate the end of the tube with a water-soluble gel.
   b. Attach the mask and lock in place.
   c. Place the patient's head in a neutral position.
   d. Grasp patient's jaw with thumb along the tongue and lift up.
   e. Insert the tube along the right side of the mouth.
   f. Seal the mask on the patient's face, attach resuscitator bag and deliver a breath; observe the chest rising.
   g. Auscultate with a stethoscope for equal breath sounds and listen over the stomach to make sure no air is entering the stomach.
   h. Inflate the cuff with no more than 30 mL of air.

Note

The cuff of the EOA must be passed below the level of the carina before it is inflated. If this is not done, the cuff could compress the trachea, resulting in an obstructed airway.

---

6. Removal of the EOA
   a. Once the patient becomes conscious or begins breathing or personnel trained in ET intubation are available, the tube should be removed.
   b. Deflate the cuff and **turn the patient's head to the side as the tube is withdrawn.** Vomiting is very common on removal of the tube, and turning the head helps prevent the aspiration of stomach contents. **Placement of a NG tube to decompress the stomach before removal of the EOA will also reduce the risk of aspiration.**
   ★ c. Intubating the patient's trachea with an ET tube before the removal of the EOA is the best method for preventing aspiration, especially if the patient requires an ET tube once the EOA is removed.
   ★ d. Suctioning equipment must be readily available when removing an EOA.
7. **Contraindications for the EOA**
   a. Conscious or semiconscious patients
   b. Children under age 16 (tubes are available in adult sizes only)
   c. Patients who can rapidly be brought out of a coma (drug overdose, hypoglycemic coma)
   d. Tube should not be in the esophagus for more than 2 hr
   e. Patients with known esophageal trauma
8. **Hazards of the EOA**
   a. Esophageal perforation
   b. Rupture of the esophagus caused by vomiting with the airway in place and the cuff inflated; rupture is recognized by chest pain,

subcutaneous emphysema, and pneumomediastinum

   c. Inadvertent tracheal intubation, recognized by absent breath sounds and no chest excursion

   d. Vomiting on removal of the EOA

9. **Problems associated with the EOA**

   a. Failure to seal the mask adequately while ventilating the patient

   b. Inability to insert the EOA

   c. EOA interferes with the placement of an ET tube

D. **Esophageal Tracheal Combitube** (ETC): also referred to as the pharyngotracheal lumen (PTL) airway

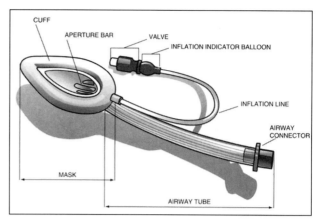

Courtesy of LMA North America, Inc.

---

1. The ETC is similar to an EOA, but it is a double-lumen tube. The tubes run parallel to each other.

2. Once the tube is inserted, a pharyngeal balloon is inflated, which occludes the pharynx to prevent air from leaking out of the nose or mouth. Because of this, a mask is not necessary.

3. Once the airway is advanced beyond the pharynx, it enters into either the trachea or the esophagus. It makes no difference which structure it enters.

4. A balloon at the distal end of the tube is inflated and seals off either the trachea or the esophagus.

   a. If the tube rests in the trachea, that lumen is used to ventilate the patient just like an ET tube.

   b. If the tube rests in the esophagus, the patient is ventilated through holes in the upper part of the tube below the pharyngeal cuff, similar to those on the EOA.

5. These airways have been shown to provide adequate ventilation in emergency resuscitation and surgery.

E. **Laryngeal Mask Airway** (LMA)

1. The LMA is designed to be used as an alternative to a face mask for achieving and maintaining control of the airway during surgery when tracheal intubation is not necessary. It is also used as a method of establishing a patent airway in an unconscious patient who needs artificial ventilation after attempts at tracheal intubation have failed.

2. For the airway to be inserted successfully, the patient must be anesthetized so that the upper airway reflexes are obtunded. Otherwise, laryngospasm may occur.

3. Before insertion, the mask is deflated so that it easily passes around the back of the tongue and behind the epiglottis. The patient is placed in the "sniff position," just as for ET intubation.

4. The posterior wall of the LMA should be lubricated (with K-Y jelly or similar product) before insertion.

5. See accompanying figures for proper insertion technique

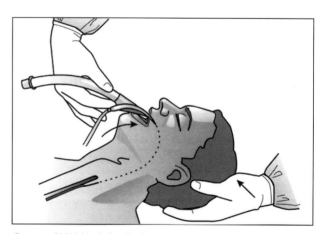

Courtesy of LMA North America, Inc.

6. Using the index finger, the LMA is advanced until resistance is met. The tip of the LMA should rest against the upper esophageal sphincter in the hypopharynx. The cuff should be inflated until no leak is heard. To determine proper position, the

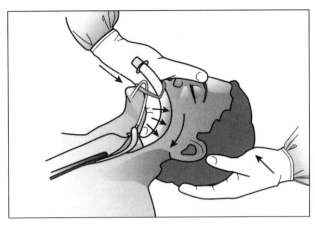

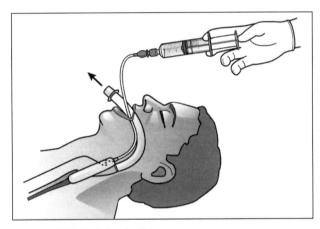

lungs should be auscultated bilaterally. Capnography may also be used to confirm an adequate airway.

7. To determine if mild laryngospasm is present as a result of light anesthesia, the anterolateral neck should be auscultated to detect wheezing.

8. Since the LMA does not protect the airway from regurgitation, the patient must not eat for several hours before its insertion.

9. Side effects include sore throat and difficulty speaking after removal of the airway.

10. The only recommended method for sterilizing the LMA is by autoclaving.

F. **ET Tubes**
 1. **Indications for ET Tubes**
  a. Relief of upper airway obstruction resulting from laryngospasm, epiglottitis, or glottic edema
  b. Protection of the airway; the airway has four protective reflexes.
   (1) Pharyngeal reflex: gag and swallowing
   (2) Laryngeal reflex: laryngospasm
   (3) Tracheal reflex: coughing when trachea is irritated

(4) Carinal reflex: coughing when carina is irritated

> **★ Note**
>
> When these reflexes are obtunded or knocked out, the airway must be protected with an ET tube. These reflexes may be obtunded by paralysis, drugs, loss of consciousness, or neuromuscular disease.

> **Note**
>
> As these reflexes become obtunded, they are lost in progression from the pharyngeal to the carinal. As they are recovered, they come back in progression from the carinal to the pharyngeal.

  c. To facilitate tracheal suctioning
  d. To assist manual or mechanical ventilation
 2. **Hazards of ET tubes**
  a. Contamination of the tracheobronchial tree
  b. Cough mechanism reduced
  c. Damage to the vocal cords
  d. Laryngeal or tracheal edema
  e. Mucosal damage leading to tracheal stenosis
  f. Tube occlusion with inspissated secretions
  g. Loss of patient's dignity

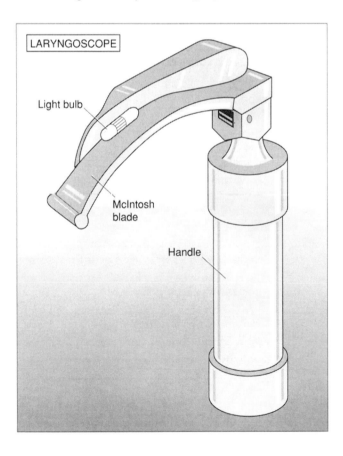

LARYNGOSCOPE

Light bulb

McIntosh blade

Handle

h. Loss of patient's ability to talk
3. **Steps to perform ET intubation**
   a. Select a laryngoscope with a **Miller (straight) blade** or a **McIntosh (curved) blade.** Make sure the light bulb is tight, because it will not light if it is loose.
   b. Place the patient in the "sniffing position." (head above shoulder level)

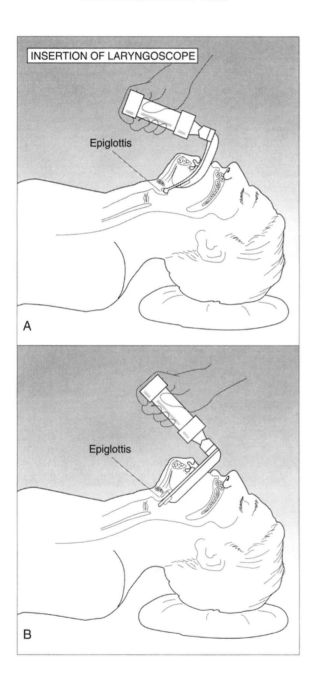

c. Select the proper size of ET tube, insert air into the cuff to make sure it holds air and then deflate the cuff.
d. Insert a stylet into the ET tube to make the tube more rigid for easier insertion. Make sure the stylet doesn't extend past the end of the tube.
e. Insert the laryngoscope blade into the right side of the mouth (if laryngoscope is in left hand) and move tongue to the left.
f. Advance the blade forward.
   (1) The curved blade (McIntosh) should be inserted between the epiglottis and the base of the tongue (vallecula); and with a forward and upward motion, the epiglottis is raised to expose the glottis and vocal cords.
   (2) The straight blade (Miller) should be placed under the epiglottis and lifted upward and forward to expose the cords

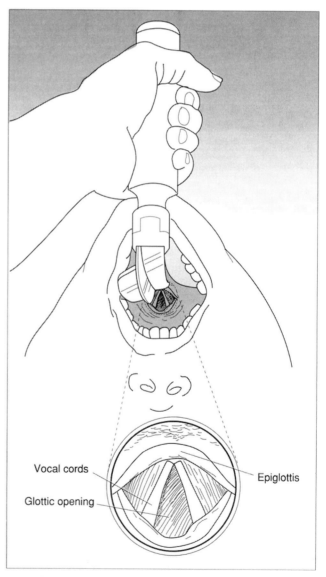

View of the larynx through the laryngoscope.

> **Note**
>
> Never exceed 15 to 20 sec per intubation attempt. The blade and tube in the back of the throat may stimulate the vagus nerve, leading to bradycardia. Remove the blade and tube and bag-mask ventilate until cardiac status has stabilized.

    g. As the cords are observed, advance the ET tube **approximately 2 cm in past the cords.**

> **Note**
>
> If the tube is inserted too far, it will enter the right mainstem bronchus.

★ h. Inflate the cuff and listen for equal and bi-lateral breath sounds. If louder sounds are heard on the right than the left, the tube probably is in the right mainstem. Deflate the cuff and withdraw the tube until equal breath sounds are heard.

    i. Another method to determine if the tube is in the airway is by exhaled CO_2 analysis, or capnometry. **If the ET tube is in the airway, CO_2 levels will begin to rise, as seen on the capnogram. End-tidal CO_2 levels are generally around 6%. If the tube is in the esophagus, the end-tidal CO_2 reading will remain near zero.**

    j. An easier and less expensive method of monitoring exhaled CO_2 levels is with the use of a disposable colorimetric CO_2 detector on the proximal end of the ET tube. The indicator on the detector changes colors when exposed to different CO_2 levels.

> **Note**
>
> During resuscitative procedures when cardiac output and blood pressure are low, gas exchange is reduced and the CO_2 detector may read near zero even if the ET tube is in the trachea.

> **Note**
>
> The average distance from the teeth to the carina is 27 cm. Note that the ET tube has markings in centimeters indicating the distance to the end of the tube from that point. Therefore, taping the tube at the 23- to 25-cm mark at the teeth will most likely place the tube in a proper position.

Appropriate ET Tube Sizes

Newborns (by body weight)

Less than 1 kg	2.5 mm
1 to 2 kg	3.0 mm
2 to 3 kg	3.5 mm
More than 3 kg	4.0 mm

Children (by age)

6 mo	3.0 – 4.0 mm
18 mo	3.5 – 4.5 mm
2 yr	4.0 – 5.0 mm
3 to 5 yr	4.5 – 5.5 mm
6 yr	5.5 – 6.0 mm
8 yr	6.0 – 6.5 mm
12 yr	6.0 – 7.0 mm
16 yr	6.5 – 7.5 mm

Adults (by gender)

Women	7.5 – 9.0 mm
Men	8.0 – 9.5 mm

    k. Obtain a stat chest x-ray film for tube placement. The end of the tube should rest 2 to 7 cm above the carina. **The carina is located on radiographs at the fourth rib or the 4th thoracic vertebra.**

    l. Tape the tube securely.

2. **Parts of the ET tube**

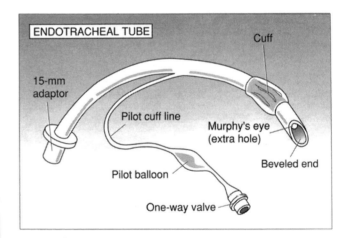

3. **ET tube markings**
    a. IT (implantation tested): Indicates the material in the tube is nontoxic and does not cause tissue reaction when implanted in rabbit tissue.

> **Note**
>
> Polyvinylchloride (PVC) is the most common material used in ET tubes.

b. Z-79: The Z-79 Committee for Anesthesia Equipment for the American National Standards Institute. This committee ensures that the tube manufacturer is using material that is not toxic to tissues.

c. ID: internal diameter of the tube in millimeters. This is how the tubes are designated by size.

d. OD: outside diameter of the tube in millimeters. Also measured in French units.

e. Numbers and marks indicating the distance in centimeters from that mark to the distal tip of the tube.

4. **Complications caused by oral ET tubes.**

a. Poorly tolerated by conscious or semiconscious patients

b. Difficult to stabilize because of the movement of the tube

c. Stimulation of oral secretions

d. Gagging caused by tube irritation

e. More difficult to pass suction catheter as a result of the curvature of the tube and poor stabilization

f. Harder to communicate

g. Harder to attach equipment to a poorly stabilized ET tube

h. Patient may bite the tube, occluding air flow and setting off the ventilator high pressure alarm, which ends inspiration prematurely.

i. Erosion of corners of mouth

5. **Nasotracheal tubes**

a. These are considered nonemergent tubes.

b. **Nasotracheal intubation**

(1) Nose should be anesthetized with lidocaine or cocaine spray. A vasoconstrictor, such as phenylphrine hydrochloride (Neo-Synephrine) drops, are used to shrink nasal mucosal blood vessels for easier tube insertion.

(2) Lubricate the tube with water soluble gel and insert through a patent nostril.

(3) If the patient is alert and breathing spontaneously, try advancing the tube as the patient is taking a deep breath or coughing. This is called "blind nasal intubation."

(4) If patient is not cooperative or is unconscious, the tube is visualized in the mouth, grasped by **McGill forceps,** and guided through the vocal cords by means of direct visualization with a laryngoscope.

(5) Tape the tube in place when proper placement is assured.

c. **Advantages of nasotracheal tubes (vs. oral tubes)**

(1) Easier to stabilize

(2) Tolerated by the patient better, because gagging is not as likely

(3) Less potential for inadvertent extubation

(4) Equipment attaches easier

(5) Easier to pass suction catheter

(6) Easier to eat or drink

d. **Complications of nasotracheal tubes**

(1) Pressure necrosis of the nasal tissue

(2) Sinus obstruction, leading to sinusitis

(3) Obstruction of eustachian tube, resulting in middle-ear infections

(4) Septal deviation

(5) Bleeding during intubation or extubation

6. **Double-lumen ET tubes**

a. There are several models of double-lumen ET tubes. Some are designed for right mainstem bronchus intubation and others for left mainstem bronchus intubation.

b. Double-lumen tubes are used for independent lung ventilation for patients with unilateral lung disease (see chapter on ventilator management) and during thoracic surgeries (e.g., pneumonectomy).

G. **Tracheostomy Tubes**

1. Tracheostomy tubes are inserted through an incision (stoma) made between the second and third tracheal rings.

2. The obturator should always be inserted into the outer cannula when the tube is being advanced into the stoma.

3. Once the tube is properly positioned, the obturator should be removed and the inner cannula inserted.

4. The cuff is then inflated and tracheostomy ties are used to secure the tube.

5. Some tubes use foam cuffs (Mikity-Wilson Fome Cuff and Kamen Fome Cuff), which are deflated during insertion; when the tube is in place, the cuff is allowed to resume its normal foam shape, which provides an effective seal against the tracheal wall. (This type of cuff exerts about 20 mm Hg pressure on the tracheal wall.

6. **Indications for tracheostomies**

a. To bypass upper airway obstruction

b. Reduce anatomic deadspace (by 50%)

c. To prevent problems posed by oral or nasal ET tubes

d. To allow patient to swallow and receive nourishment

e. For long-term airway care (ET tubes should be left in no longer than 3 to 4 wk)

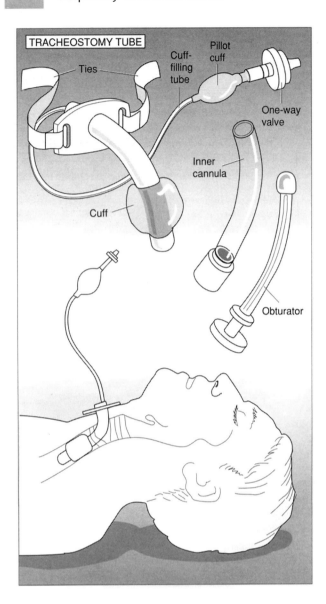

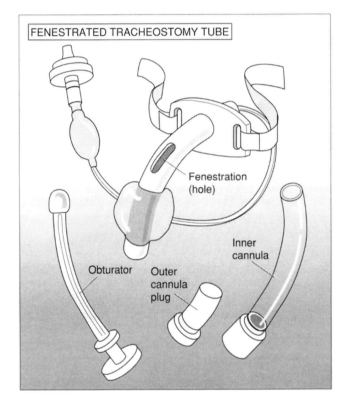

9. **Special tracheostomy tubes**
   a. **Fenestrated tracheostomy tube**

(1) This tube is used to aid in weaning the patient from a tracheostomy tube and to allow the patient to talk.
(2) With the inner cannula removed, air may pass through the hole (fenestra-tion) in the outer cannula, allowing for weaning from the tracheostomy tube and enabling speech.
(3) The outer cannula may be plugged with the cap on the proximal end of the tube. With the cuff deflated, air will flow through the tube, out the fenestra-tion, and through the patient's upper airway.
(4) Should ventilation be necessary, the inner cannula may be reinserted and the cuff reinflated.

b. **Tracheostomy button**
(1) Consists of a short, hollow tube, which is used to replace the tracheostomy

7. **Immediate complications of tra-cheostomy tubes:** occurring within the first 24 hr and associated with the tracheotomy procedure
   a. Pneumothorax
   b. Bleeding
   c. Air embolism from tearing of pleural vein
   d. Subcutaneous emphysema
8. **Late complications of tracheostomy tubes:** occurring more than 2 days after the tracheotomy
   a. Hemorrhage
   b. Infection
   c. Airway obstruction
   d. Tracheoesophageal fistula
   e. Interference with swallowing
   f. Rupture of innominate artery
   g. Stomal stenosis
   h. Tracheitis

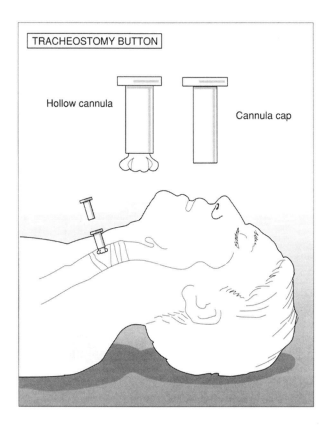

tube but still maintain the stoma patent, in case problems arise.

(2) The patient has complete use of the upper airway.

c. **Kistner tracheostomy tube**

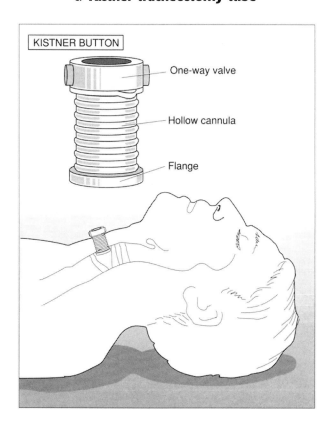

(1) Used to wean patients from tracheostomy tubes and yet maintain a patent stoma
(2) Kistner tubes are much like tracheostomy buttons, except that they have a one-way valve on the proximal end of the tube.
(3) Air enters through the one-way valve and the tube during inspiration. As the patient exhales, the valve closes and the air flows up through the vocal cords and out the nose and mouth.

d. **Speaking tracheostomy tubes**

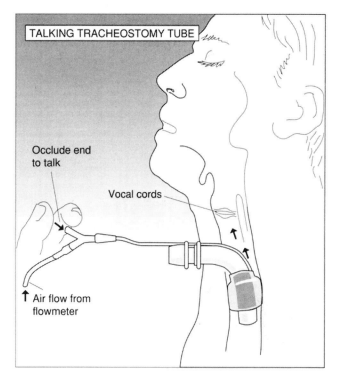

(1) A constant gas flow is available above the cuff and around the vocal cords to allow speech.
(2) The cuff remains inflated.

III. **MAINTENANCE OF ARTIFICIAL AIRWAYS**
A. **Cuff Care**
1. Tubes should employ **high-volume, low-pressure cuffs only,** because they cause less occlusion to tracheal blood flow, since they apply less pressure. They are also called "floppy cuffs." If excessive air is placed in the cuff, it will act as a **high-pressure cuff.**
2. To ensure that the cuff is exerting the least amount of pressure on the tracheal wall and still providing an adequate seal, **the minimal leak technique or minimal occluding volume technique** should be used.

a. **Minimal leak technique:** With the stethoscope beside the larynx, listen for air flow as the cuff is inflated. Inflate the cuff until no air flow is heard, then withdraw air slowly until a slight leak is heard.

b. **Minimal occluding volume technique:** Accomplished the same way as the minimal leak technique, except the cuff is slowly inflated just to the point where no leak is heard.

> **Note**
>
> If the peak inspiratory pressure (PIP) on the ventilator decreases after the minimal leak has been determined, the leak technique should be redone at the lower pressure. For example, the minimal leak test is done when the PIP is 40 cm H_2O. Let's say the patient is suctioned and the PIP drops to 30 cm H_2O. Since the cuff was inflated to create a slight leak at 40 cm H_2O, and the PIP has dropped to 30 cm H_2O, there is now excessive air in the ET tube cuff. There should no longer be a leak at this lower PIP; therefore, the minimal leak technique should be determined again at 30 cm H_2O.

c. **Cuff pressures should be kept below 20 mm Hg (27 cm H_2O) to prevent tracheal wall damage.**

d. If the cuff is inflated above 20 mm Hg and a leak is still heard, continue inflating the cuff using the minimal leak or occluding volume technique. It may be that the ET tube is too small, and it is taking more air in the cuff to adequately seal the airway. In this case, the cuff pressure does not relate to the pressure on the tracheal wall. **To be safe, the ET tube should be replaced with a larger one.**

e. **Effects of cuff pressure on the tracheal wall**
   (1) More 30 mm Hg obstructs arterial flow, leading to ischemia
   (2) More than 20 mm Hg obstructs venous flow, leading to congestion
   (3) More than 5 mm Hg obstructs lymphatic flow, leading to edema

B. **Suctioning the Airway**
   1. **Technique of suctioning**
      a. Hyperoxygenate and hyperinflate the patient. This is done to help prevent hypoxemia, which may lead to bradycardia.
      b. Instill 3 to 5 mL of normal saline to help thin secretions; in infants, use 0.3 to 0.5 mL.
      c. Insert the catheter without applying suction and advance until an obstruction (the

carina) is met. Do not jab with the catheter, because this may cause carinal damage and bradycardia (vagal stimulation).

d. Withdraw the catheter approximately 1 to 2 cm and **apply suction,** while rotating the catheter between the thumb and finger. **(This decreases mucosal damage.)**

e. Never leave the catheter in the airway for more than **15 seconds.**

f. Upon removal of the catheter, reoxygenate and hyperinflate the patient; wait 30 sec to 1 min before entering the airway again.

> **Note**
>
> Monitor ECG and stop procedure if complications occur; hyperoxygenate and ventilate (if patient is on a ventilator).

g. Repeat steps until secretions are removed by suctioning and airway sounds clear.

h. Suctioning the nasal and oral pharynx may now be done, remembering to never re-enter the ET tube with this catheter.

> **Note**
>
> When nasotracheal suctioning is performed, the above steps should be followed in addition to the following techniques:
> (1) Lubricate catheter with water-soluble gel.
> (2) Instruct patient to take a deep breath or cough as the catheter advances to the oropharynx. This aids in inserting the catheter through the glottic opening.

2. **Selecting the proper size of catheter**
   a. The suction catheter should not occupy more than **one-half to two-thirds** of the internal diameter of the tube. (Suction catheters are sized by French [Fr] units.)
   b. To estimate the proper catheter size, multiply the internal diameter of the ET tube by 2, then use the next smallest catheter size.

EXAMPLE:

What is the proper size of catheter to use to suction an 8.0-mm ET tube?

$$8.0 \times 2 = 16$$

The next smallest size catheter is 14 Fr. (Suction catheters come in the following sizes: $6\frac{1}{2}$ Fr, 8 Fr, 10 Fr, 12 Fr, 14 Fr, 16 Fr.)

3. Other types of catheters
   a. Yankauer suction (tonsil): used to suction the oropharynx

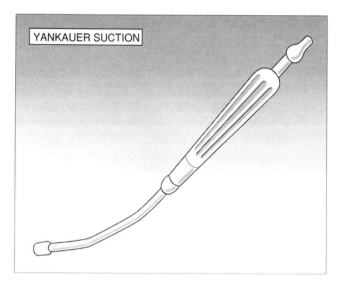

YANKAUER SUCTION

   b. **Coudé suction catheter:** angled-tip catheter used to suction the left mainstem bronchus
4. **Indications for tracheal suctioning**
   a. To remove retained secretions that the patient cannot mobilize
   b. To maintain patency of artificial airways
   c. To obtain sputum for culture and sensitivity testing
5. **Hazards of tracheal suctioning**
   a. Hypoxemia: **increase F_{IO_2} before suctioning**
   b. Arrhythmias: caused by hypoxemia and vagal nerve stimulation. **Vagus nerve is stimulated as catheter irritates the oral or nasal mucosa, tracheal mucosa, and carina, causing bradycardia.**
   c. Hypotension: caused by bradycardia and prolonged coughing episodes
   d. Atelectasis: caused by using a suction catheter that is too large or excessive suction pressure
   e. Tissue trauma: caused by jabbing catheter during insertion and improper lubrication during nasal suctioning.

Note

Suctioning may suddenly stop as a result of a kinked suction catheter, a mucus plug lodged in the catheter, or a suction collection bottle that is full.

6. **Vacuum systems and collection bottles**
   a. The suction catheter is attached to a connecting tube, which attaches to the outlet of a collection bottle. This bottle attaches to a DISS connection on the suction or vacuum regulator, which is either a portable pump or a 50-psi vacuum wall outlet at the bedside.
   b. The vacuum regulator supplies the negative (subatmospheric) pressure necessary to suction the airway.
   c. The secretion collection bottle is generally equipped with a system that interrupts suction when the bottle becomes full of secretions.
   d. Most suction or vacuum systems provide up to -200 mm Hg pressure, but the desired vacuum level can be adjusted by occluding the suction regulator outlet and turning a vacuum control knob on the regulator. Most systems use locking mechanisms to prevent excessive suction pressures from being used.
   e. Appropriate suction levels
      Adults: -80 to -120 mm Hg
      Children: -80 to -100 mm Hg
      Infants: -60 to -80 mm Hg

IV. **ET TUBE EXTUBATION**
   A. Procedure of Extubation
      1. Explain procedure to the patient.
      2. Increase the F_{IO_2} level.
      3. Suction down the ET tube.
      4. Suction the mouth and back of throat.
      5. Untape the ET tube, deflate the cuff and instruct the patient to take a deep breath. **At peak inspiration, withdraw the tube.**

Note

A resuscitator bag may be used to deliver the deep breath and to better ensure that the tube is removed at peak inspiration.

Note

It is permissible to withdraw the tube while suctioning because this clears the airway while extubating.

   B. **Complications of Extubation**
      1. **Laryngospasm**
         a. Spasm of the vocal cords caused by irritation of the tube, resulting in airway obstruction. This is detected by observing

respiratory difficulty immediately after extubation.
  b. If laryngospasm occurs, administer a high FIO₂ concentration and, if it persists for more than 1 to 2 min, administer a bronchodilator via a handheld nebulizer.
2. **Glottic edema** (see later section in chapter)

> **Note**
>
> Intubation equipment should be readily available at the bedside during extubation in case reintubation becomes necessary.

V. **LARYNGEAL AND TRACHEAL COMPLICATIONS OF ET TUBES**
  A. **Sore Throat and Hoarseness**
    1. Common result of tube irritation
    2. Usually subside within 2 to 3 days
    3. Treat with cool aerosol
  B. **Glottic Edema**
    1. **Inspiratory stridor** is the major clinical sign
    2. Caused by:
      a. Traumatic intubation
      b. Insertion with oversized ET tube
      c. Poor ET tube maintenance
      d. Allergic response to material in the ET tube
    3. Stridor should be treated with
      ★ a. Cool aerosol to decrease swelling
      ★ b. Vasoconstrictor, such as racemic epinephrine, via handheld nebulizer to constrict mucosal blood vessels reducing swelling
      ★ c. Corticosteroids, such as dexamethasone (Decadron), may be used to reduce swelling
  C. **Subglottic Edema**
    1. Edema that occurs below the glottis at the level of the cricoid cartilage.
    ★ 2. A serious complication after extubation, which may lead to reintubation.
    3. If postextubation distress cannot be relieved, subglottic edema must be suspected.
  D. **Vocal Cord Ulceration**
    1. Suspected if hoarseness continues for more than 1 wk.
    2. Caused by:
      a. Traumatic intubation
      b. Tight-fitting tube
      c. Allergic reaction to material in tube
      d. Excessive movement of the tube
  E. **Tracheal Mucosal Ulceration**
    1. Common after extubation.
    2. Occurs at the area of the cuff site.
  F. **Vocal Cord Paralysis**
    1. Caused by damage to the recurrent laryngeal nerve.

2. Usually occurs secondary to upper chest or neck surgery.
  G. **Laryngotracheal Web**
    1. Caused by necrotic tissue at the glottic or subglottic level that leads to fibrin formation, which combines with secretions and cellular debris to form a membrane, or web.
    2. Stridor and acute airway obstruction generally occur.
    3. The web should be suctioned from the airway immediately.
    4. Often occurs several days after extubation.
  H. **Tracheal Stenosis**
    1. A lesion found at the cuff site or the level of the cricoid membrane.
    2. As the lesion heals, it constricts, leading to a narrowing of the airway.
    3. A narrowing of less than 50% of the diameter of the airway will not be symptomatic.
    4. To help prevent tracheal stenosis, maintain cuff pressure by use of the **minimal leak technique.**
  I. **Tracheal Malacia**
    1. Loss of the cartilaginous support of the trachea.
    2. After extubation, the trachea collapses, leading to respiratory distress.

POST-CHAPTER STUDY QUESTIONS

1. To prevent venous congestion on the trachea wall, the ET tube cuff should be maintained below what level of pressure?
2. Inspiratory stridor is a major clinical sign of what airway condition?
3. What is the name of the airway that may be placed in either the esophagus or the trachea to manually ventilate a patient?
4. Describe the purpose of an oropharyngeal airway.
5. What is the primary purpose of a fenestrated tracheostomy tube?
6. List the problems associated with the use of oral ET tubes.
7. How would you determine that an ET tube is resting in the right mainstem bronchus before a chest x-ray film is obtained?
8. What is a Yankauer suction device used for?
9. What is the maximum amount of suction pressure that may be used to suction an adult patient's airway?
10. When extubating a patient, the ET tube should be withdrawn at what point in the breathing cycle?

Answers are at the end of the chapter.

REFERENCES

Branson RD, Hess DR, and Chatburn RL, Respiratory care equipment, ed 2, Philadelphia, 1999, JB Lippincott Co.

Eubanks DH and Bone RC: Comprehensive respiratory care, ed 2, St. Louis, 1990, The CV Mosby Co.

McPherson SP: Respiratory therapy equipment, ed 5, St. Louis, 1995, Mosby-Yearbook Inc.

Scanlan CL, Wilkins RL, and Stoller JK: Egan's fundamentals of respiratory care, ed 7, St. Louis, 1999, Mosby Inc.

Shapiro BT et al: Clinical application of respiratory care, ed 4, St. Louis, 1991, The CV Mosby Company.

PRE-TEST ANSWERS

1. D
2. D
3. A
4. B
5. C
6. C

ANSWERS TO POST-CHAPTER STUDY QUESTIONS

1. 20 mm Hg (27 cm H_2O)
2. Glottic edema
3. Esophageal tracheal combitube (ETC)
4. The oropharyngeal airway is used to prevent upper airway obstruction, mainly from the tongue, in unconscious patients only. It may be used as a bite block for unconscious intubated patients.
5. A fenestrated tracheostomy tube is used to wean a patient from a conventional tracheostomy tube and allow the patient to speak.
6. Poorly tolerated by conscious or semiconscious patients, biting the tube, increased production of oral secretions, easier inadvertent extubation, harder to communicate, gagging, tube not as stable, difficulty passing suction catheter because of curvature of tube
7. Diminished breath sounds in the left lung, asymmetrical chest movement
8. To suction the oropharynx
9. -120 mm Hg
10. At peak inspiration

Chapter 5

Special Respiratory Care Procedures

PRE-TEST QUESTIONS

Answer the pre-test questions before studying the chapter. This will help you determine your strong and weak areas regarding the material covered.

1. Which of the following are complications associated with bronchoscopy?

   I. pulmonary hemorrhage
   II. pneumothorax
   III. hypoxemia

   A. I only
   B. II only
   C. I and III only
   D. I, II, and III

2. While assisting with a bronchoscopy, you note that the physician is having difficulty entering the trachea. This may be the result of which of the following?

   A. Pneumothorax
   B. Hypoxemia
   C. Laryngospasm
   D. Pulmonary hemorrhage

3. After a bronchoscopy, the respiratory therapist notes that it is taking more ventilator pressure to ventilate the patient than before the procedure. This could be caused by which of the following?

   I. Bronchospasm
   II. Pneumothorax
   III. Hypoxemia
   IV. Pulmonary hemorrhage

   A. I and II only
   B. II and III only
   C. I, II, and IV only
   D. II, III, and IV only

4. During a thoracentesis, the patient suddenly complains of chest pain and becomes dyspneic. This is most likely the result of which of the following?

   A. Atelectasis
   B. Myocardial infarction
   C. Empyema
   D. Pneumothorax

5. To aid in the evacuation of air from the pleural space, a chest tube should be inserted at what level?

   A. Supraclavicular space
   B. Second intercostal space anteriorly
   C. Sixth intercostal space anteriorly
   D. Eighth intercostal space anteriorly

6. The respiratory therapist notices on a patient's chest tube drainage system that there is fluctuation of the water level in the water seal chamber with each patient breath and air bubbles seen only in the suction control chamber, which has a suction pressure of -15 cm H_2O. The most appropriate action is which of the following?

   A. Clamp the chest tube and check for leaks.
   B. Insert the chest tube farther, until bubbling stops in the vacuum chamber.
   C. Withdraw the chest tube until bubbling starts in the water seal chamber.
   D. Recommend a chest radiograph to determine whether the pneumothorax has resolved.

7. The respiratory therapist observes that, during a patient's breathing cycle, there is no fluctuation in the water seal chamber of the pleural drainage system. The most appropriate action is which of the following?

   A. Withdraw the tube until fluctuation is seen.
   B. "Strip" the chest tube to clear a possible obstruction.
   C. Increase the vacuum pressure.
   D. Clamp the chest tube and observe for leaks.

Answers are at the end of the chapter.

REVIEW

I. BRONCHOSCOPY
   A. A technique for assessing and examining the bronchi by means of a bronchoscope, which

is used for both therapeutic and diagnostic purposes.

B. **Types of Bronchoscopes**

1. Rigid bronchoscope

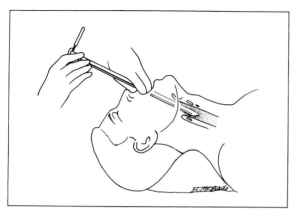

From Scanlan CL and Simmons KF: Airway management. In Scanian CL, Wilkins RL, Stoller JK, editors: Egan's Fundamentals of Respiratory Care, ed. 7, St. Louis, 1999, Mosby, Inc.

   a. Consists of a hollow metal tube with a light on its distal end.
   b. Tube is inserted orally, then passed between the vocal cords into the trachea.
   c. Useful for removing aspirated foreign bodies and thick secretions from the lungs.

2. Fiberoptic bronchoscope

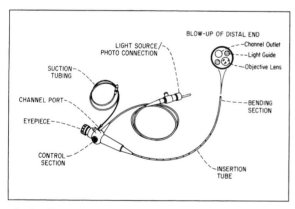

From Scanlan CL and Simmons KF: Airway management. In Scanian CL, Wilkins RL, Stoller JK, editors: Egan's Fundamentals of Respiratory Care, ed. 7, St. Louis, 1999, Mosby, Inc.

   a. Consists of a collection of thin, thread-like glass strands called fiberoptic filaments with a light source projected to its distal end for visualization.
   b. Because of its more flexible nature, it is better tolerated by patients than the rigid bronchoscope and is therefore more commonly used.
   c. Preparatory regimen for fiberoptic bronchoscopy
      (1) Because bronchoscopy is uncomfortable, a mild sedative should be admin-

istered to the patient 1 to 2 hr before the procedure. Commonly, **diazepam (Valium)** or **midazolam (Versed)** is used for this purpose. Level of sedation, referred to as **conscious sedation,** should be just enough to allow the patient to follow commands, yet still be comfortable.
      (2) The airway must be dry during the procedure to aid in visualization, which is usually achieved by administering **atropine** 1 to 2 hr before the procedure. Atropine may also decrease vagal tone, resulting in a decreased potential for bradycardia and hypotension, which can occur during the procedure.
      (3) The tube may be inserted orally, nasally, or through the ET tube. The bronchoscopic tube should be lubricated with a water-soluble jelly for easier nasal insertion. Often, **lidocaine (Xylocaine)** jelly is used both as a lubricant and for its anesthetic effects. In some cases, the RCP administers aerosolized lidocaine before the procedure.
      (4) Because of its flexibility, a fiberoptic bronchoscope can be advanced farther into the airway than a rigid one, thereby allowing more visualization of the conducting airways.
      (5) Biopsy forceps and brushes may be inserted through the bronchoscope to obtain tissue samples.

C. **Indications for Bronchoscopy**

1. Removal of foreign bodies
2. Removal of mucus plugs and thick secretions
   a. Normally performed if secretions cannot be removed by routine suctioning techniques.
   b. Once the site of the secretions is visualized, the area should be lavaged with saline before suctioning.
3. Atelectasis that affects a lobe or an entire lung
4. Pulmonary hemorrhage
   a. To locate the area of bleeding
   b. To control bleeding by instillation of epinephrine or iced saline lavage at the bleeding site
5. To enable difficult tracheal intubation as a result of upper airway trauma, obesity, tumors, or spinal deformity
   a. The ET tube is slipped over the fiberoptic bronchoscope, with the scope protruding well past the end of the ET tube.
   b. The vocal cords are visualized, and the scope is advanced through the cords to the midtracheal level, where the ET tube is

then advanced over the scope to the proper position. The scope is then withdrawn.
6. For biopsy of suspected tumors
7. To obtain sputum for culture and sensitivity studies

D. **Complications of Bronchoscopy**
1. Hypoxemia
   a. Monitor oxygen saturation during procedure
   b. Increase oxygen percentage during procedure
2. Laryngospasm
   a. Makes advancing the tube more difficult
   b. Bronchodilator should be readily available
3. Bronchospasm
   a. Results from irritation of the airway
   b. Bronchodilator should be readily available
4. Arrhythmias
   a. Result from vagal stimulation
   b. Monitor ECG and remove bronchoscope until cardiac status is stabilized
5. Hemorrhage
   a. May occur during insertion
   b. May occur after biopsy
6. Respiratory depression
   a. Results from sedatives given before the procedure
   b. Monitor respiratory status closely
7. Hypotension
   a. Results from vagal nerve stimulation
   b. May result from sedatives given before the procedure
8. Pneumothorax
   a. Results from inadvertent puncture of the lung
   b. Monitor respiratory status closely

E. **RCP Responsibilities during Bronchoscopy**

Note

Responsibilities of the RCP vary according to the institution's protocols. Those listed below are among the most common responsibilities.

1. Prepare the patient and explain the procedure.
2. Administer aerosolized local anesthetic to the patient's upper airway.
3. Conduct patient monitoring throughout the procedure.
   a. Pulse/Blood pressure
   b. Respiratory rate
   c. ECG
   d. Oxygen saturation
   e. Level of consciousness

4. Collect sputum and tissue samples that the physician has obtained and prepare them for laboratory analysis.
5. Clean the bronchoscope properly after the procedure. The CDC recommends that bronchoscopes be disinfected by immersion in glutaraldehyde (Cidex) for 3 to 10 hr.

II. **THORACENTESIS**
A. A procedure in which a needle is inserted into the chest wall to obtain material from the lung or to drain fluid from the pleural space (pleural effusion or empyema).
B. **Technique of Thoracentesis**
1. A local anesthetic is injected into the skin at the area where the fluid has been detected.
2. A local anesthetic is also injected into the periosteum of the rib with a 22-gauge needle.
3. With the patient in a sitting position, a needle (usually 22-gauge or larger) is inserted into the pleural space and the fluid is aspirated.
4. Thoracentesis is generally performed by the physician while the RCP assists with obtaining the specimen and preparing it for laboratory analysis.
5. After the fluid is removed, it is analyzed for:
   a. Odor
   b. Color
   c. RBC count
   d. WBC count
   e. Characteristics shown by Gram's stain
   f. Identification of the infecting organism by culture and sensitivity tests

Note

Pus in the pleural space (empyema) should be drained before chest physical therapy.

★ 6. Thoracentesis may be performed in cases of pneumonia in which consolidation has occurred. The needle may be inserted into the affected area of the lung and the secretions withdrawn so that culture and sensitivity tests may be done to identify the infecting organism.
7. Lung tissue may also be obtained by inserting a needle into the affected area to sample lung morphology of suspected tumors. Technique is referred to as **percutaneous lung biopsy.**
C. **Complications of Thoracentesis**
1. Pneumothorax
2. Bacterial infection
3. Subcutaneous emphysema

III. TRANSTRACHEAL ASPIRATION

A. Obtaining sputum for culture and sensitivity tests via nasotracheal suctioning may not accurately identify the organisms within the trachea and lower airway, because the sample is contaminated by "normal bacterial flora" located in the nasal and oral pharynx.

B. To avoid contamination of the lower respiratory tract with nasal and oral suctioning, transtracheal aspiration may be performed.

C. **Technique of Transtracheal Aspiration**

1. This procedure is performed by introducing a thin polyethylene needle catheter into the trachea through the cricoid membrane under local anesthesia.

2. The needle is removed while the catheter remains in place, and saline is instilled into the trachea through the catheter.

3. This usually stimulates a strong cough, and the product of the cough is aspirated through the catheter with a syringe.

4. Only a small amount of sputum is needed for analysis.

5. This procedure is performed by a physician while the RCP assists with obtaining the sputum sample and preparing it to be sent to the laboratory for analysis.

D. **Complications of Transtracheal Aspiration**

1. Patient discomfort
2. Subcutaneous emphysema
3. Esophageal damage
4. Damage to the nerves and blood vessels surrounding the area of entrance into the trachea

IV. CHEST TUBE INSERTION AND MONITORING

A. Chest tubes are used to drain substances that accumulate in the pleural space.

B. Substances that may accumulate in the pleural space and their diagnoses include:

1. Air: pneumothorax
2. Blood: hemothorax
3. Lymph: chylothorax
4. Serous fluid: pleural effusion
5. Pus: pyothorax or empyema

> *Note*
>
> The term hydrothorax is often used to refer to lymph, serum, or plasma in the pleural space.

C. To help evacuate air (pneumothorax) from the pleural space, the chest tube is usually inserted in the second, third, or fourth intercostal space. To remove fluids, the tube is placed lower, usually in the seventh or eighth intercostal space.

D. Chest tube insertion is done under local anesthesia; for large tubes, regional anesthesia with an intercostal block is used.

E. Chest tubes are sutured in and the insertion distance should be monitored daily to ensure the tube is not migrating outward. If the proximal hole on the chest tube slips out of the chest, air will enter the tube resulting in bubbling in the system, which will appear to be a persistent leak in the lung.

> *Note*
>
> Once the air is evacuated from the pleural space, spontaneous healing or sealing of the leak in the lung will usually occur.

F. **Chest Tube Drainage Systems**
   1. **One-bottle system**

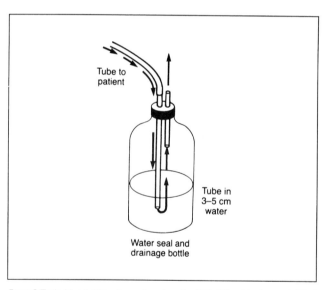

From O'Toole M, ed: Miller-Keane Encyclopedia of Medicine, Nursing, and Allied Health, 5 ed. Philadelphia: WB Saunders, 1992.

a. Fluid or air drains from the pleural space through the chest tube and enters the drainage bottle through a glass tube, which is submerged under water. This forms a seal that acts like a one-way valve to prevent air from entering the pleural cavity.

b. Air entering the bottle is then vented out the short tube in the top of the bottle.

c. The one-bottle setup is both a water-seal container and a collection container.

2. Two-bottle system

a. In this system, a second bottle is added to collect air exiting the pleural space. Liquid drains into the first bottle.

b. The purpose of this system is to better control the amount of suction applied. A suction source may be connected to the vent of the water-seal bottle.

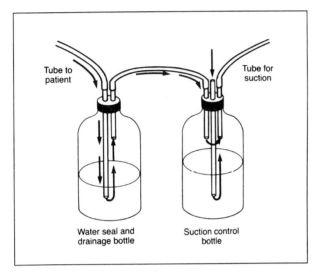

From O'Toole M, ed: Miller-Keane Encyclopedia of Medicine, Nursing, and Allied Health, 5 ed. Philadelphia: WB Saunders, 1992.

3. Three-bottle system

a. A third bottle may be added to determine the amount of subatmospheric pressure in the water-seal bottle.

b. The amount of suction is determined by how far under the water the tube is submerged.

c. A suction source may be attached to the third bottle's vent to maintain a desired constant subatmospheric pressure.

> **Note**
>
> Most chest tubes today are attached to chest tube collection systems, commercially called Pleur-Eval systems. It is equivalent to the three-bottle system mentioned above. Chambers are used instead of bottles to accomplish drainage.

G. Important Points Concerning Chest Tube Drainage

1. The water level in the water seal bottle will fluctuate with changes in pleural pressure that occur with normal breathing. **If no fluctuation is occurring in the water-seal bottle, obstruction of the tube should be suspected.**

2. Chest tubes may become obstructed as a result of blood clots or kinks in the tube itself. **Obstructed chest tubes may result in a tension pneumothorax.**

★ 3. To assure adequate drainage and tube patency, the tube should be "stripped" or "milked" every 1 to 2 hr. This is accomplished by compressing and releasing the tubing, which creates a sudden gush of suction, thereby keeping the tube clear of obstruction caused by a clot.

★ 4. Occasional bubbling in the water-seal bottle is normal as air enters from the pleural space. Excessive or persistent bubbling may indicate air leaks in the system. The absence of bubbling indicates that no air is being removed from the pleural space, a sign of the patient's improvement.

★ 5. If an air leak is suspected, the chest tube should be clamped to identify the source of the leak.

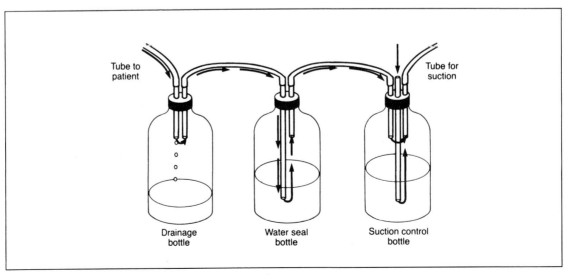

From O'Toole M, ed: Miller-Keane Encyclopedia of Medicine, Nursing, and Allied Health, 5 ed. Philadelphia: WB Saunders, 1992.

★ 6. Clamping of the tube is required when changing drainage bottles, but must be done with caution on patients with pleural air leaks, because a tension pneumothorax may result.

7. The drainage and collection bottles must be kept at a level below the chest to prevent backflow.

8. The drainage and collection system must be kept airtight with no leaks around the connections. The glass tube **must always** be kept submerged under the water.

9. If a suction source is connected to the vent tube in the suction bottle, a negative pressure (not to exceed -15 cm H_2O) is usually necessary.

10. After the lung re-expands, the chest tube should remain in place for another 1 to 2 days. After the tube is removed, the wound should be covered with a sterile petroleum jelly dressing to prevent air from entering the pleural space.

POST-CHAPTER STUDY QUESTIONS

1. List five indications for bronchoscopy.
2. List eight complications of bronchoscopy.
3. Name one medication that is commonly used to achieve conscious sedation before bronchoscopy.
4. What is the purpose of administering atropine before bronchoscopy?
5. How should the bronchoscope be cleaned after the procedure?
6. After a thoracentesis is performed, for what is the fluid analyzed?
7. List three complications of thoracentesis.
8. What is the purpose of transtracheal aspiration?
9. What is the purpose of insertion of a chest tube?
10. If the water in the water-seal bottle is not fluctuating, what should be suspected?
11. If a chest tube becomes obstructed, what may occur?
12. If an air leak from a chest tube is suspected, what should be done first?
13. How much negative pressure is generally required to help evacuate fluid or air from the pleural space?

Answers are at the end of the chapter.

REFERENCES

Des Jardins T: Cardiopulmonary anatomy and physiology: essentials for respiratory care, ed 3, Albany, 1998, Delmar Publishers.

Des Jardins T and Burton G: Clinical manifestations of respiratory disease, ed 2, Chicago, 1990, YearBook Medical Publishers.

Kacmarek R and Stoller J: Current respiratory care, Philadelphia, 1988, BC Decker Inc.

Levitzky M, Cairo J, and Hall S: Introduction to respiratory care, Philadelphia, 1990, WB Saunders Co.

O'Toole M: Encyclopedia and dictionary of medicine, nursing, and allied health, ed 5, Philadelphia, 1992, WB Saunders Co.

Scanlan CL, Wilkins RL, and Stoller JK: Egan's fundamentals of respiratory care, ed 7, St. Louis, 1999, Mosby Inc.

Weinberger S: Principles of pulmonary medicine, ed 2, Philadelphia, 1992, WB Saunders Co.

PRE-TEST ANSWERS

1. D
2. C
3. C
4. D
5. B
6. D
7. B

ANSWERS TO POST-CHAPTER STUDY QUESTIONS

1. Removal of foreign bodies and mucus plugs to treat atelectasis; pulmonary hemorrhage; difficult tracheal intubation; biopsy of airway tumors; sputum collection for culture and sensitivity
2. Hypoxemia, laryngospasm, bronchospasm, arrhythmias, hemorrhage, respiratory depression, hypotension, pneumothorax
3. Diazepam (Valium) or midazolam (Versed)
4. To dry out the airway
5. Soak in glutaraldehyde (Cidex) solution for 3 to 10 hr to disinfect or sterilize
6. Odor, color, RBC count, WBC count, Gram's stain, identification of organisms
7. Pneumothorax, bacterial infection, subcutaneous emphysema
8. To obtain a "clean" sample by avoiding the normal flora in the upper airway
9. To drain fluid or air from the pleural space so the lung may re-expand
10. Obstruction of the tube
11. Tension pneumothorax
12. Clamp the tube and identify the source of the leak
13. -15 cm H_2O

Cardiopulmonary Resuscitation Techniques

Answer the pre-test questions before studying the chapter. This will help you determine your strong and weak areas regarding the material covered.

1. You enter a patient's room to give a treatment and observe the patient is unconscious and not breathing. Your **first** action should be which of the following?

   A. Deliver two breaths
   B. Begin chest compressions
   C. Perform abdominal thrusts
   D. Open the airway

2. After 10 min of CPR, an infant's pulse returns but no ventilatory effort is present. The RCP should do which of the following?

   A. Continue compressions and rescue breathing at a ratio of 5:1.
   B. Stop compressions and deliver one breath every 6 sec.
   C. Deliver five back blows, until breathing resumes.
   D. Stop compressions and deliver one breath every 3 sec.

3. A patient has been intubated and CPR is being performed. The patient's ECG strip indicates asystole, and the physician is unable to start an IV line. The respiratory therapist should recommend which of the following immediately?

   A. Instill sodium bicarbonate directly down the ET tube.
   B. Continue to attempt to start an IV in a peripheral vein.
   C. Instill epinephrine directly down the ET tube.
   D. Inject epinephrine directly into the myocardium.

4. Which of the following drugs is used to treat ventricular fibrillation during CPR?

   I. Epinephrine
   II. Lidocaine
   III. Atropine sulfate

   A. I only
   B. II only
   C. I and II only
   D. II and III only

5. During CPR, the patient's ECG strip indicates ventricular fibrillation. The patient has been defibrillated with 200 joules with no change in the ECG reading. The respiratory therapist should recommend which of the following?

   A. Repeat defibrillation with 300 joules.
   B. Repeat defibrillation with 450 joules.
   C. Instill sodium bicarbonate directly down the ET tube.
   D. Continue two rescuer CPR with a compression/ventilation ratio of 5:2.

6. A patient's ECG strip indicates atrial fibrillation and cardioversion should be attempted. The defibrillator should be set at what level to return the heart to normal function?

   A. 50 joules
   B. 150 joules
   C. 250 joules
   D. 400 joules

Answers are at end of the chapter.

I. **CARDIOPULMONARY RESUSCITATION**
   A. **Obstructed Airway (in a Conscious Adult)**
      1. Determine whether there is an airway obstruction by asking the patient if he or she is choking and can speak or cough.
      2. Perform **abdominal thrusts** until the foreign body is expelled or the patient loses consciousness.
      3. If the patient loses consciousness, place the patient on his or her back and call for help.

4. Use the tongue/jaw lift to open the mouth and perform a finger sweep with the patient's head turned to the side.
5. Open the airway by using the head tilt/chin lift method.
6. Give two breaths.
7. If the ventilation attempts fail (determined by observing the chest not rising or difficulty in expelling air into the patient), reposition the airway and ventilate again. If there is still no air movement, straddle the patient's thighs and perform up to five abdominal thrusts.
8. Again, perform a finger sweep and re-attempt ventilations.
9. Repeat this sequence until the airway is cleared.

B. **Obstructed Airway (in an Unconscious Adult)**
1. Determine unresponsiveness.
2. Call for help.
3. Position the patient on his or her back.
4. Open the airway using the head tilt/chin lift method.
5. **Determine breathlessness** by placing ear over the patient's mouth and **look, listen, and feel for air movement.**
6. Attempt to ventilate.
7. If no air movement, reposition the airway and reattempt to ventilate.
8. If still no air movement, straddle the patient's thighs and perform up to five abdominal thrusts.
9. Perform a finger sweep with the patient's head turned to the side.
10. Attempt ventilation.
11. Repeat the sequence until the airway is cleared.

C. **One-Rescuer CPR (Adult Patient)**
1. Determine unresponsiveness.
2. Call for help.
3. Position patient on back.
4. Open the airway using the head tilt/chin lift method.
5. Determine breathlessness by placing ear over the patient's mouth and look, listen, and feel for air movement.
6. Give two breaths while observing chest rise. (Allow lungs to deflate between breaths.)
7. Determine pulselessness by palpating the **carotid artery.** (Palpate **brachial artery** in an **infant.**)
8. Begin chest compressions at a rate of 80 to 100/min (15 compressions to 2 breaths).
9. Continue until patient responds, help arrives, or you can physically no longer continue.

D. **Two Rescuer CPR (Adult Patient)**
1. When second rescuer arrives, he or she should take over as the new compressor, while the first rescuer gets into position to be the breather. Palpate for a spontaneous pulse at this time.
2. If no pulse is present, the breather delivers one breath and signals the compressor to resume CPR **(5 compressions per breath).**
3. The compressor should pause briefly after the fifth compression so the breather can administer a breath.
4. The patient should be intubated as soon as possible to provide a more effective airway and to prevent air from entering the stomach during ventilation.
5. As the compressor begins to tire, he or she may signal the breather to change positions by altering the pmnemonic from "one, one thousand" to "change, one thousand." After the next 5:1 sequence, the compressor moves to the head to begin ventilations (but first checking the pulse), while the breather gets into position to begin compressions.

E. **Neonatal Resuscitation (Immediately after Delivery)**
1. Dry and warm the infant.
2. Suction the nose and mouth with a bulb syringe or DeLee suction catheter.
3. If meconium is seen, intubate the infant and suction the trachea.
4. Provide tactile stimulation to stimulate breathing.
5. If the infant is not breathing or the heart rate is less than 100/min, begin positive pressure ventilation with 100% oxygen with a bag and mask.
   a. Initial ventilation rate should be 40/min.
   b. Initial ventilation pressure should be 30 to 40 cm H_2O, with all the breaths thereafter at 15 to 20 cm H_2O. (When resuscitating an infant hours after delivery who has respiratory problems resulting in decreased lung compliance, higher pressures may be necessary for ventilation.)

Note

The manual resuscitator should have a manometer attached to measure peak inspiratory pressure.

---

6. After ventilating for 15 to 30 sec, the pulse should be reassessed, and if the heart rate is

less than 60/min, or 60/min to 80/min and
not increasing, ventilation should continue
and chest compressions should be started.
a. The compression rate should be approximately 120/min.
b. Once the heart rate is 80/min or higher,
compressions should be discontinued
while manual ventilation is maintained.
c. If the heart rate stays below 80/min, the
infant should be intubated. Positive pressure ventilation and chest compressions
should continue, and the infant should be
reassessed periodically.
7. Drugs used during neonatal resuscitation
a. **Epinephrine** is a cardiac stimulant that
should be administered either via IV drip
or **directly down an ET tube**
(1) If the heart rate remains below 80/min
after 30 sec of chest compressions and
manual ventilation
(2) If a heart rate cannot be detected
(3) See section on pharmacological intervention during CPR on page 70.
b. **Volume expanders** are administered to
increase vascular fluid volume to reverse
relative hypovolemia; they include:
(1) Whole blood (type O-negative blood
cross-matched with mother's blood)
(2) Normal saline solution
(3) Saline solution with 5% albumin
(4) Ringer's lactate solution
c. **Sodium bicarbonate** is indicated in the
presence of documented metabolic acidosis, which is caused by increased lactic
acid production as a result of prolonged
asphyxia.
d. **Naloxone hydrochloride (Narcan)** is a
narcotic antagonist that reverses narcotic-
induced respiratory depression. In infants,
this most commonly occurs when narcotics
are administered to the mother within 4 hr
of delivery. **Narcan administration is
indicated when severe respiratory
depression is present and the
mother is known to have had narcotics in the past 4 hr.**

> *Note*
> Narcan may be administered intravenously, intramuscularly,
> subcutaneously, or instilled down the ET tube.

II. **ADULT, CHILD, AND INFANT CPR
MODIFICATIONS**
A. **Compression/Ventilation Ratios (for One
Rescuer)**

1. Adult: compression/ventilation ratio is 15:2;
80 to 100 compressions per minute
2. Child: compression/ventilation ratio is 5:1;
100 compressions per minute
3. Infant: compression/ventilation ratio is 5:1;
more than 100 compressions per minute
B. **Compression/Ventilation Ratios (for Two
Rescuers)**
1. Adult: compression/ventilation ratio is 5:1
2. Child: compression/ventilation ratio is 5:1
3. Infant: compression/ventilation ratio is 5:1
C. **Rescue Breathing for Patient who has
Pulse**
1. Adult: 1 breath every 5 sec
2. Child: 1 breath every 3 sec
3. Infant: 1 breath every 3 sec
D. **Compression Depth**
1. Adult: **1½ to 2 in** with two hands stacked
and heel of one hand on lower half of the
patient's sternum
2. Child: **1 to 1½ in** with one hand on the
lower half of the patient's sternum
3. Infant: **½ to 1 in** with two or three fingers a
finger's breadth below the nipple line.

III. **CPR: SPECIAL CONSIDERATIONS**
A. **Do not** hyperextend the neck of an infant to
open the airway because this may close the
airway off.
B. If a manual resuscitator bag and mask are not
available for rescue breathing, **a mask with a
one-way valve should be used to prevent
contamination from the patient's exhaled
air.** Mouth-to-mouth ventilation is used only if
no other means is available.
C. **Never compress the chest of a patient
who has even the weakest pulse.**
1. A weak pulse more than likely delivers a higher
cardiac output than do manual compressions.
2. Manual compressions achieve only about
25% to 35% of normal cardiac output.
D. On entering a room where one-rescuer CPR is
being performed, the first step to take before
changing to two-rescuer CPR is to establish the
presence or absence of a pulse.
E. The best indicator of adequate cerebral blood
flow while performing chest compressions is
pupillary reaction.
F. Patients with suspected **neck injury** should
have their airway opened by the **jaw-thrust
maneuver without head tilt.**
G. **Hazards of CPR**
1. Rib fracture (especially in infants and elderly
persons); may lead to pneumothorax or lacer-
ated liver
2. Fat embolism (microfractures of the ribs or
sternum lead to leaking of fat from bone

marrow; this fat finds its way into the venous circulation)

3. Gastric distention (from air entering the stomach from rescue breathing); air should be removed from the stomach with a naso-gastric (NG) tube, since a distended abdomen interferes with lung expansion

IV. MANUAL RESUSCITATORS
A. Uses of Manual Resuscitators
1. Rescue breathing
2. Hyperinflation of lungs before tracheal suctioning
3. During transport of patient who requires artificial ventilation

B. Manual Resuscitator

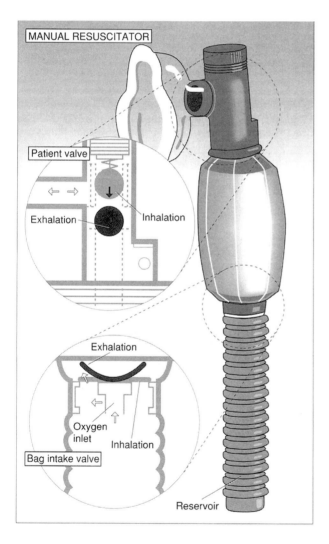

MANUAL RESUSCITATOR

Patient valve

Exhalation — Inhalation

Exhalation

Oxygen inlet   Inhalation

Bag intake valve

Reservoir

C. Design of Resuscitators: all are basically the same
1. A non-rebreathing valve with a standard universal adaptor, consisting of a 22-mm OD that fits standard resuscitation masks and a 15 mm ID that connects to standard ET or tracheostomy tubes.

2. The non-rebreathing valve also houses the exhalation valve and ports, which prevent the rebreathing of exhaled air.
3. The resuscitators use **self-inflating bags** by means of a bag intake valve. **(The bag may still be used to ventilate, even without gas flowing to it.)**
★ 4. A reservoir attachment should be connected to the bag intake valve so that, as the bag reinflates, it fills with supplemental oxygen instead of room air. This ensures higher oxygen levels (approaching 100%) being delivered to the patient.
5. Most resuscitator bags have pressure-relief devices that open to the atmosphere at a pressure of 40 cm H_2O to prevent excessive pressures from being delivered to the patient's lungs.
6. Some resuscitators come equipped with PEEP valves for "bagging" patients who are on PEEP while on the ventilator. This is very beneficial, because it has been shown that patients taken off PEEP to be "bagged" have drastic reductions in their PaO_2 if ventilated without PEEP.
7. **To achieve the highest delivered O_2 levels possible, follow these criteria.**
★ a. Always use a reservoir attachment, if available.
★ b. Use the highest flow rate available (10 to 15 L/min).
★ c. Use the longest possible bag refill time; this means a slower ventilation rate. Allow the bag to fully refill before the next breath. A faster ventilation rate decreases the percentage of delivered O_2.
★ d. Do not use large stroke volumes (i.e., the volume squeezed from the bag), if possible. High volumes delivered from the bag mean more room air entrained, thus lower levels of O_2. **(This is not significant if a reservoir attachment is used.)**

D. Hazards of Using Manual Resuscitators
1. Leaks during inspiration caused by improperly fitted face mask or inadequately filled ET-tube cuff.
2. Equipment malfunction caused by sticking valves, missing parts, improper assembly, or dirty valve mechanisms.
3. Poor ventilation technique.

> **Note**
>
> Whenever the bag is squeezed, little or no resistance is met, and the chest does not rise adequately, suspect a leak around the exhalation valve, O_2 intake valve, or ET-tube cuff or a poor-fitting mask.

E. **Gas-Powered Resuscitators**

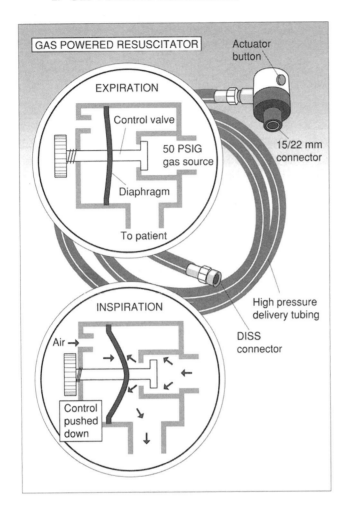

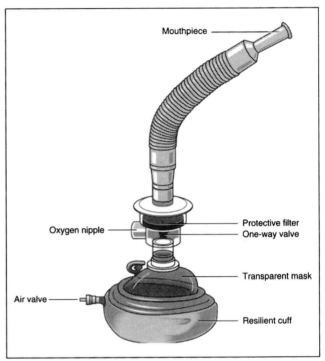

on a mask. The other end has a mouthpiece attached. The rescue breather may now manually ventilate the patient through the mouthpiece; the patient's exhaled air passes around the exhalation ports to the outside.

3. This one-way valve system for rescue breathing protects the breather from cross-contamination from the patient's exhaled air.

1. These are usually pressure-limited devices.
2. Some use demand valves, which open and deliver gas if the patient creates a negative pressure.
3. They usually have manual control buttons to initiate inspiration if the patient is apneic.
4. They are able to deliver 100% O_2.
5. Volume delivery decreases if the pressure needed to ventilate the patient's lungs is higher than the capacity of the unit.
6. The unit is powered from a 50-psi O_2 wall outlet. If the diaphragm in the unit breaks, the patient's airway could be exposed to this high pressure.
7. These units have pressure-relief devices that vent pressures above 50 cm H_2O.

F. **Mouth-to-Valve Mask Ventilation**
1. This method of ventilation provides an option to mouth-to-mouth ventilation, which should be avoided, unless no other means is available.
2. Mouth-to-valve mask rescue breathing involves placing one end of the one-way valve

V. **PHARMACOLOGIC INTERVENTION DURING CPR**
A. **Routes of Administration**
1. Central venous line: ideal route if available
2. Peripheral IV line: best route if central venous line is not available
3. **ET tube:** drugs such **lidocaine, epinephrine, and atropine** may be instilled directly into the tracheobronchial tree via the ET tube for rapid absorption.

Note

When using this route, administer the drugs at 2 to 2.5 times the recommended IV dose with 10.0 mL of normal saline.

---

4. Intracardiac: epinephrine is the only drug that may be injected directly into the heart, but only if the ET tube or IV route is not available or administration via those routes has failed to elicit a response.

B. **Drugs Commonly Administered During CPR**
  1. **Epinephrine**
     a. Indications
        (1) Asystole
        (2) Sinus arrest
        (3) Ventricular fibrillation
     b. Route of administration
        (1) IV bolus
        (2) **ET tube**
        (3) Intracardiac
     c. Dosage is one of the following
        (1) 0.1 mL/kg IV every 5 min (to a 10 mL maximum) of a 0.1 mg/mL (1 : 10,000) preparation
        (2) 10 mL down ET tube
        (3) 0.1 mL/kg intracardiac dose every 5 min (to a 10 mL maximum) of a 0.1 mg/ml (1 : 10,000) preparation
     d. Pharmacologic actions
        (1) Increased heart rate
        (2) Increased force of contraction of the heart
        (3) Increased coronary perfusion pressure
        (4) Vasoconstriction
  2. **Lidocaine**
     a. Indications
        (1) Ventricular fibrillation
        (2) Ventricular tachycardia
        (3) PVCs
     b. Route of administration
        (1) IV bolus
        (2) IV drip
        (3) **ET tube**
     c. Dosage: 1 mg/kg IV bolus followed by additional boluses of 0.5 to 1.5 mg/kg every 3–5 minutes, up to a total of 3 mg/kg. Continuous infusion (drip) may be started at a rate of 2.0 to 4.0 mg/min when perfusion is restored following ventricular fibrillation.
     d. Pharmacologic actions
        (1) Decreases ventricular activity
  3. **Atropine sulfate**
     a. Indications
        (1) Sinus bradycardia
        (2) Asystole
        (3) Nodal bradycardia
     b. Route of administration
        (1) IV bolus
        (2) **ET tube**
     c. Dosage
        (1) 1.0 mg IV every 5 min for asystole
        (2) 0.5 mg IV every 5 min (to a 2.0-mg maximum) for bradycardia
     d. Pharmacologic actions
        (1) Increased heart rate
        (2) Increased force of contraction of the heart
  4. **Procainamide**
     a. Indications
        (1) Ventricular tachycardia
        (2) Ventricular fibrillation
        (3) PVCs
     b. Route of administration
        (1) IV bolus
        (2) IV drip
     c. Dosage:
        (1) 50 mg IV bolus every 5 min
        (2) 1 to 4 mg/min IV drip of a 100 mg/mL preparation
     d. Pharmacologic actions
        (1) May cause hypotension
        (2) Increases electrical stimulation threshold
        (3) Decreases electrical activity of the ventricles
  5. **Bretylium tosylate**
     a. Indications
        (1) Ventricular tachycardia
        (2) Ventricular fibrillation
        (3) PVCs
     b. Route of administration
        (1) IV bolus
     c. Dosage: 5 mg/kg in 50 mL diluent over 5 to 10 min
     d. Pharmacologic actions
        (1) May cause hypotension
        (2) Increases electrical stimulation threshold
        (3) Decreases the electrical activity of the ventricles
  6. **Propranolol hydrochloride**
     a. Indications
        (1) MI
        (2) Angina pectoris
        (3) Supraventricular arrhythmias
        (4) Ventricular tachycardia
     b. Route of administration
        (1) IV bolus
     c. Dosage: 1 to 5 mg (to a maximum of 1 mg/min) of a 1 mg/mL preparation
     d. Pharmacologic actions
        (1) Decreased heart rate
        (2) Decreased stroke volume
        (3) Increased left ventricular end-diastolic pressure (LVEDP)
  7. **Dobutamine hydrochloride**
     a. Indications
        Depressed myocardial contractility
     b. Route of administration
        IV drip

c. Dosage: 2.5 to 10 μg/kg/min
d. Pharmacologic actions
  (1) Increased cardiac output
  (2) Enhanced atrioventricular conduction

8. **Isoproteronol hydrochloride**
  a. Indications
    (1) Bradycardia
    (2) Heart block
    (3) Hypotension
  b. Route of administration
    IV drip
  c. Dosage: 1 mg/500 mL of 5% dextrose
    (2 μg/mL)
  d. Pharmacologic actions
    (1) Increased heart rate
    (2) Increased force of contraction of the heart

9. **Dopamine hydrochloride**
  a. Indications
    Hypotension
  b. Route of administration
    IV drip
  c. Dosage: 2 to 30 μg/kg/min
  d. Pharmacologic actions
    (1) Increased cardiac output
    (2) Increased blood pressure

10. **Sodium nitroprusside (Nipride)**
  a. Indications
    Hypertension
  b. Route of administration
    IV drip
  c. Dosage: 0.5 to 8.0 μg/kg/min
  d. Pharmacologic actions
    (1) Peripheral vasodilation
    (2) Decreased blood pressure

11. **Calcium chloride**
  a. Indications
    (1) Hypocalcemia
    (2) Hyperkalemia
  b. Route of administration
    IV (do not mix with other medications)
  c. Dosage: 0.2 mL/kg
  d. Pharmacologic actions
    Increased force of contraction of the heart

Note

The use of sodium bicarbonate ($NaHCO_3$) is no longer recommended during CPR. It has been found to cause adverse effects, including a shift of the HbO_2 curve to the left (decreased release of O_2 by Hb), depression of cerebral and myocardial function, and the deactivation of catecholamines (e.g., isoproterenol, epinephrine) used during the resuscitative effort.

VI. **DEFIBRILLATION AND CARDIOVERSION**
A. **Defibrillation**
  1. Defibrillation is a nonsynchronized current of electricity delivered to the heart during ventricular fibrillation.
  2. It is administered by means of paddles placed on specific areas of the chest. After conducting gel is applied to the paddles, one paddle is placed below the clavicle and to the right of the upper part of the sternum. The other paddle is placed on the midaxillary line just to the left of the left nipple.
  3. The initial electric current delivered should be **200 joules (W/sec) for adults** and 2 joules/kg of body weight in infants and children. Should this level not be effective in restoring normal ventricular activity, it may be increased to **no more than 360 joules for adults** or 4 joules/kg in infants and children.
  4. This high charge of electricity delivered to the myocardium is intended to reverse life-threatening ventricular arrhythmias and accomplishes this by causing complete depolarization of the cardiac muscle, thereby disrupting the electrical circuits in the heart that are causing the ventricular fibrillation.
  5. Lidocaine and epinephrine may be administered, since they improve the success of defibrillation.
  6. It is essential that appropriate levels of electric current be used to prevent myocardial damage and cardiac arrhythmias.

B. **Cardioversion**
  1. Cardioversion is a synchronized current of electricity delivered to the heart during ventricular depolarization (QRS complex).
  2. Cardioversion is used to terminate the following arrhythmias:.
    a. Atrial flutter
    b. Atrial fibrillation
    c. Ventricular tachycardia
    d. Paroxysmal supraventricular tachycardia
    e. Ventricular fibrillation (defibrillation is usually indicated)
  3. Cardioversion delivers a lower energy level than does defibrillation. Normal levels for cardioversion are a charge of between 25 to 100 joules to restore normal cardiac rhythm in adults and 0.2 to 1.0 joules/kg in infants and children.
  4. A RCP's duties in assisting with this procedure should include the following:
    a. Monitor heart rate and respiratory rate
    b. Monitor O_2 saturation
    c. Have O_2 delivery device readily available

d. Have manual resuscitator and intubation equipment readily available

> ### Note
>
> See chapter 9: Cardiac Monitoring, for further information on ECGs and specific arrhythmias.

VII. TRANSPORTING THE CRITICALLY ILL PATIENT

> ### ★ Exam Note
>
> Questions relating to transporting patients via land or air appear on the RRT examination only.

A. Patients may be transported by either land or air.
B. Important points concerning the transport of patients by land or air
  1. Unstable patients must be transported with great care to avoid worsening of the their condition.
  2. The practitioner should hold the ET tube with one hand and bag with the other. This better stabilizes the tube and helps avoid inadvertent extubation.
  3. Sudden changes in speed or direction may cause a drop in the patient's blood pressure.
  4. Special attention must be given to monitoring lines that could become dislodged in transport.
  5. Ventilators used for transport should have demand valves to conserve gas.
  6. Patients should be adequately sedated to help prevent anxiety and allow safer transport.
  ★ 7. During transport in an unpressurized aircraft, rapid increases in altitude result in decreased atmospheric pressure and P_{O_2}. This may be managed by increasing delivered O_2 concentrations.
  ★ 8. Higher altitudes (lower atmospheric pressure) may increase the size of an untreated pneumothorax and increase ET-tube cuff pressure, which may decrease capillary perfusion to the trachea.
  9. Lightweight equipment (such as transport ventilators) is necessary for air transportation.
  10. Patient monitoring is more difficult in aircraft, especially helicopters.
  11. Heated humidity or aerosol for ventilators or masks during transport is not necessary for such short-term use.

C. Respiratory care equipment needed during transport:
  1. O_2 system (tanks or liquid)
  2. Portable suction machine and catheters
  3. Portable ventilator
  4. Portable ECG unit
  5. Arterial pressure monitor
  6. Pulse oximeter
  7. Intubation equipment
  8. Manual resuscitator

POST-CHAPTER STUDY QUESTIONS

1. List three medications that are commonly instilled directly down the ET tube.
2. What is the major indication for the administration of dopamine?
3. List three indications for lidocaine.
4. Sodium nitroprusside (Nipride) is indicated for the treatment of what condition?
5. Describe the proper airway management of a post-term neonate in whom meconium aspiration is suspected.
6. When resuscitating a neonate immediately after delivery, what is the proper ventilation rate and peak inspiratory pressure for manual ventilation?
7. List four criteria that aid in delivering the highest O_2 concentration with a manual resuscitator.
8. What is the initial current delivered during defibrillation of an adult?
9. What is the maximum current used to defibrillate an adult?
10. List two drugs that may be administered to improve the success of defibrillation.
11. List five arrhythmias that cardioversion is used to terminate.
12. How many joules are delivered to the patient during cardioversion?
13. List three potential consequences that could affect a patient during an air transport at high altitude.

Answers are at the end of the chapter.

REFERENCES

American Heart Association: CPR Guidelines, 1997.

Barnes T: Respiratory care practice, Chicago, 1988, Year Book Medical Publishers.

Eubanks D and Bone R: Comprehensive respiratory care, ed 2, St. Louis, 1990, The CV Mosby Co.

Levitzky M: Introduction to respiratory care, Philadelphia, 1990, WB Saunders Co.

McPherson S: Respiratory therapy equipment, ed 5, St. Louis, 1995, Mosby-Yearbook Inc.

Miller-Keane: Encyclopedia and dictionary of medicine, nursing and allied health, ed 5, Philadelphia, 1992, WB Saunders Co.

Scanlan CL, Wilkins RL, and Stoller JK: Egan's fundamentals of respiratory care, ed 7, St. Louis, 1999, Mosby Inc.

PRE-TEST ANSWERS

1. D
2. D
3. C
4. C
5. A
6. A

ANSWERS TO POST-CHAPTER STUDY QUESTIONS

1. Atropine, epinephrine, lidocaine
2. Hypotension
3. Ventricular fibrillation, ventricular tachycardia, PVCs
4. Hypertension
5. Intubate and suction the airway
6. Ventilatory rate: 40/min, peak inspiratory pressure initially 30 to 40 cm H_2O, with subsequent pressure of 15 to 20 cm H_2O
7. Add O_2 reservoir, use high O_2 flow rate (10 to 15 L/min), slower ventilation rate (10 to 20/min), avoid excessive volumes if reservoir attachment is not used
8. 200 joules
9. 360 joules
10. Lidocaine, epinephrine
11. Atrial flutter, atrial fibrillation, ventricular tachycardia, paroxysmal supraventricular tachycardia, ventricular fibrillation
12. 25 to 100 joules
13. Decreased PaO_2, increased size of pneumothorax, increased ET-tube cuff pressure

Chapter 7

IPPB Therapy

PRE-TEST QUESTIONS

1. Which of the following increases the delivered V_T to a patient taking an IPPB treatment with the Bird Mark 7 IPPB machine?

       I. Increasing flow rate
       II. Increasing inspiratory pressure
       III. Decreasing sensitivity
       IV. Decreasing flow rate

   A. I and II only
   B. I and III only
   C. II and IV only
   D. I, II, and III only

2. During an IPPB treatment the patient suddenly complains of chest pain and becomes short of breath. On assessing the patient, you auscultate the chest and hear decreased breath sounds on the left. These findings are consistent with which of the following?

   A. Atelectasis
   B. Left-sided pneumothorax
   C. Pulmonary embolism
   D. Pleural effusion

3. The respiratory therapist is administering IPPB, and the patient complains of feeling lightheaded and dizzy. What should the therapist do to correct this?

   A. Instruct the patient to pause longer between breaths.
   B. Instruct the patient to take deeper breaths.
   C. Increase the inspiratory pressure.
   D. Decrease the inspiratory flow.

4. While the respiratory therapist is administering IPPB, the patient begins coughing up large amounts of blood. The therapist should

   A. Continue the treatment and notify the physician that a chest radiograph is needed.
   B. Decrease the inspiratory pressure.

   C. Stop the treatment briefly, and resume it when the patient is feeling better.
   D. Stop the treatment and notify the physician.

5. Which of the following are hazards of IPPB therapy?

       I. Excessive ventilation
       II. Increased cardiac output
       III. Decreased ICP

   A. I only
   B. II only
   C. I and III only
   D. II and III only

6. The respiratory therapist has received an order to deliver IPPB to a patient with head trauma. What modifications in therapy may benefit this patient?

       I. Use a higher flow rate.
       II. Use lower peak pressures.
       III. Set the sensitivity to -5 cm H_2O.

   A. I only
   B. II only
   C. I and II only
   D. II and III only

Answers are at end of the chapter.

REVIEW

I. **INTRODUCTION TO IPPB THERAPY**
   A. IPPB is defined as a short-term (10- to 15-min) breathing treatment in which pressures above atmospheric pressure are delivered to the patient's lungs via a pressure-cycled ventilator.
   B. Effective IPPB depends on four factors:
      1. An RCP who has been well trained and has a knowledge of the equipment, medications used, reasons for therapy, and side effects and goals of therapy.
      2. A relaxed, informed, and cooperative patient.

3. A pressure-limited IPPB machine with a means of measuring V_T.
4. Proper instruction of the patient on breathing patterns and cough techniques by the RCP.

II. PHYSIOLOGIC EFFECTS OF IPPB

A. Increased Mean Airway Pressure

1. During normal spontaneous inspiration, airway pressure drops below atmospheric pressure (-2 cm H_2O), thereby setting up a pressure gradient between the atmosphere (at nose and mouth) and the airways. Air flows into the airways, gradually building pressure back up to atmospheric level. Air flow stops and passive exhalation occurs as a result of the natural recoil properties of lung tissue. The lung is never subjected to significant positive pressure.
2. During an IPPB machine breath, positive pressure is applied to the airways to improve the ventilation status of the lung. This is what is meant by "increased mean airway pressure"; it is the average (mean) pressure in the airways during one breathing cycle.

B. Increased V_T

1. IPPB should deliver V_T of 12 to 15 mL/kg of ideal body weight.
2. Delivered V_T depends on the patient's lung status (e.g., compliance, airway resistance).
   a. Decreased compliance results in a decreased delivered V_T
   b. Increased compliance results in an increased delivered V_T
   c. Decreased airway resistance results in an increased delivered V_T
   d. Increased airway resistance results in a decreased delivered V_T
3. Delivered V_T may be measured with a respirometer or gas-collection bag on the exhalation port.
4. The inspiratory pressure control adjusts the delivered V_T.
   a. Increase pressure to increase delivered V_T
   b. Decrease pressure to decrease delivered V_T

C. Decreased Work of Breathing

1. A patient experiencing acute hypoventilation may avoid intubation and placement on mechanical ventilation (possibly only temporarily) by administration of frequent IPPB treatments.
2. The practitioner must encourage the patient to relax and allow the IPPB unit to do all the work for the patient's work of breathing to decrease.
3. IPPB may increase the patient's work of breathing if:

a. The machine sensitivity is set too low, making it difficult for the patient to cycle the machine into inspiration. **The patient should be required to pull no more than -2 cm H_2O of pressure to initiate inspiration.**
b. The flow rate is inadequate to meet the patient's inspiratory flow demands. Increase the flow rate if inspiratory time is prolonged and you notice the manometer needle is **rising slowly** to peak pressure.
c. The delivered V_T is inadequate. Monitor V_T and listen to basilar breath sounds to ensure adequate volumes are being delivered.
d. Adequate time is not allowed for passive exhalation to occur. The machine **sensitivity** may be set **too high, resulting in self-cycling.**

D. Alteration of the Inspiratory and Expiratory Time

1. By placing a patient with respiratory difficulties on IPPB, the alveolar ventilation should be improved, thereby making the patient more comfortable, less "air hungry," and returning the I/E ratio and respiratory rate to normal.
2. Normal I/E ratio for an adult is 1:2.

E. Mechanical Bronchodilation

1. A patient with respiratory disease experiences an **increased resistance to air flow** as the diameter of the airways decreases as a result of **bronchospasm, secretions,** and other factors.
2. When positive pressure is applied to constricted airways, dilation of these airways can occur to a greater degree than with spontaneous breathing.

> **Note**
>
> Some studies show that higher flow rates and pressures may cause a bronchoconstrictive reflex in the airways. This may be counteracted by administering bronchodilating agents.

F. Cerebral Blood Flow Alteration

1. A patient receiving IPPB may experience lightheadedness, dizziness, or faintness from reduced $PaCO_2$ levels and the resultant alkalemia. **Decreased $PaCO_2$ levels result in cerebral vasoconstriction, thus decreasing cerebral blood flow.**
2. To prevent reduced $PaCO_2$ levels, encourage the patient to breathe slowly and to pause between breaths.

3. A 50 mL flex tube should be connected between the mouthpiece and manifold; this allows a slight rebreathing of CO_2, preventing decreased Pa_{CO_2} levels.

III. INDICATIONS FOR IPPB THERAPY

A. Increased work of breathing
B. Hypoventilation
C. Inadequate cough
D. Increased airway resistance
E. Atelectasis: especially sedated post-operative patients and patients recovering from chest or abdominal surgery who are reluctant to breathe deeply
F. Pulmonary edema
G. Aid in weaning from continuous mechanical ventilation

IV. HAZARDS OF IPPB THERAPY

A. **Excessive Ventilation**
   1. Leads to decreased Pa_{CO_2} levels causing cerebral vasoconstriction, resulting in dizziness
   2. Patient should be instructed not to stand or walk immediately after the treatment.
B. **Excessive Oxygenation**
   1. Patients with moderate to severe COPD breathe by the "hypoxic drive" mechanism. If the IPPB treatment is given with O_2, it may elevate the Pa_{O_2} above their normal level (50–65 mm Hg) knocking out their drive to breathe.
   2. Hypoxic drive potential will be indicated by the following ABG levels: pH, 7.35 to 7.40 (compensated); Pa_{CO_2}, more than 50 mm Hg; Pa_{O_2}, less than 65 mm Hg
C. **Decreased Cardiac Output**
   1. Positive pressure applied to the airways is likewise exerted on blood vessels returning blood to the heart. This restricts venous blood return to the heart, which in turn decreases cardiac output from the left ventricle.
   2. Avoiding high inspiratory pressures and long inspiratory times minimizes this hazard.
   3. If there is a decreased venous return during the therapy, the patient may experience **tachycardia** and a **drop in systemic blood pressure,** caused by decreased left ventricular filling pressure.
D. **Increased ICP**
   1. Blood flow from the head is restricted as positive pressure is exerted on the superior vena cava, which is returning blood to the heart from the upper body. This keeps more blood in the cerebral vessels, elevating ICP levels.
   2. Normal ICP is less than 10 mm Hg.

3. Using lower pressures and shorter inspiratory times (increased flows), and having the patient positioned in Fowler's position or sitting on the edge of the bed, will minimize this hazard.
4. This is not a common hazard, except in patients with closed head injuries or CNS disease.

E. **Pneumothorax**
   1. Most common in patients with COPD with bullous disease or emphysema with bleb formation.
   ★ 2. Patients who complain of sudden chest pain, shortness of breath, or other breathing difficulties and who have tachycardia during IPPB must be suspected of having a pneumothorax.
   3. Listen with stethoscope for bilateral breath sounds and observe for asymmetric chest movement.
   ★ 4. If pneumothorax is suspected, the treatment must be stopped immediately.
F. **Hemoptysis**
   1. The coughing up of blood during or after IPPB may not be caused by IPPB itself but may be related to a strong cough accompanying the treatment.
   2. The treatment must be stopped immediately, because air could be forced into a blood vessel, resulting in an air embolism.
G. **Gastric Distention**
   1. Caused by swallowing air during the treatment.
   2. May cause the patient to complain of nausea during or after the treatment.
H. **Nosocomial Infection**
   1. Circuits should be changed every 24 hr.
   2. Appropriate filters should be used on the IPPB unit to prevent machine contamination.
   3. The practitioner should wash his or her hands before and after every treatment.

V. CONTRAINDICATIONS TO IPPB THERAPY

A. **Untreated Pneumothorax: Absolute Contraindication**
   1. IPPB should not be administered under any circumstances with this condition, because it only worsens the problem.
   2. IPPB is safe for patients with a pneumothorax who have a chest tube in place.
B. **Pulmonary Hemorrhage: Absolute Contraindication**
   1. If IPPB is administered in this situation, air may enter a blood vessel, resulting in an air embolism.
C. **Relative Contraindications** (under certain circumstances IPPB may be administered or the therapy modified)

1. **Tuberculosis**
   a. May lead to the spread of the disease, if patient isn't receiving anti-tuberculosis medications.
   b. IPPB is safe if patient is receiving such drugs.

2. **Subcutaneous Emphysema**
   a. Indicates an air leak from the lung, and further positive pressure would worsen the condition.
   b. This condition is not a danger in itself, but it may be an indication of a more severe condition, such as pneumothorax or pneumomediastinum.

3. **Hemoptysis**
   a. This condition indicates an open pulmonary blood vessel, which could lead to an air embolism.
   b. The origin of the bleeding must be determined.

4. **Closed Head Injury**
   a. IPPB may increase ICP, therefore ICP must be monitored closely during IPPB in these patients.
   b. To lessen the potential of increasing ICP, use **higher flow rates (decreased inspiratory time) and lower peak pressures.**

5. **Bullous Disease**
   a. Patients with bullae or bleb formation, such as those with COPD, are more prone to a pneumothorax. Bullae and blebs constitute weak air spaces and rupture easily.
   b. Lower peak inspiratory pressures help to alleviate this problem.
   c. Rupturing of blebs or bullae may result from a strong cough effort during the treatment. These patients must be monitored closely.

6. **Cardiac Insufficiency**
   a. Patients with decreased blood pressure, decreased cardiac output, or other such cardiac problems must be monitored closely for further cardiac side effects.
   b. Further cardiac problems may result from:
      (1) Positive pressure causing decreased venous return
      (2) Cardiac side effects of bronchodilating agents

7. **COPD Patient with Air Trapping**
   a. IPPB may lead to an increase in air trapping in these patients, causing an inadvertent PEEP, which may decrease cardiac output.
   b. These patients already have hyperinflated lungs, and IPPB may worsen this condition.

8. **Uncooperative Patient**
   a. Patient must be cooperative for treatment to be effective.
   b. Alternative therapy should be considered.

VI. **IPPB IN THE TREATMENT OF PULMONARY EDEMA**
Positive Effects of IPPB in Pulmonary Edema
A. Decreases venous return.
B. Increases V_T to improve ventilation and oxygenation, resulting in improved cardiac activity.
C. Improves oxygenation by increasing the diameter of the fluid-filled alveoli, so that more surface area is available for gas exchange.
D. Delivers aerosolized ethanol (40% to 50% concentration in water), which results in the dissipation of foamy edematous fluid.
E. Increases oxygenation by delivering the treatment on 100% oxygen.

VII. **PROPER ADMINISTRATION OF IPPB**
A. Assemble all equipment and check machine for leaks.
B. Affirm physician order: If there is a question about the order, such as medication dosage, contact the physician for clarification.
C. Briefly review patient chart
   1. Last treatment given
   2. Latest chest film interpretation
   3. Latest ABG results
D. Wash hands
E. Identify patient by wristband, introduce yourself, and explain the reasons for administering the treatment.
F. Connect the circuit to the IPPB unit and plug into gas source.
G. Place medications in nebulizer.
H. Auscultate breath sounds to locate problem areas (e.g., atelectasis, secretions).
I. Determine heart rate and respiratory rate.
J. Position patient in an upright position because this allows better ventilation.
K. Place the mouthpiece in patient's mouth and encourage the patient to keep their lips sealed tight and breathe only through the mouth. (Use nose clips if patient has difficulty)
L. Instruct the patient to "sip" on the mouthpiece and allow the machine to fill their lungs until it cycles off. **Tell patient to hold his or her breath for a count of three before exhaling** to better distribute medications and improve gas exchange. **Tell the patient to pause before the next breath.**
M. Set Machine Parameters.
   ★1. Inspiratory pressure: Start lower than desired pressure and gradually increase as treatment

continues. (Increase flow rate as pressure is increased to maintain same inspiratory time.)
2. Flow rate
3. Nebulization
4. Sensitivity
N. Check vital signs halfway through the treatment. Allow a brief rest period.

O. After 10 min or when the medication is completely nebulized, encourage the patient to cough.
P. Check vital signs again.
Q. Encourage patient to cough periodically for the next 30 min to 2 hr as the effect of the medications peaks.
R. Wash hands.
S. Record vital signs, tolerance to treatment, cough effort, sputum characteristics (i.e., color, amount, consistency), and measured exhaled IPPB V_T in the patient's chart.

VIII. CHARACTERISTICS OF SPECIFIC IPPB UNITS
A. **Bird Mark 7**
  1. The Bird Mark 7 is a pneumatically powered and controlled ventilator. It is designed to

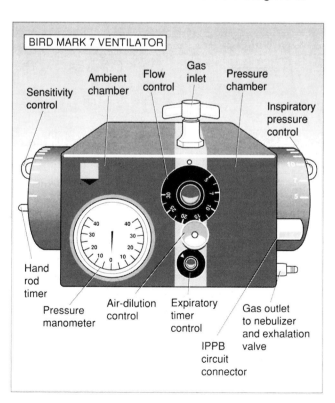

operate with oxygen or air at a pressure of 50 psig. It is pressure-cycled and may be set to patient-cycle, time-cycle, or manually cycle.
2. **Gas flow through the Bird Mark 7**
  a. Gas enters the unit from the 50-psig wall outlet through a brass filter.
  b. The first control that the gas travels to is the **flow rate control,** which is a simple needle valve.
  c. From the flow rate control, gas travels to the **ceramic switch,** which is positioned between the ambient chamber and pressure chamber of the unit. Depending on the position of the ceramic switch, flow is either blocked or is allowed to pass through.
  d. For the patient to cycle the unit into inspiration, he or she must create enough negative pressure to separate a metal clutch plate from a magnet in the ambient chamber. This pulls the ceramic switch to the right, allowing gas flow to continue through the unit.
  e. As gas flows past the ceramic switch, the gas splits, with part of the flow supplying the expiratory drive line and nebulizer, and the other part flowing into the ambient chamber through a Venturi tube, which entrains ambient air. This increases flow and decreases percentage of O_2.
  f. The "mixed" gas now travels through the Venturi gate and into the pressure chamber, where the patient circuit is connected and flow continues on to the patient.
  g. Inspiration ends as gas in the patient's lungs builds up to a pressure that overcomes the magnetic force between another magnet and metal clutch plate located in the pressure chamber.
3. **Bird Mark 7 Controls**
  a. **Flow control**
    (1) The scale is simply made up of reference numbers and does not represent liters per min.
    (2) Flow rates available are 0 to 80 L/min on air mix and 0 to 50 L/min on 100% O_2.
  ★ (3) To decrease inspiratory time, increase flow rate; to increase inspiratory time, decrease flow rate.
    (4) Flow wave patterns on Bird Mark 7
      (a) Square wave (constant flow) on 100% O_2
      (b) Tapered wave (decelerating flow) on air mix

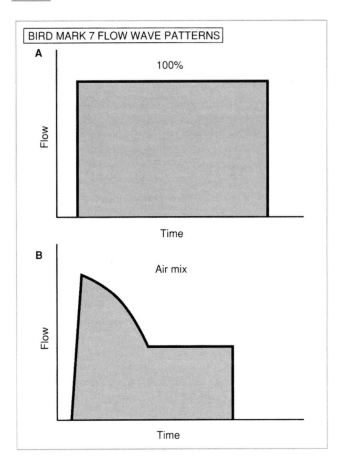

BIRD MARK 7 FLOW WAVE PATTERNS

A — 100% — Flow / Time

B — Air mix — Flow / Time

sure is required by the patient to cycle the machine into inspiration (and vice versa)

(3) The position of the magnet should be such that the patient is required to generate a pressure of no more than -2 cm H_2O to initiate inspiration

e. **Expiratory timing device**
(1) This is a needle valve that controls a leak from the expiratory timer cartridge and is used to automatically cycle the unit.
(2) It should always be turned off while administering IPPB, or the unit will self-cycle.

f. **Hand timer rod**
Located on the left side of the unit (ambient pressure side) and is used to manually cycle the unit off or on

B. **Bennett PR-2 Ventilator**

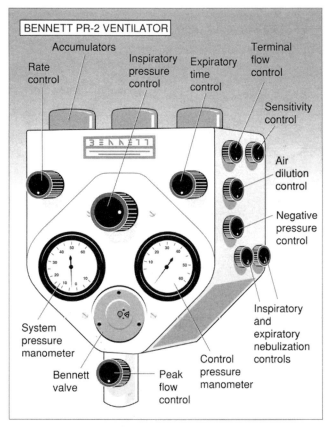

BENNETT PR-2 VENTILATOR

Accumulators — Rate control — Inspiratory pressure control — Expiratory time control — Terminal flow control — Sensitivity control — Air dilution control — Negative pressure control — Inspiratory and expiratory nebulization controls — Control pressure manometer — Peak flow control — Bennett valve — System pressure manometer

b. **Air mix control**
(1) When pulled out, allows flow into ambient chamber, then through a Venturi tube, resulting in air entrainment and delivery of 40% to 90% O_2.
(2) When pushed in, blocks the flow to the ambient chamber, not allowing for air entrainment, and therefore delivering 100% O_2.
(3) Air mix-setting creates higher flow rate; 100% O_2 creates lower flow rate.

c. **Inspiratory pressure control**
(1) Adjusts the position of the magnet in the pressure chamber closer to or farther away from the metal clutch plate
(2) The closer the magnet is to the metal clutch plate, the higher the inspiratory pressure required to move the clutch plate and to end inspiration.
(3) Increasing pressure will increase V_T; decreasing pressure will decrease V_T

d. **Sensitivity control**
(1) Adjusts the position of the magnet in the ambient chamber closer to or farther away from the metal clutch plate
(2) The closer the magnet is to the metal clutch plate, the more negative pres-

1. The PR-2 is a pneumatically powered, pressure-cycled ventilator that may be patient- or time-cycled and is flow- or time-limited.

2. **Diluter regulator**
a. This is an adjustable reducing valve that controls the pressure generated in the patient circuit

b. It is adjustable from 0 to 50 cm H_2O

3. **Bennett valve**
   a. This is the heart of the PR-2. Gas comes from the diluter regulator to this valve and rotates it to the opened position. Gas then travels on to the patient via the circuit. The valve also opens in response to the patient's negative pressure.
   b. As inspiratory pressure increases, the flow begins to decrease (resulting from decrease in pressure gradient) and this rotates the Bennett valve to the closed position, stopping gas flow and ending inspiration.

4. **PR-2 controls**
   a. **Inspiratory pressure control**
      (1) Adjusts the peak inspiratory pressure
      (2) Adjustable from approximately 0 to 50 cm H_2O
   b. **Dilution control**
      (1) When dilution control knob is pushed in, air entrainment is allowed and percentage of delivered O_2 varies from 40% to 90%.
      (2) When dilution control knob is pulled out, no air entrainment is allowed and 100% O_2 is delivered
   c. **Terminal flow control**
      (1) Adds an additional 12 to 15 L/min of flow below the Bennett valve to help cycle the unit off in case leaks are present
      (2) This added flow goes to a Venturi tube, which decreases the percentage of O_2 (especially important if patient is on 100% O_2).
   d. **Sensitivity control**
      (1) Turning this control counterclockwise increases the sensitivity, making it easier for the patient to cycle the unit into inspiration (and vice versa).
      (2) When the sensitivity control is turned off, the unit is factory-set for the patient to initiate inspiration by generating a pressure of $-\frac{1}{2}$ cm H_2O.
   e. **Peak flow control**
      (1) In its fully open position (all the way to the left), the flow rate is approximately 90 to 100 L/min with air dilution and 20 cm H_2O of pressure
      (2) In the fully closed position (all the way to the right), the flow is approximately 15 L/min
   f. **Nebulization control**
      (1) Separate controls for inspiratory or expiratory nebulization

      (2) Gas that is sent to the nebulizer is source gas (100% O_2 if unit is plugged into an O_2 outlet); therefore percentage of O_2 increases when using nebulizer for medications.
   g. **Rate control and expiratory time**
      (1) Used to automatically cycle the unit on
      (2) Turning rate control to the right sets the rate (adjustable from 0 to 50 breaths/min).
      (3) Expiratory time control lengthens expiratory time.
      (4) These controls should be turned off during the administration of IPPB, or the unit self-cycles.

C. **Bennett AP-5**

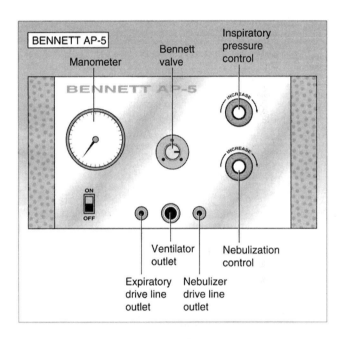

1. This IPPB unit is **electrically powered,** and inspiratory flow is powered by a compressor.
★ 2. Compressed gas is not necessary for the functioning of this IPPB machine; therefore, it is a popular model for use in the home.
3. It is pressure-limited and patient-cycled, with a continuous flow for nebulization that comes from the compressor to the jet of the nebulizer.
4. Maximum peak pressure is approximately 30 cm H_2O.

IX. **FACTORS TO CONSIDER WHEN USING A PRESSURE-LIMITED IPPB MACHINE**
A. **Effects on delivered V_T**
   1. Increased airway resistance results in decreased V_T

2. Decreased airway resistance results in increased V_T
3. Increased lung compliance results in increased V_T
4. Decreased lung compliance results in decreased V_T
5. Increased inspiratory pressure results in increased V_T
6. Decreased inspiratory pressure results in decreased V_T
7. Increased flow results in decreased V_T
8. Decreased flow results in increased V_T

B. **Effects on inspiratory time**
   1. Increased flow results in decreased inspiratory time
   2. Decreased flow results in increased inspiratory time
   3. Increased lung compliance results in increased inspiratory time
   4. Decreased lung compliance results in decreased inspiratory time
   5. Increased airway resistance results in decreased inspiratory time
   6. Decreased airway resistance results in increased inspiratory time

X. **PROBLEMS WITH IPPB AND CORRECTIVE ACTIONS**
   A. The patient is having difficulty cycling the IPPB machine into the inspiratory phase. **Corrective actions:**
      1. Adjust the sensitivity so that the patient has to generate a pressure of $-.5$ to -2 cm H_2O to start inspiration.
      2. Make sure machine is plugged into wall gas outlet.
      3. Ensure machine tubing connections are all tight.
      4. Ensure the patient has lips sealed tightly around the mouthpiece or, if a mask is used, that there are no leaks around it.
      5. If the Bird Mark 7 is used, ensure the flow control is turned on.
   B. The patient complains of dizziness and tingling in the extremities during the treatment with no appreciable increase in heart rate. **Corrective action:**
      Instruct the patient to breathe slower and to pause longer between breaths.
   C. Patient's heart rate increases more than 20 beats/min during the treatment. **Corrective action:**
      Stop treatment immediately and notify the physician. This is most likely the result of the nebulized bronchodilating agent stimulating the heart.
   D. The patient cannot cycle the IPPB machine off. **Corrective actions:**

      1. Tighten all tubing connections.
      2. Ensure that there are no leaks around the mouthpiece or mask.
      3. Ensure that the ET tube or tracheostomy-tube cuff is inflated adequately.
      4. If using the Bennett PR-2, check to make sure that the Bennett valve is not stuck.
      5. If using the PR-2, turn on the terminal flow control to help compensate for leaks.
      6. Check the expiratory valve function.
   E. As the patient inhales, there is no nebulization of the medication. **Corrective actions:**
      1. Ensure that the capillary tube of the nebulizer is connected.
      2. If using the Bennett PR-2, ensure that the nebulization control is turned on.
      3. Ensure that the nebulizer drive line is connected.
      4. Ensure that there is medication in the nebulizer.
      5. Ensure that the nebulizer is positioned in an upright position.
   F. During inspiration the manometer needle stays in the negative area for the first half of the breath and then rises to the positive area during the last half. **Corrective action:**
      Increase the machine flow rate.
   G. The IPPB machine repeatedly cycles on shortly after the patient has begun the expiratory phase. **Corrective actions:**
      1. Decrease the machine sensitivity.
      2. If using the Bird Mark 7, ensure that the expiratory time for apnea control is turned off.
      3. If using the Bennett PR-2, ensure that the rate control is turned off.

POST-CHAPTER STUDY QUESTIONS

1. List five physiologic effects of IPPB.
2. List seven indications for IPPB.
3. List eight hazards of IPPB.
4. List two absolute contraindications to IPPB.
5. The pulse rate must not exceed how many beats per minute before the treatment must be terminated?
6. What effect does an increased airway resistance have on delivered V_T on a pressure-limited IPPB machine?
7. What effect does an increased lung compliance have on the delivered V_T on a pressure-limited IPPB machine?
8. How does a decreased lung compliance effect inspiratory time?
9. List ways to help correct a situation where the patient has difficulty cycling the IPPB machine into the expiratory phase.

10. How should an IPPB treatment be modified for a patient with a closed head injury?

Answers are at the end of the chapter.

REFERENCES

Eubanks D and Bone RI: Comprehensive respiratory care, ed 2, St. Louis, 1990, The CV Mosby Co.

McPherson SP: Respiratory therapy equipment, ed 5, St. Louis, 1995, Mosby-Yearbook Inc.

Scanlan CL, Wilkins RL, and Stoller JK: Egan's fundamentals of respiratory care, ed 7, St. Louis, 1999, Mosby Inc.

Shapiro BA: Clinical application of respiratory care, ed 4, St. Louis, 1990, Mosby Year-Book Publishers.

PRE-TEST ANSWERS

1. C
2. B
3. A
4. D
5. A
6. C

ANSWERS TO POST-CHAPTER QUESTIONS

1. Increased mean airway pressure, increased V_T, decreased work of breathing, alteration of I/E times, mechanical bronchodilation, reduced cerebral blood flow
2. Increased work of breathing, hypoventilation, inadequate cough effort, increased airway resistance, atelectasis, pulmonary edema, weaning from ventilator
3. Hyperventilation, hyperoxygenation, decreased cardiac output, increased ICP, pneumothorax, hemoptysis, gastric distention, nosocomial infection
4. Pulmonary hemorrhage, untreated pneumothorax
5. 20 beats/min
6. Decreased V_T
7. Increased V_T
8. Decreased inspiratory time
9. Tighten tubing connections; check for leaks around mouthpiece, mask, or ET tube; check expiratory valve function
10. Increased inspiratory flow, decreased peak inspiratory pressure.

Chapter 8

Bronchopulmonary Hygiene Techniques And Incentive Spirometry

PRE-TEST QUESTIONS

1. Postural drainage and percussion are not indicated in which of the following conditions?

   A. Bronchiectasis
   B. Cystic fibrosis
   C. Pulmonary edema
   D. Acute atelectasis

2. In which of the following airway clearance techniques is the patient instructed to alter V_T in three phases before a cough effort?

   A. Intrapulmonary percussive ventilation
   B. Autogenic lung drainage
   C. Positive expiratory pressure (PEP) therapy
   D. Chest percussion or vibration

3. The respiratory care practitioner receives an order for postural drainage on a patient to mobilize secretions from the anterior segment of the right upper lobe of the lung. How should the patient be positioned for the lung to drain most effectively?

   A. Patient lying supine with pillows under the knees.
   B. Patient lying on right side in Trendelenburg position.
   C. Patient lying on stomach in Trendelenburg position.
   D. Patient lying on left side, rotated back 25°, with the bed flat.

4. Which statement is FALSE regarding incentive spirometry?

   A. The patient should be positioned upright.
   B. The initial goal should be twice the patient's V_T.
   C. The patient's inspiratory time should be 3 to 5 sec long.
   D. The patient should be instructed to hold his or her breath at peak inspiration for 2 to 3 sec.

Answers are at end of the chapter.

REVIEW

I. CHEST PHYSICAL THERAPY

> ★ *Exam Note*
>
> Conducting postural drainage, percussion, and vibration to remove pulmonary secretions appear on the CRT examination only. Other areas relating to these procedures (e.g., modifying the technique, altering position, coordinating the sequence of therapies) appear on both the examinations.

A. Chest physical therapy (CPT) is a variety of techniques aimed at the mobilization of pulmonary secretions and promotion of greater use of the respiratory muscles, resulting in an increase in the distribution of ventilation. **Techniques included in CPT are**
   1. Postural drainage
   2. Chest percussion
   3. Chest vibration
   4. Cough techniques
   5. Breathing exercises (see chapter on respiratory home care)

B. **Goals of CPT**
   1. To prevent the accumulation of pulmonary secretions
   2. To improve the mobilization of retained secretions
   3. To improve the distribution of ventilation
   4. To decrease airway resistance

C. **Indications for CPT**
   1. Lung conditions that cause increased difficulty in mobilizing pulmonary secretions:
      a. Bronchiectasis
      b. Cystic fibrosis
      c. Lung abscess
   2. Acute respiratory failure with retained pulmonary secretions

3. Acute atelectasis
4. Ventilation and perfusion abnormalities resulting from retained pulmonary secretions
5. COPD patients with inefficient breathing patterns
6. Prevention of postoperative respiratory complications

D. **Postural Drainage Positions**
E. **Percussion**
   1. A means of improving the mobilization of pulmonary secretions by manually striking the chest wall with a cupped hand or placing a mechanical percussor on the chest wall. Both of these techniques are generally performed with the patient in postural drainage positions.
   2. Mechanical percussors operate on either compressed air or electricity and are thought to be more effective than manual hand percussion.
   3. Percussion should be performed over each specified area for 2 to 5 min.
   4. Percussion should not performed over the following areas:
      a. Spine
      b. Sternum
      c. Scapulae
      d. Clavicles
      e. Surgical sites
      f. Areas of trauma
      g. Bare skin
         Although some practitioners advocate manually percussing over bare skin, the energy wave produced by the air trapped under the hand is not significantly reduced by a light covering, such as a hospital gown.
      h. Female breasts
F. **Vibration**
   1. Manual vibration is accomplished by the therapist placing one hand on top of the other over a specified lung segment and, with a vibrating motion, applying moderate pressure.
★ 2. The patient should be instructed to take a deep breath and vibration should be applied during exhalation.
   3. Mechanical vibrators may be used by placing the vibrator attachment over specified areas. The vibrator should not be applied to one area for more than 45 to 60 sec at a time.
   4. Vibration helps to mobilize retained pulmonary secretions.
G. **Complications of CPT**
   1. Hypoxemia
      a. Especially in patients with COPD or cardiac disease or obese patients
      b. Modification of drainage position makes CPT more tolerable for these patients

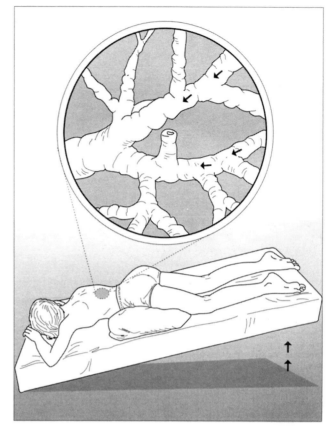

Position to drain the posterior basal segment of the lower lobe of the lung.

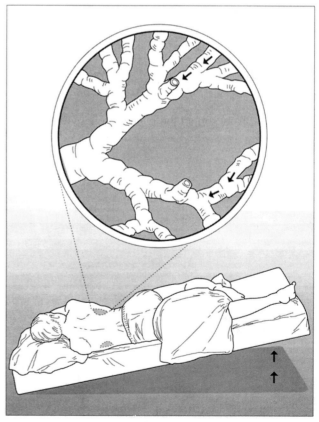

Position to drain the lateral basal segment of the lower lobe of the lung.

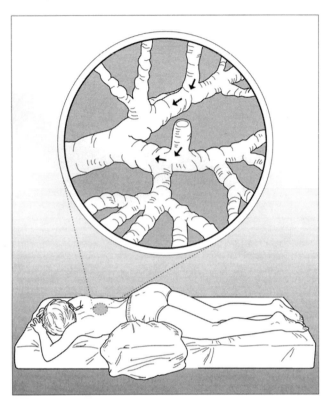

Position to drain the anterior basal segment of the lower lobe of the lung.

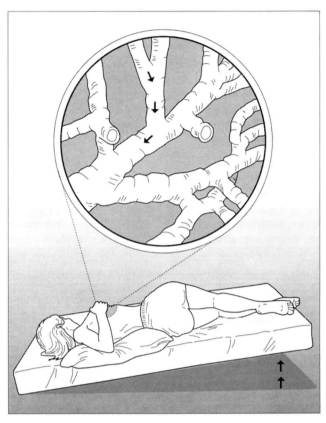

Position to drain the lateral and medial segments of the right middle lobe of the lung.

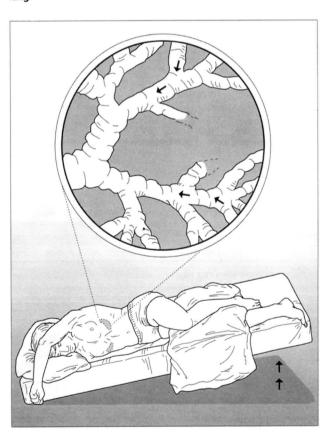

Position to drain the superior segment of the lower lobe of the lung.

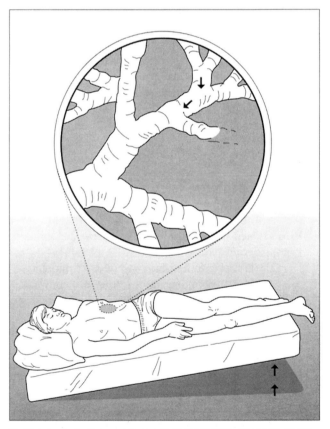

Position to drain the superior and inferior lingular segments of the left lung.

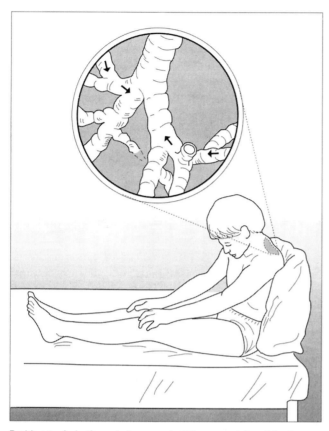

Position to drain the apical segment of the upper lobe of the lung.

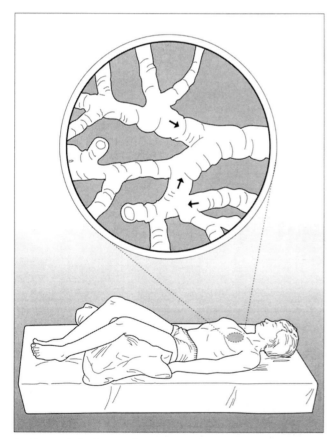

Position to drain the anterior segment of the upper lobe of the lung.

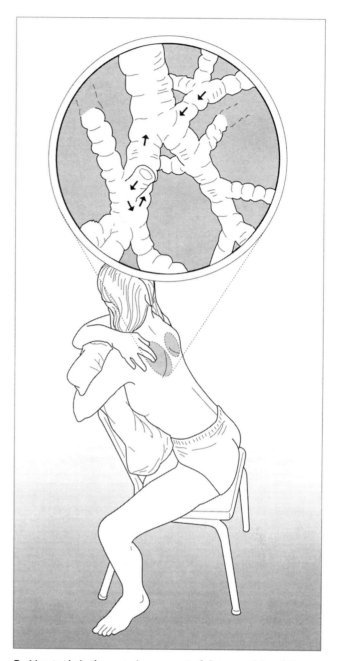

Position to drain the posterior segment of the upper lobe of the lung.

c. May be minimized by administration of a bronchodilating agent before CPT and delivery of supplemental O_2 during the treatment
2. Rib fractures
   a. Caused from overly vigorous percussion
   b. Most common in neonates and elderly patients
3. Increased airway resistance
   a. Patient should be instructed to cough periodically throughout the treatment.
   b. Suction equipment should be readily available for patients having difficulty expectorating secretions.

4. Increased ICP
   a. Patients with head trauma should not be placed in the Trendelenburg (head down) position
   b. Increased ICP may result from prolonged coughing during CPT
5. Hemorrhage
6. Decreased cardiac output
   a. Often the result of positional hypotension
   b. Check heart rate periodically during the treatment
7. Aspiration
   a. Caused by vomiting during the treatment
   b. CPT should be performed no sooner than 1 hr after a meal

H. **Cough Technique**
1. While sitting, the patient should be instructed to inhale deeply through the nose and hold the breath for 3 to 5 sec.
2. Instruct the patient to clasp his or her arms across the abdomen and produce 2 to 3 sharp coughs without taking a breath, while pressing the arms into the abdomen.
3. A pillow should be used to splint thoracic or abdominal incisions to decrease pain and improve the cough effort.

II. **OTHER BRONCHOPULMONARY HYGIENE TECHNIQUES**

A. **Autogenic Drainage**
1. Autogenic drainage is a modified coughing technique that has been shown in some studies to be comparable in secretion clearance to postural drainage and percussion techniques.
2. The patient should be placed in a sitting position and instructed to use a breathing pattern that varies lung volume and expiratory flow in three different phases:
   a. Phase 1: From the resting expiratory level, the patient is instructed to take the deepest breath possible (inspiratory capacity maneuver) followed by breathing at low lung volumes for several breaths.
   b. Phase 2: The patient is instructed to increase V_T to low to middle volumes for several breaths. (These breaths are slightly larger the than normal V_T.)
   c. Phase 3: The patient then increases V_T to moderate volumes for several breaths. After this phase is completed, the patient is instructed to cough.
3. This type of breathing pattern helps loosen secretions, moving them into larger airways, so that they may be mobilized with an effective cough.
4. This technique has shown some promise in patients with cystic fibrosis. It appears to mobilize secretions in a way comparable to postural drainage and percussion but without the degree of O_2 desaturation, and it is tolerated better by this type of patient.
5. This technique is difficult to teach the patient, and can pose a problem because it is taught for the patient's independent use.

B. **Intrapulmonary Percussive Ventilation**
1. This is another airway clearance technique that uses a pneumatic ventilator to deliver a series of small V_Ts at high frequency (110- to 225 cycles/min).
2. The length of each percussive cycle is controlled either by the practitioner or by the patient, using a thumb control button.
3. These pressurized bursts of gas are delivered to the patient via a mouthpiece. Bronchodilating or mucolytic agents may be administered through a pneumatic nebulizer during this 15 to 20 min treatment.
4. It has been demonstrated that the pulsed gas flow is as effective in breaking up secretions for easier mobilization as postural drainage and percussion are in cystic fibrosis patients.
5. This procedure has the advantage over conventional CPT in that fatigue and practitioner technique are not a factor.

C. **High-Frequency Chest Wall Oscillation**
1. This is a new technique to improve sputum clearance from the airways.
2. An inflatable vest is wrapped around the patient's chest and is attached to an air-pulse generator, which intermittently injects small volumes of air in and ejects them out of the vest at a high rate. This creates oscillatory movement that has been shown to aid in the mobilization of secretions.
3. The duration of therapy is usually about 30 min, using an oscillation frequency of between 5 and 25 Hz (300 to 1500 cycles/min).
4. As of this writing, this technique has not proven to be as effective as postural drainage or percussion in cystic fibrosis patients.

> **Note**
>
> An alternative to this device uses a chest shell, instead of an inflatable vest, that is attached to a negative/positive pressure generator that administers oscillations at a frequency of up to 900 cycles/min. Currently, there are no studies regarding the effectiveness of this airway clearance device.

D. **PEP Therapy**

> ### *Exam Note*
>
> The selection, assembly, function, and cleaning of the PEP device appears on the RRT examination only. All other areas relating to PEP therapy (e.g., modifying treatment techniques, altering duration of treatment) appear on both examinations.

1. Positive expiratory pressure (PEP) is a bronchial hygiene therapy used in the management of airway secretions and postoperative atelectasis.
2. It is becoming increasingly popular as an alternative to chest physical therapy and incentive spirometry, especially in pediatric patients with cystic fibrosis and bronchiectasis.
3. It has also been found effective for preventing postoperative atelectasis by opening airways and improving gas exchange.
4. PEP is achieved by having the patient exhale through a mask or mouthpiece with a resistance valve. The valve creates back pressure into the patient's airway. Different sizes of resistors or adjustable resistors are used to increase or decrease the amount of PEP. **Generally, PEP levels of 10 to 20 cm H_2O are used.**
5. **Therapeutic effects of PEP**
   a. Improved distribution of inspired volume in the lung by means of collateral air channels (pores of Kohn).
   b. Prevention of expiratory airway collapse.
   c. Generation of pressure on exhalation in an area distal to the site of mucus obstruction.

6. **Contraindications to PEP**
   a. Acute sinusitis
   b. Middle ear infection
   c. Epitaxis (nose bleed)
   d. Recent facial, oral, or skull injury or surgery
   e. Active hemoptysis
7. **Steps in performing PEP mask therapy**
   a. Assemble equipment and select appropriate expiratory resistor (10- to 20-cm H_2O)
   b. Position patient sitting up with elbows resting on table, with mask applied tightly (to prevent leaks) over the nose and mouth.
   c. Instruct patient to inhale a larger-than-normal volume, but not quite as deep as possible, and then actively exhale, but not forcefully, with expiration lasting two to three times longer than inspiration.
   d. The patient should perform 10 to 20 of these PEP breaths, and then remove the mask and perform two to three "huff" coughs, also referred to as the FET, which require forceful exhaling from a middle to low lung volume with an open glottis. This has been proven very effective for secretion clearance.
   e. Patient should cough normally to mobilize secretions as needed.
   f. Repeat procedure four to six times per session.
8. PEP therapy may be an effective alternative to postural drainage and percussion, with the added benefit that the patient can perform this simple task independently with fewer side effects.
9. PEP therapy may also be combined with aerosolized bronchodilator therapy by

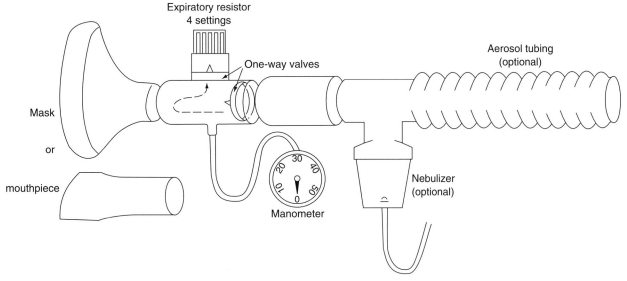

Mask or mouthpiece — Expiratory resistor 4 settings — One-way valves — Manometer — Nebulizer (optional) — Aerosol tubing (optional)

(Redrawn from Malmeister MJ, Fink JB, Hoffman GL: Positive expiratory pressure mask therapy: theoretical and practical considerations and a review of the literature. *Respir Care* 36:1218, 1991.)

attaching a nebulizer or an inhaler to the one-way inspiratory valve of the PEP device.

10. If while assessing the patient during therapy, the pressure being used appears to be ineffective, increase the PEP level by 3 to 5 cm H_2O and continue to monitor.

E. **Flutter Valve**

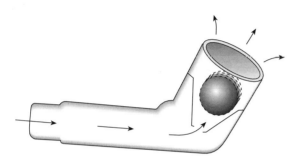

From Scanlan C, Wilkins R, Stoller J, Egan's Fundamentals of Respiratory Care, ed 7, St. Louis, 1999, Mosby.

1. The flutter valve is a pipe-shaped device (see diagram) through which the patient exhales to produce a PEP of between 10 and 25 cm H_2O.
2. The patient should be instructed to inhale slowly, just a bit more than a normal breath (not totally filling the lungs), and hold the breath for 2 to 3 sec. The patient should then exhale reasonably fast, but not forcefully, through the flutter device, which causes a stainless steel ball to be pushed up into the angled portion of the device to produce PEP. The angle causes the ball to oscillate, or "flutter," up and down. The oscillations are transmitted down the respiratory tract, creating vibrations that result in mobilization of secretions.
3. This technique should be repeated 5 to 10 times to help loosen secretions and should be followed by coughing to aid in the removal of sputum. The treatment should last 5 to 15 min.
4. The effectiveness of the device is controversial, but some studies have shown improved secretion clearance in cystic fibrosis patients.
5. The flutter valve may be disassembled after each use and rinsed in tap water and dried before reassembly. In the home, the device should be cleaned every 2 days in a soap solution and disinfected at regular intervals

by soaking in a 1:3 solution of vinegar and water for 15 min, dried, and reassembled for future use.

III. INCENTIVE SPIROMETRY (SUSTAINED MAXIMAL INSPIRATORY THERAPY)

A. **Goals of Incentive Spirometry**
1. To treat atelectasis
2. To improve the cough mechanism
3. To maintain the airway during the preoperative period
    a. Strengthens lung muscles before surgery
    b. Improves mobilization of secretions
4. To prevent postoperative atelectasis; **this therapy is most effective in treating this condition.**
5. To provide early detection of atelectasis or pneumonia by observing decreasing inspiratory capacity levels.

B. **Hazards of Incentive Spirometry**
1. Hyperventilation
2. Pneumothorax (unlikely; higher incidence in COPD patients)
3. Increased intrapleural pressure and stimulation of the vagal reflex, causing bradycardia if the sustained maximal inspiratory pause is performed against a closed glottis (Valsalva's maneuver)

C. **Requirements for Effective Incentive Spirometry**
1. Cooperative patient
2. Motivated patient
3. Patient's respiratory rate should be less than 25/min
4. Patient's VC should be more than 15 mL/kg of body weight; **IPPB may be indicated if VC is less than 15 mL/kg.**

D. **Important Points Concerning Incentive Spirometry**

1. Patient should be positioned upright in Fowler's or semi-Fowler's position.
2. The initial inspiratory goal should be twice the patient's V_T.
3. The inspiratory time should be 5 to 15 sec with a 2- to 3-second pause at end inspiration.
4. Incentive spirometry is an alternative to IPPB in treating atelectasis if the patient is able to achieve a VC of more than 15 mL/kg of body weight.

E. **Incentive Spirometry Devices**

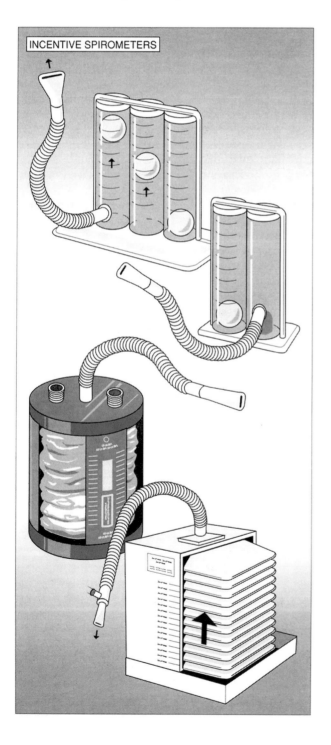

INCENTIVE SPIROMETERS

POST-CHAPTER STUDY QUESTIONS

1. What is the most appropriate pressure range for PEP therapy?
2. What is the range of pressure used for flutter valve therapy?
3. What types of patients seem to benefit the most from intrapulmonary percussive ventilation?
4. Intrapulmonary percussive ventilation, flutter valve therapy, and PEP therapy may be alternatives for what other popular therapy?
5. For incentive spirometry to be effective, the patient must be able to achieve a VC of at least how many milliliters per kilogram of body weight?
6. List five complications of chest physical therapy.
7. To drain the posterior basal segment of the lower lobe of the lung, how should the patient be positioned?
8. List four contraindications to PEP therapy.

★ **Answers are at the end of the chapter.**

REFERENCES

Branson R, Hess D, and Chatburn R: Respiratory care equipment, Philadelphia, 1995, JB Lippincott Co.

Eubanks D and Bone R: Comprehensive respiratory care, ed 2, St. Louis, 1990, The CV Mosby Co.

Scanlan C, Wilkins R, and Stoller J: Egan's fundamentals of respiratory care, ed 7, St. Louis, 1999, Mosby Inc.

Shapiro B: Clinical application of respiratory care, ed 4, St. Louis, 1990, The CV Mosby Co.

PRE-TEST ANSWERS

1. C
2. B
3. A
4. C

ANSWERS TO POST-CHAPTER STUDY QUESTIONS

1. 10 to 20 cm H_2O
2. 10 to 25 cm H_2O
3. Patients with cystic fibrosis
4. Postural drainage and percussion
5. 15 mL/kg
6. Hypoxemia, rib fractures, increased airway resistance, increased ICP, hemorrhage, decreased cardiac output, aspiration
7. Prone, with head down
8. Sinusitis; middle ear infection; epitaxis; facial, oral, or skull surgery or trauma

Chapter 9

Cardiac Monitoring

PRE-TEST QUESTIONS

Answer the pre-test questions before studying the chapter. This will help you determine your strong and weak areas regarding the material covered.

1. Which statement about the P wave on ECG is *FALSE?*

   A. *It represents atrial depolarization.*
   B. *It is a positive wave on the graph.*
   C. *Normal duration time is 0.06 to 0.10 sec.*
   D. *It represents ventricular repolarization.*

2. Artifacts found on an ECG may be caused by which of the following?

   I. Electrical interference at the bedside.
   II. Poor electrode contact with the skin.
   III. Excessive movement of the patient.

   A. *I only*
   B. *II only*
   C. *I and III only*
   D. *I, II, and III*

3. In which of the following cardiac arrhythmias is the QRS complex abnormally shaped as well as wider than normal?

   A. *Sinus tachycardia*
   B. *PVCs*
   C. *Atrial fibrillation*
   D. *PACs*

4. A patient with a blood pressure of 110/50 mm Hg and a pulse rate of 75 beats/min has which of the following pulse pressures?

   A. *40 mm Hg*
   B. *50 mm Hg*
   C. *60 mm Hg*
   D. *70 mm Hg*

5. A weak pulse is detected distal to the arterial catheter in a patient. This is indicative of which of the following?

A. *Infection*
B. *Hemorrhage*
C. *Thrombosis*
D. *Tachycardia*

6. Which of the following conditions results in a decreased CVP reading?

   I. Hypovolemia
   II. Vasoconstriction
   III. Air bubbles in the CVP line

A. *I only*
B. *II only*
C. *I and II only*
D. *I and III only*

Answers are at end of the chapter.

REVIEW

I. **ELECTROCARDIOGRAPHY**
   A. **Electrical Conduction of the Heart**
      1. The SA node is the pacemaker of the heart; it usually initiates about 75 impulse/min.
      2. Once an impulse has been initiated by the SA node, the impulse travels down to the AV node.
      3. From the AV node, the impulse travels on to the bundle of His, located in the interventricular septum.
      4. The bundle of His divides into the right and left bundle branches, which deliver the impulses to the right and left sides of the heart.
      5. The bundle branches divide even further into the Purkinje fibers, which send the impulse to individual muscle fibers of the ventricles, causing ventricular contraction.
      6. Once the SA node sends an impulse, the conduction system depolarizes, sending the impulse through the conduction system to the heart muscle, which depolarizes and contracts. After contraction, repolarization occurs, which is the heart in a resting state, called **diastole.**

The term used for the heart in contraction is **systole.**

B. **ECG Leads:** Through the use of various numbers of electrodes (leads) placed on the patient's body, the electrical activity of the heart can be monitored. The device to which the electrodes are attached is the **electrocardiograph** (ECG). The electrical activity of the heart recorded on graph paper is called the **electrocardiogram** (ECG) and may be displayed continuously on an ECG monitor, called an **oscilloscope.**

C. **Standard 12-Lead ECG Has Three Lead Systems**

1. Standard limb leads (three leads) (+ = positive pole; − = negative pole)
   a. The leads are placed on the right arm, left arm, and left leg.
   b. **Limb lead I** measures the electrical potential between the right arm (−) and left arm (+).
   c. **Limb lead II** measures the electrical potential between the right arm (−) and left leg (+).
   d. **Limb lead III** measures the electrical potential between the left arm (−) and the left leg (+).
   e. A ground is placed on the right leg.

2. Augmented leads (three leads)
   a. The same electrodes used in the standard leads are used for augmented lead composition, but in different combinations.
   b. **Lead aVR:** Leads are connected to right arm (+), left arm and left leg. The right arm is the positive electrode and records electrical activity from the direction of the right arm.
   c. **Lead aVL:** Leads are connected to left arm (+), right arm and left leg. The left arm is the positive electrode and views the electrical activity from the direction of the left arm.
   d. **Lead aVF:** Leads are connected to left leg (+), right arm and left arm. The left leg is the positive electrode and views the electrical activity from the direction of the bottom of the heart.

3. Precordial (chest) leads (six leads)
   a. **Lead 1 (V$_1$):** positioned at the **4th** intercostal space at the **right** border of the sternum
   b. **Lead 2 (V$_2$):** positioned at the **4th** intercostal space at the **left** border of the sternum
   c. **Lead 3 (V$_3$):** positioned in a straight line between lead 2 and lead 4
   d. **Lead 4 (V$_4$):** positioned at the midclavicular line and at the **5th** intercostal space
   e. **Lead 5 (V$_5$):** positioned at the anterior axillary line, level with lead 4 horizontally
   f. **Lead 6 (V$_6$):** positioned at the midaxillary line, level with lead 4 and 5 horizontally

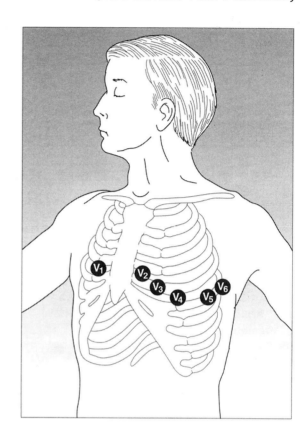

Note

The 12-lead ECG is not normally used for long-term ECG monitoring, such as that seen in ICU or CCU.

D. **Long-Term ECG Monitoring**
1. Lead placements (three leads)
   a. The first electrode is placed on the upper right side of the chest (−).
   b. The second electrode is placed on the lower left side of the chest (+).
   c. The third electrode is used as a ground and may be attached to any location that is convenient.
2. To obtain a clear ECG reading, there must be good skin contact with the electrode. An electrode gel is used to improve conduction. Hair should be shaved from the chest if an electrode is to be attached in that area.

E. **ECG Graph Paper**
1. The ECG paper is made up of very small squares, which represent 0.04 sec horizontally and 0.5 mV vertically (voltage axis).

TIME

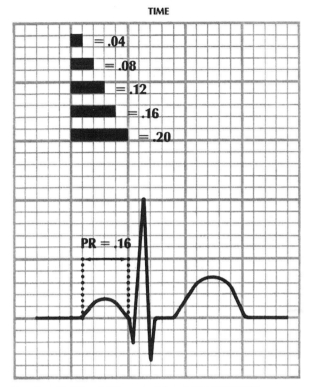

From Davis D. Differential Diagnosis of Arrhythmias. Philadelphia: WB Saunders, 1992.

2. To make counting time easier, there is a darkened line at every fifth small square; from one darkened line to the next is 0.20 sec (0.04 sec × 5 squares).
3. Most ECG paper has short vertical lines at the top to designate 3-sec intervals, making it easier to calculate the heart rate.

F. **Normal ECG Pattern**

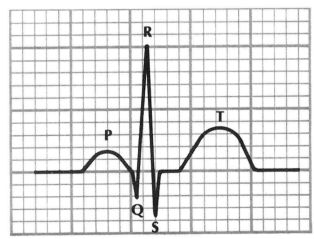

From Davis D. Differential Diagnosis of Arrhythmias. Philadelphia: WB Saunders, 1992.

The ECG strip shows a baseline and positive and negative deflections from it.

G. **ECG Waves:** One cardiac cycle consists of a series of waves, represented by the letters P, Q, R, S, and T.
  1. **P wave**
     a. Positive wave
     b. **Represents atrial depolarization (contraction)**
     c. Duration: 0.06 to 0.10 sec
  2. **Q wave**
     a. Negative wave that follows the P wave
     b. May be absent even in healthy people
  3. **R wave**
     Positive wave that follows the Q wave
  4. **S wave**
     Negative wave that follows the R wave
  5. **QRS complex**
     a. **Represents ventricular depolarization (contraction).** Atrial repolarization occurs during the QRS complex, and therefore is not seen on the ECG.
     b. Duration: 0.06 to 0.12 sec
     c. **Widened QRS seen in right bundle-branch block**

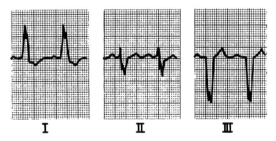

ECG tracing showing the widened QRS complex
From Levitsky MG, Cairo JN, Hall SM: Introduction to Respiratory Care. Philadelphia: WB Saunders, 1990.

  6. **T wave**
     a. Positive wave
     b. Represents ventricular repolarization
     c. **Inverted (negative-wave) T waves indicate coronary artery disease is present.**
  7. **PR interval**
     a. Measured from the beginning of the P wave to the beginning of the Q wave.
     b. Represents the time it takes for the impulse to travel from the SA node through the AV node.
     c. Duration: 0.12 to 0.20 sec
     d. May be prolonged in first- and second-degree heart block
  8. **ST segment**
     a. Measured from the end of the S wave to the beginning of the T wave.

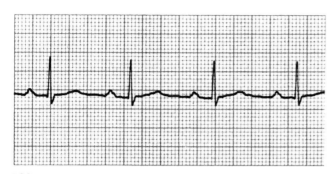

ECG tracing showing a prolonged PR interval.
From Davis D. Differential Diagnosis of Arrhythmias. Philadelphia:
WB Saunders, 1992.

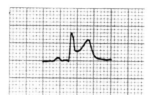

**ECG tracing showing ST
segment depression.**
From Davis D. Differential Diagnosis
of Arrhythmias. Philadelphia:
WB Saunders, 1992.

b. Measures the time that is required for ventricular repolarization to begin.
c. The ST segment may be elevated above the baseline or depressed below the baseline. This is an indication of **cardiac ischemia.** Cardiac ischemia results from a decreased amount of oxygenated blood delivered to the left ventricle because of narrowed coronary arteries. If the blood supply is not restored, ventricular muscle may die; this is called **infarction. ST segment elevation or depression is a sign of coronary artery disease.**

H. **Normal Heart Rhythm**
1. Atrial depolarization (contraction): represented on ECG as P wave

> ### Note
>
> Blood supply to the heart is supplied by two main arteries, the right and left coronary arteries, which originate from the aorta. The right coronary artery extends down to feed the right ventricle and then separates into several branches. The left coronary artery divides into two major branches,: the circumflex branch, which feeds the upper lateral wall of the left atrium and left ventricle, and the left anterior descending branch (anterior interventricular artery), which feeds the anterior portion of the heart.

2. Cardiac impulse travels to the AV node, bundle of His, and the Purkinje fibers: represented on ECG as the PR interval
3. Cardiac impulse reaches muscles in the ventricles, causing ventricular depolarization (contraction): represented on ECG as the QRS complex

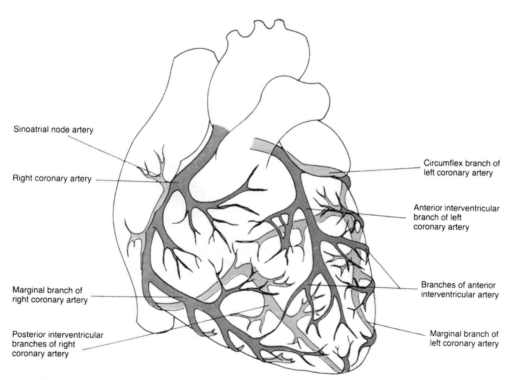

From O'Toole M, ed. Miller-Keane Encyclopedia of Medicine, Nursing and Allied Health, 5th ed. Philadelphia: WB Saunders, 1992.

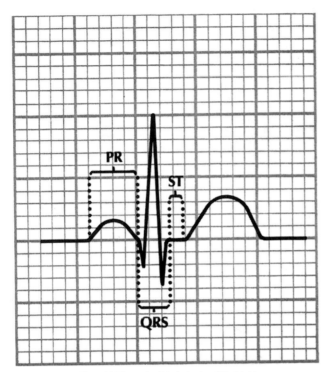

From Davis D. Differential Diagnosis of Arrhythmias. Philadelphia: WB Saunders, 1992.

4. Ventricular repolarization: represented on ECG as the ST segment and T wave

I. **Basic Steps to ECG Interpretation**
1. **Calculate heart rate**
   a. As mentioned, most ECG paper has 3-sec intervals marked off at the top of the paper. **Count the number of R waves in a 6-sec period and multiply by 10 to obtain the number of beats per minute.**
   b. Normal rate: 60 to 100 beats/min
   c. Bradycardia: less than 60 beats/min
   d. Tachycardia: more than 100 beats/min
2. **Determine regularity of the rhythm**
   a. Using calipers, measure the distance between a pair of R waves. Leave the calipers at that distance and measure the next pair of R waves to see if the distance is the same.
   b. Continue measuring the distance between successive pairs of R waves to see if it is constant. If the distances remain constant, the rhythm is regular.
3. **Observe P waves and PR interval**
   a. Make sure that there is a P wave before every QRS complex and that they are of the same shape.
   b. Using calipers, measure several P-R intervals to determine if they are consistent.
   c. As stated earlier, the normal PR interval is 0.12 to 0.20 sec. If the PR interval is longer

than 0.20 sec, first-degree heart block is present.
4. **Determine length of the QRS complex**
   a. Remember, that the QRS complex represents the time it takes for ventricular depolarization to occur. With the normal QRS complex taking 0.06 to 0.12 secs, any longer duration would indicate heart block.

Note

If all the above observations are within normal limits, the ECG shows normal sinus rhythm.

J. **Cardiac Arrhythmias:** most often encountered by RCPs
1. **Sinus bradycardia**

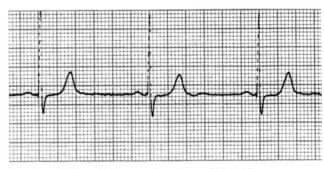

From Davis D. Differential Diagnosis of Arrhythmias. Philadelphia: WB Saunders, 1992.

   a. Rate: less than 60 beats/min
   b. Rhythm: regular
   c. Wave pattern abnormalities: none
   d. Cause: stimulation of vagus nerve (during tracheal suctioning for example), hypothermia, increased ICP; sinus bradycardia may be normal in well-conditioned athletes
   e. Treatment: If accompanied by shortness of breath, hypotension, or abnormal beats, atropine is used; a pacemaker may also be indicated.
2. **Sinus tachycardia**

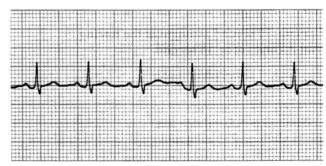

From Davis D. Differential Diagnosis of Arrhythmias. Philadelphia: WB Saunders, 1992.

a. Rate: 100 to 160 beats/min
b. Rhythm: regular
c. Wave pattern abnormalities: none
d. Cause: hypoxemia, increased sympathetic nervous system stimulation (e.g., fear, anxiety), medication
e. Treatment: stop underlying cause; administration of digitalis or beta blockers

3. **Sinus arrhythmia**

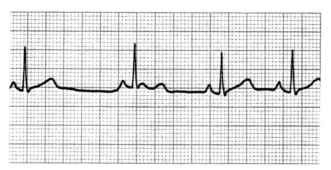

From Davis D. Differential Diagnosis of Arrhythmias. Philadelphia: WB Saunders, 1992.

a. Rate: 60 to 100 beats/min
b. Rhythm: irregular
c. Wave pattern abnormalities: R to R cycles vary more than 0.16 sec. **In Figure 9.11, note how the distance between the R wave of the QRS complex varies and is inconsistent.**
d. Cause: none; normal in young, healthy individuals; heart rate may increase during inspiration and decrease during expiration
e. Treatment: none necessary

4. **Premature Atrial Contraction (PAC)**

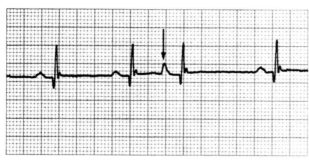

From Davis D. Differential Diagnosis of Arrhythmias. Philadelphia: WB Saunders, 1992.

a. Rate: 60 to 100 beats/min. **If there are less than 6 PACs/min, it's considered a minor arrhythmia, but more than 6/min is considered major arrhythmia.**
b. Rhythm: regular, except for PAC
c. Wave pattern abnormalities: the premature P wave looks different than the sinus P wave; the PAC occurs sooner than the next beat would be expected.
d. Cause: atrial irritability caused by organic heart disease, CNS disturbances, sympathomimetic drugs, tobacco, caffeine
e. Treatment: if more than 6/min, lidocaine may be used

5. **Premature Ventricular Contraction (PVC)**

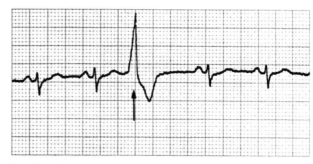

From Davis D. Differential Diagnosis of Arrhythmias. Philadelphia: WB Saunders, 1992.

a. Rate: 60 to 100 beats/min; less than 6 PVCs/min is considered minor and more than 6/min is considered major.
b. Rhythm: regular, except for PVCs

> **Note**
>
> When every other beat is a PVC, the arrhythmia is termed bigeminy, which is considered a dangerous arrhythmia.

c. Wave pattern abnormalities: the shape of the QRS complex is abnormal and wider than 0.12 sec
d. Cause: ventricular irritability caused by hypoxia, acid-base disturbances, electrolyte abnormalities, excessive dose of digitalis, CHF, myocardial inflammation, coronary artery disease
e. Treatment: lidocaine IV or other antiarrhythmia drugs, such as procainamide or propranolol if more than 6 PVCs/min.

6. **Atrial fibrillation**
a. Rate: variable; atrial rate greater than 350/min
b. Rhythm: irregular
c. Wave pattern abnormalities: P waves cannot be distinguished and have an uneven baseline; P-R interval is also indistinguishable
d. Cause: hypoxia, arteriosclerotic heart disease, mitral stenosis, valvular heart disease
e. Treatment: cardioversion, propranolol, digitalis

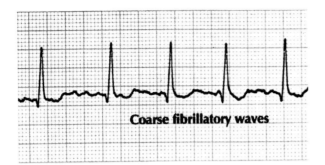

Coarse fibrillatory waves

From Davis D. Differential Diagnosis of Arrhythmias. Philadelphia: WB Saunders, 1992.

> **Note**
>
> This is considered a major arrhythmia, whereby the atria fail to pump blood adequately to the ventricles resulting in a significant decrease in cardiac output.

7. Atrial flutter

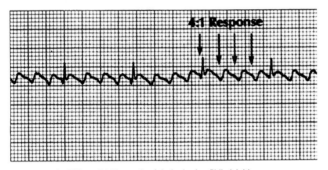

4:1 Response

From Davis D. Differential Diagnosis of Arrhythmias. Philadelphia: WB Saunders, 1992.

a. Rate: atrial, 200 to 400/min; ventricular, 60 to 150/min
b. Rhythm: regular or irregular
c. Wave pattern abnormalities: P waves have a characteristic sawtooth pattern and thus are often referred to as "F" waves
d. Cause: hypoxia, arteriosclerotic heart disease, MI, rheumatic heart disease
e. Treatment: cardioversion, carotid artery massage, procainamide, digitalis, tranquilizers

> **Note**
>
> This arrhythmia results in blockade of atrial impulses in what is called a 2:1, 3:1, or 4:1 block. In a 2:1 block, there are two atrial impulses for each ventricular beat, and there are 3 or 4 impulses to each ventricular beat in a 3:1 or 4:1 block, respectively.

8. Ventricular tachycardia (lethal)
a. Rate: 140 to 200 beats/min

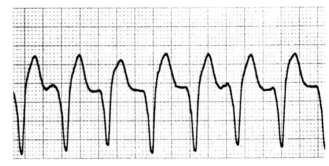

From Davis D. Differential Diagnosis of Arrhythmias. Philadelphia: WB Saunders, 1992.

b. Rhythm: regular
c. Wave pattern abnormalities: P waves and P-R intervals are absent or hidden in the QRS complex; each QRS is wider than normal and is a run of three or more PVCs
d. Cause: arteriosclerotic heart disease, coronary artery disease, myocardial ischemia, mitral valve prolapse, hypertensive heart disease
★ e. Treatment: lidocaine, defibrillation, CPR

9. Ventricular fibrillation (lethal)

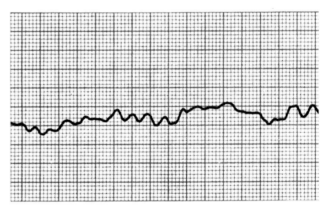

From Davis D. Differential Diagnosis of Arrhythmias. Philadelphia: WB Saunders, 1992.

a. Rate: cannot be determined
b. Rhythm: cannot be determined
c. Wave pattern abnormalities: no distinguishable waves
d. Cause: coronary artery disease, hypertensive heart disease, acute MI, digitalis overdose
★ e. Treatment: defibrillation, CPR. If this arrhythmia is not reversed, death soon results, since there is essentially no blood being pumped out of the heart.

10. First degree heart block
a. Rate: 60 to 100 beats/min
b. Rhythm: regular
c. Wave pattern abnormalities: PR interval longer than 0.20 sec

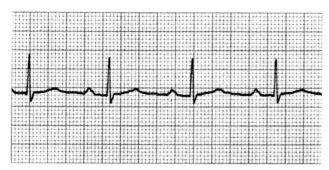

From Davis D. Differential Diagnosis of Arrhythmias. Philadelphia: WB Saunders, 1992.

d. Cause: complication of digoxin or beta-blockers, ischemia of the A-V node
e. Treatment: atropine, isoproterenol

11. **Second degree heart block**

Dropped beat

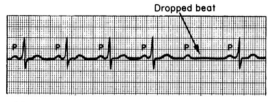

ECG tracing showing the widened QRS complex
From Levitsky MG, Cairo JN, Hall SM: Introduction to Respiratory Care. Philadelphia: WB Saunders, 1990.

a. Rate: 60 to 100 beats/min
b. Rhythm: regular or irregular
c. Wave pattern abnormalities: the QRS complex is normal, but may be preceded by two to four P waves
d. Cause: myocardial ischemia; may be a progression from first-degree block
e. Treatment: isoproterenol, atropine; pacemaker

12. **Third-degree heart block**
a. Rate: atrial rate, normal; ventricular rate, less than 40/min

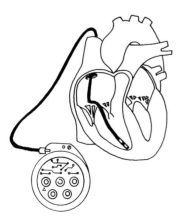

From Eubanks D and Bone R: Comprehensive Respiratory Care, ed. 2, St. Louis, 1990, Mosby, Inc.

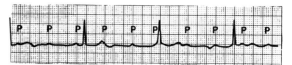

ECG tracing showing the widened QRS complex
From Levitsky MG, Cairo JN, Hall SM: Introduction to Respiratory Care. Philadelphia: WB Saunders, 1990.

b. Rhythm: atrial and ventricular rhythm are regular but are independent of each other
c. Wave pattern abnormalities: PR interval cannot be determined; QRS complex may be normal or widened
d. Cause: myocardial ischemia, AV node damage
e. Treatment: pacemaker

13. **Electromechanical dissociation (EMD)** (also referred to as pulseless electrical activity (PEA)).
a. A condition in which there is dissociation between the electrical and mechanical activity of the heart. The ECG pattern that appears on the oscilloscope (or ECG monitor) does not reflect the actual mechanical activity of the heart.
★ b. For example, the ECG may show regular QRS complexes, but the patient has no pulse. Certainly, the tracing should be ignored and chest compressions started.
c. While EMD is not common, it is often associated with cardiac trauma, tension pneumothorax, severe electrolyte disturbances, and severe acid-base imbalances.

K. **Electric Cardiac Pacemakers**
1. Electric pacemakers are devices used to replace the heart's natural pacemaker (SA node); they control the contractions of the heart by a series of rhythmic electrical discharges.

2. External pacemaker: the electrodes that deliver the discharges are placed on the outside of the chest.
3. Internal pacemaker: the electrodes are placed inside the chest wall.
4. The transvenous pacemaker, a **temporary** internal pacer, is introduced into a peripheral vein and, with the use of fluoroscopy and ECG monitoring, is advanced through the superior vena cava and right atrium and positioned in the right ventricle.
   Indications for the temporary transvenous pacemaker are second- and third-degree heart blocks, ventricular asystole, and other arrhythmias resulting in symptomatic bradycardia.
5. A pacer spike is a straight line observed on the ECG strip.
6. To treat permanent arrhythmias, permanent pacemakers are surgically implanted.
7. The electrodes are attached to a battery-operated pace generator, which fires impulses at a specific rate continuously, or to a demand-type pacer, which fires if the patient's heart rate slows to a pre-set rate.
8. The RCP must know whether the patient has a temporary pacemaker before beginning a treatment, such as chest physical therapy, because this type of pacemaker can be dislodged with vigorous movement.

L. **Holter Monitoring**
1. A Holter monitor is a portable, battery-powered recording device that records the patient's ECG tracing while the patient conducts daily activities. The monitoring is generally done over 24 hr.
2. The patient keeps a diary of activity throughout the day, so that it can be compared to the ECG recording. The patient records any symptoms in the diary, which are later correlated to the ECG at that specific time.
★ 3. Since arrhythmias and inadequate blood flow to the heart may occur only briefly or unpredictably, this method of monitoring is very useful in patients experiencing irregular heart beats on an inconsistent basis.

II. **HEMODYNAMIC MONITORING**

Exam Note

Hemodynamic monitoring appears on both examinations. More basic questions appear on the CRT examination; more advanced questions appear on the RRT examination. Below is a description of what areas are covered on each examination, according to the matrix for each examination.

CRT Exam

Questions referring to hemodynamic monitoring are limited to reviewing the patient chart for hemodynamic values; recommending the use of arterial, central venous, and pulmonary artery lines; and determining the proper position of these lines or catheters.

RRT Exam

Questions appear relating to the areas covered for the CRT examination as well as questions on performing the procedures (assisting the physician in the insertion of the lines or catheters); evaluating, monitoring, calculating, and interpreting the results of the data; and recommending modifications to therapy based on this data. Questions relating to the selection, cleaning, function, and malfunctions of the equipment used to obtain hemodynamic data appear on the RRT examination only.

A. **Arterial Catheter (arterial "line")**
1. Systemic arterial blood pressure is most accurately measured by placing a catheter directly into a peripheral artery.
2. Peripheral arterial lines should be used in patients with hemodynamic instability. Along with the measurement of blood pressure, these lines provide a direct route for the frequent blood samples drawn from these patients.
3. The most common peripheral artery sites
   a. Radial: most common because of easy access and good collateral circulation (with ulnar artery). **The Allen's test must be performed before puncture to determine if collateral circulation is present.** (Description of this procedure is in the chapter on ABG interpretation.)
   b. Brachial
   c. Femoral
4. Using sterile technique, the 18- or 20-gauge catheter may be placed into the artery by either surgical cutdown or percutaneous puncture. The catheter is connected to a system that delivers a continuous flow of fluid from an IV bag to maintain patency of the system. The IV bag, which should contain normal saline with added heparin, is pressurized by a hand-bulb pressure pump.
5. The system is also equipped with stopcocks to allow for calibration with atmospheric pressure as well as for arterial sampling.
6. A **strain gauge pressure transducer** (the most commonly used transducer) is connected to the system to provide a display of the

pressure waveform and a digital reading of the arterial pressure in millimeters of mercury.

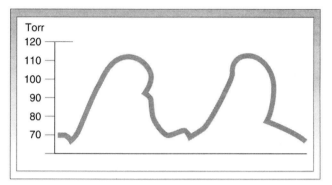

Normal arterial waveform

7. Pressures measured on the arterial waveform
   a. **Systolic pressure:** equal to the peak of the waveform **(normally 90 to 140 mm Hg).** Systole occurs as the heart contracts, forcing blood through the aorta (to the systemic circulation) and pulmonary arteries (to the lungs).
   b. **Diastolic pressure:** measured at the lowest point of the waveform **(normally 60 to 90 mm Hg).** Diastole occurs in between the contractions of the atria and ventricles (or while the heart is at rest), as these chambers begin refilling with blood.
   c. **Pulse pressure:** the difference between the systolic and diastolic pressures **(normally about 40 mm Hg)**
   d. Mean arterial pressure: represents the average pressure during the cardiac cycle **(normally 80 to 100 mm Hg).**
8. **Complications of arterial catheters**
   a. Infection: risk may be reduced with removal of the catheter within 4 days
   b. Hemorrhage: make sure all connections in the system are tight
   c. Ischemia: note the color and temperature of the skin distal to the insertion site to determine distal perfusion
   d. Thrombosis and embolization: a weak pulse distal to the puncture site may indicate thrombosis. A continuous flush of saline and heparin through the system helps to avoid clot formation.

> **Note**
>
> The catheter site and points distal to it should be assessed frequently by the respiratory care practitioner for signs of the above complications.

9. **Troubleshooting for arterial lines**

> **Note**
>
> In many instances, the RCP is responsible for the maintenance and troubleshooting of arterial lines.

   a. "Damped" pressure tracing; causes include
      (1) **Occlusion of the catheter tip by a clot;** correct by aspiration of the clot and flushing with heparinized saline
      (2) **Catheter tip resting against the wall of the vessel;** correct by repositioning catheter while observing waveform
      (3) **Clot in transducer or stopcock;** correct by flushing system and, if no improvement in the waveform tracing, change the stopcock and transducer
      (4) **Air bubbles in the line;** correct by disconnecting transducer and flushing out air bubbles
   b. Abnormally high or low pressure readings; causes include
      (1) **Improper calibration;** correct by recalibration of monitor and strain gauge
      (2) **Improper transducer position;** correct by ensuring the transducer is kept at the level of the patient's heart
   c. No pressure reading; causes include
      (1) **Improper scale selection;** correct by selecting appropriate scale
      (2) **Transducer not open to catheter;** correct by checking system and making sure the transducer is open to the catheter
B. **4-Channel Swan-Ganz Catheter**
   1. The Swan-Ganz catheter is a balloon-tipped catheter made of polyvinyl chloride that is used to measure **CVP, PAP, and PAWP,** which is sometimes referred to as PCWP.
   2. The catheter also allows for the aspiration of blood from the pulmonary artery for **mixed venous blood gas sampling** and injection of fluids to determine cardiac output.
   3. The distal channel (lumen) is used for the measurement of PAP and for obtaining mixed venous blood from the pulmonary artery.
   4. The proximal channel (lumen) is used for the measurement of CVP or right atrial pressure and for the injection of fluids to determine cardiac output.
   5. The balloon inflation channel controls the inflation and deflation of a small balloon, located

about 1 cm from the distal tip of the catheter, and is used to measure PAWP.

6. The fourth channel is an extra port for the continuous infusion of fluid when necessary.

7. This catheter is also equipped with a computer connector to measure cardiac output using the thermodilution technique.

> **Note**
>
> Some catheters are equipped with only two channels, the distal channel and the balloon inflation channel.

8. **Insertion of the Swan-Ganz catheter:**
   a. The catheter is inserted through the brachial, femoral, subclavian, or internal or external jugular vein.
   b. Continuous monitoring of the catheter pressure and waveform is necessary along with ECG monitoring.
   c. Once the vein is entered, the catheter is advanced into the right atrium, at which time the balloon is inflated and the catheter flows through the right atrium, right ventricle, and into the pulmonary artery, where it "wedges" into a distal branch.
   d. Pressures and pressure waveform tracings are recorded as the catheter passes through the right side of the heart.
   e. Once the catheter "wedges" in a distal branch of the pulmonary artery, the PAWP may be measured, and the balloon should

then be deflated, allowing blood flow past the tip of the catheter. Since blood flow is stopped distal to the wedge position when the balloon is inflated, it should not be inflated any longer than **15 to 20 sec or pulmonary infarction may occur.**

C. **Monitoring of CVP, PAP, and PAWP**
   1. **CVP** may be monitored with a Swan-Ganz catheter or from a separate CVP catheter that is inserted through the subclavian, jugular, or brachial vein. The CVP catheter is connected to a water manometer, which reads the pressure in cm H_2O. Measuring the CVP with a Swan-Ganz catheter gives the pressure in mm Hg.

> **Note**
>
> When monitoring CVP with a water manometer, the manometer must be level with the heart while the patient is lying flat. This method of monitoring CVP is not as accurate as using a Swan-Ganz catheter and is not commonly used.

   a. CVP is a measurement of right atrial pressure which reflects systemic venous return and right ventricular preload. **The normal value is less than 8 cm H_2O or less than 6 mm Hg.**
   ★ b. Conditions that increase CVP
      (1) Hypervolemia (volume overload)
      (2) Pulmonary hypertension
      (3) Right ventricular failure

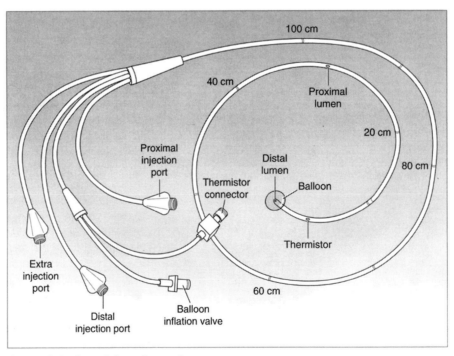

Quadruple (4-channel) Swan-Ganz catheter

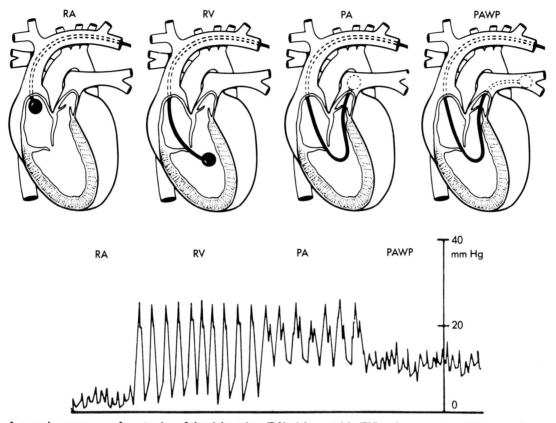

RA   RV   PA   PAWP

A normal pressure waveform tracing of the right atrium (RA), right ventricle (RV), pulmonary artery (PA), and pulmonary artery wedge pressure (PAWP).
From Scanlan C, Wilkins C, and Stoller J: *Egan's fundamentals of respiratory care*, ed 7, St. Louis, 1999, Mosby, Inc.

(4) Pulmonary valve stenosis

(5) Tricuspid valve stenosis

(6) Pulmonary embolism

(7) Arterial vasodilation, resulting in increased blood volume in the venous system

(8) Left heart failure

(9) Improper transducer placement (below the level of the right atrium)

(10) Positive pressure ventilator breath (measure CVP at end of expiration)

(11) Severe flail chest or pneumothorax: these conditions may compress the superior and inferior vena cavae, decreasing venous return and increasing CVP as a result of compression of the heart.

Note

To determine what effect PEEP has on venous return and CVP, measure CVP while patient is on PEEP. To determine CVP without the effects of PEEP, some patients may be taken off PEEP for the measurement. However, remember that patients with critical lung conditions on high levels of PEEP cannot tolerate being removed from PEEP; therefore, CVP must be measured while the patient remains on PEEP.

c. Conditions that decrease CVP

(1) Hypovolemia (inadequate circulating blood volume)

(2) Vasodilation (from decreased venous tone)

(3) Leaks or air bubbles in pressure line

(4) Improper transducer placement (above the level of the right atrium)

2. **PAP** is a very important measurement in the care of critically ill patients with sepsis, ARDS, pulmonary edema, and myocardial infarction.

★ a. It is especially important to monitor PAP and Pv_{O_2} values on patients that are on at least 10 cm H_2O of PEEP since high levels of PEEP may compromise the cardiac status of the patient by decreasing cardiac output and oxygen delivery to the tissues.

b. Mixed venous blood sampling (to measure Pv_{O_2}) is achieved by obtaining blood from the pulmonary artery. **Normal Pv_{O_2} is 35 to 45 mm Hg.** Pv_{O_2} reflects tissue oxygenation; should this level drop after the initiation of or increase in PEEP, a decrease in tissue oxygenation has occurred, caused by a drop in cardiac output because of PEEP. PEEP should be decreased to maintain an adequate Pv_{O_2}. (See Chapter 11: Ventilator Management.)

c. **Normal systolic PAP is 20 to 30 mm Hg. Normal diastolic PAP is 5 to 15 mm Hg. Normal mean PAP is 10 to 20 mm Hg.**
★ d. Conditions that increase PAP
(1) Pulmonary hypertension (resulting from hypercapnia, acidemia, or hypoxemia, for example)
(2) Mitral valve stenosis
(3) Left ventricular failure
★ e. Conditions that decrease PAP
(1) Decreased pulmonary vascular resistance (pulmonary vasodilation); caused by improved oxygenation, for example
(2) Decreased blood volume
3. **PAWP**
a. When the balloon at the distal end of the catheter is inflated, it "wedges" in a branch of the pulmonary artery, blocking blood flow from the right side of the heart. The transducer measures the back pressure through the pulmonary circulation, which is equal to pressure in the **left atrium and the left ventricular end-diastolic pressure (LVEDP).**
★ b. PAWP (also called PCWP), therefore, is a measurement of pressure in the left side of the heart.
c. As stated, the balloon should not be inflated any longer than 15 to 20 sec, since blood flow obstructed for any longer may cause pulmonary infarction.
d. **Normal PAWP value is 4 to 12 mm Hg.** PAWP of more than 18 mm Hg usually indicates impending pulmonary edema.

> **Note**
>
> PAWP is elevated in patients with cardiogenic pulmonary edema and normal in patients with noncardiogenic pulmonary edema.

★ e. Conditions that increase PAWP
(1) Left ventricular failure
(2) Mitral valve stenosis
(3) Aortic valve stenosis
(4) Systemic hypertension
★ f. Conditions that decrease PAWP
(1) Hypovolemia
(2) Pulmonary embolism (PAWP may be normal or decreased)
D. **Complications of Swan-Ganz Catheter Insertion**
1. Damage to tricuspid valve

2. Damage to pulmonary valve
3. Pulmonary infarction
4. Pneumothorax
5. Cardiac arrhythmias
6. Air embolism
7. Ruptured pulmonary artery
E. **Measurement of Cardiac Output**
1. Cardiac output may be measured through the Swan-Ganz catheter using the **thermodilution technique.** A cold saline or dextrose solution is injected through the proximal port of the catheter. Heat loss occurs from the injection port to the distal tip of the catheter. The rate of blood flow determines the amount of heat loss and is measured on the cardiac output computer.
2. Cardiac output may be calculated using the **Fick equation**

$$QT = \frac{V_{O_2}}{[C_{aO_2} - C_{vO_2}] \times 10}$$

QT = cardiac output (L/min)
V_{O_2} = oxygen consumption (mL/min)
$[C_{aO_2} - C_{vO_2}]$ = arterial and mixed venous oxygen content difference (mL of oxygen per dL of blood), also called vol%

> **Note**
>
> mL/dL must be converted to mL/L to express the cardiac output in L/min. This is accomplished by multiplying the oxygen content difference by 10. Normal cardiac output is 5 L/min.

EXAMPLE:

Calculate a patient's cardiac output given the following information.
V_{O_2} = 250 ml/min
$C_{aO_2} - C_{vO_2}$ = 5 vol%

$$QT = \frac{250 \text{ mL/min}}{5 \times 10} = \frac{250}{50} = 5 \text{ L/min}$$

F. **Measurement of Arterial and Venous O_2 Content**
1. O_2 content refers to the total amount of O_2 dissolved in the plasma and bound to Hb in arterial or mixed venous blood.
2. The difference between arterial and venous O_2 content (arteriovenous O_2 content difference)

is used to calculate cardiac output and cardiopulmonary shunting.

3. Total O_2 content of arterial blood (CaO_2) is calculated by using the following formula

$$CaO_2 = 1.34 \times Hb \times SaO_2 \text{ (i.e., mL of } O_2 \text{ bound to Hb)} + PaO_2 \times 0.003 \text{ (mL of } O_2 \text{ dissolved in plasma)}$$

Note

1.34 mL of O_2 is capable of binding with 1 g of Hb and 0.003 mL of O_2 is dissolved in the plasma for each 1 mm Hg of PaO_2.

EXAMPLE:

Calculate the total arterial O_2 content from the following data.
Hb   15 g%
SaO_2 98%
PaO_2 86 mm Hg

$1.34 \times 15 \times 0.98 = 19.7$ mL of O_2 (bound to Hb)
$86 \times 0.003 = 0.26$ mL of O_2 (dissolved in the plasma)
$CaO_2 = 19.7$ mL $+ 0.26$ mL $=$ **19.96 mL/dL (or vol%)**

4. CvO_2 is calculated with the following formula

$$(1.34 \times Hb \times SvO_2) + (PvO_2 \times .003)$$

EXAMPLE:

Calculate the total venous O_2 content, given the following data.
Hb   15 g%
SvO_2 75%
PvO_2 40 mm Hg

$1.34 \times 15 \times 0.75 = 15$ mL of O_2 (bound to Hb)
$40 \times 0.003 = 0.12$ mL of O_2 (dissolved in plasma)
$CvO_2 = 15$ mL $+ 0.12$ mL $= 15.12$ mL/dL (or vol%)

Note

The normal $C(a-v)O_2$, or arteriovenous O_2 content difference is 4 to 6 mL/dL (or vol%).
In the above calculations, the $C(a-v)O_2$ is

$19.96 - 15.12 = 4.84$ mL/dL (vol%)

An arteriovenous O_2 content difference of less than 4 vol% may be the result of increased cardiac output (less time for tissues to

extract O_2, therefore arterial and venous O_2 closer in value); septic shock; or anemia. **An arteriovenous O_2 content difference of more than 6 vol%** may be the result of decreased cardiac output (more time for tissues to extract O_2 because of slower blood flow), therefore a greater difference between arterial and venous O_2 values-increasing fluid intake may be indicated in this case; or increased O_2 consumption.

★ Note

$C(a-v)O_2$ is useful in determining the effects that PEEP and mechanical ventilation have on the patient's cardiac output and also in evaluating the patient's need for more circulatory support.

G. **Intrapulmonary Shunting**
   1. Intrapulmonary shunting is defined as the portion of the cardiac output that perfuses through the lungs without coming in contact with ventilated alveoli. This portion of the cardiac output, therefore, passes through the lungs and into the left side of the heart without being oxygenated.
   2. In the normal, healthy person, intrapulmonary shunting occurs. This results from blood flow through the bronchial, pleural, and thebesian veins. These veins return blood back to the left atrium, therefore bypassing the oxygenation process in the lungs (called an anatomic shunt). **Normally, intrapulmonary shunting is about 2% to 5% of the cardiac output** and is primarily caused by anatomic shunting.
   3. Physiologic shunting represents only a small portion of the normal anatomic shunt. Increased physiologic shunting results in a worsening cardiopulmonary status.
   ★ 4. Conditions that **increase** physiologic shunting
      a. Pneumonia
      b. Pneumothorax
      c. Pulmonary edema
      d. Atelectasis
   5. The amount of shunt may be determined using the clinical shunt formula:

$$\frac{QS}{QT} = \frac{(PAO_2 - PaO_2)(0.003)}{(CaO_2 - CvO_2) + (PAO_2 - PaO_2)(0.003)}$$

Note

This formula requires a 100% Hb saturation of O_2 in arterial blood.

6. If measurement of $P\overline{v}O_2$ is not available (via pulmonary artery catheter), the modified shunt equation may be used:

$$\frac{QS}{QT} = \frac{(PAO_2 - PaO_2)(0.003)}{(4.5 \text{ vol}\%) + (PAO_2 - PaO_2)(0.003)}$$

4.5 vol% represents a normal $CaO_2 - C\overline{v}O_2$

EXAMPLE:

Calculate a patient's percentage of shunt given the following data

pH	7.37
$PaCO_2$	45 mm Hg
PaO_2	60 mm Hg
FIO_2	0.40
PB	747 torr

$$PAO_2 = (PB - 47) (FIO_2) - (PaCO_2 \times 1.25)^*$$
$$747 - 47) (.4) - (45 \times 1.25)$$
$$280 - 56 = \mathbf{224 \text{ torr}}$$

$$\frac{QS}{QT} = \frac{(PAO_2 - PaO_2)(0.003)}{(4.5 \text{ vol}\%) + (PAO_2 - PaO_2)(0.003)}$$

$$= \frac{(224 - 60) \times 0.003}{4.5 + (224 - 60)(0.003)} = \frac{0.49}{4.5 + .49}$$

$$= \frac{0.49}{5.0} = .098$$

$$\frac{QS}{QT} = .098 \times 100 = \mathbf{9.8\ \%}$$

This means that almost 10% of the patient's cardiac output is not being oxygenated in the lungs.

7. **Interpreting calculated shunt values**
   a. Less than 10% is normal
   b. 10% to 20% is abnormal intrapulmonary status that is usually of no significance clinically
   c. 20% to 30% is significant intrapulmonary disease, which may be life-threatening and require cardiopulmonary support
   d. More than 30% is a serious, life-threatening condition, which requires aggressive cardiopulmonary support

---

*To simplify the math ($PaCO_2 + 10$) may be used with similar results.

> **Exam Note**
>
> The following sections pertaining to cardiac index, stroke volume, systemic vascular resistance, and pulmonary vascular resistance appear on the RRT examination only.

H. **Measuring Cardiac Index (CI)**
   1. Cardiac output varies according to the patient's BSA. The CI correlates the patient's cardiac output for their specific body surface area.
   2. Formula for calculation

   $$CI = \frac{\text{cardiac output (L/min)}}{\text{body surface area (m}^2)}$$

   3. Normal CI is 2.6 to 4.3 $L/min/m^2$
   4. Factors that **increase** cardiac index:
      a. Drugs that increase cardiac contractility (e.g., dopamine, epinephrine, digitalis)
      b. Hypervolemia
      c. Decreased vascular resistance
      d. Septic shock (early stages)
   5. Factors that **decrease** cardiac index
      a. Drugs that decrease cardiac contractility (propranolol, metoprolol)
      b. Hypovolemia
      c. CHF
      d. Increased vascular resistance
      e. MI
      f. Septic shock (late stages)
      g. Positive pressure ventilation
      h. PEEP and CPAP
I. **Measuring Stroke Volume** (SV)
   1. SV is the amount of blood ejected from the ventricle during ventricular contraction.
   2. Formula for calculation

   $$SV = \frac{\text{cardiac output (mL/min)}}{\text{heart rate (beats/min)}}$$

   3. Normal SV is 60 to 120 mL/beat.
J. **Measuring Systemic Vascular Resistance** (SVR)
   1. SVR is a measurement of the resistance that the left ventricle must overcome to eject its volume of blood. This is known as **afterload.**
   2. SVR is calculated using the following formula

   $$SVR = \frac{MSAP - CVP \text{ (mm Hg)}}{QT \text{ (L/min)}}$$

MSAP = mean systemic arterial pressure

3. Normal SVR is 10 to 18 mm Hg/L/min, or 900 to 1450 dyne $\times$ sec $\times$ cm^{-5}.
4. Factors that **increase** SVR
   a. Vasocontrictors (dopamine, epinephrine)
   b. Hypovolemia
   c. Hypocapnia
5. Factors that **decrease** SVR
   a. Vasodilators (nitroprusside sodium, morphine, nitroglycerin)
   b. Hypercapnia
   c. Septic shock (early stages)
K. **Measuring Pulmonary Vascular Resistance** (PVR)
   1. PVR is a reflection of the afterload of the right ventricle.
   2. PVR is calculated using the following formula

$$PVR = \frac{MPAP - PAWP \ (mm \ Hg)}{QT \ (L/min)}$$

MPAP = mean pulmonary artery pressure
QT = cardiac output (L/min)
PAWP = pulmonary artery wedge pressure

3. Normal PVR is 1.5 to 3.0 mm Hg/L/min, or 150 to 250 dyne $\times$ sec $\times$ cm^{-5}.
4. Factors that **increase** PVR
   a. Vasoconstrictors (dopamine, epinephrine)
   b. Hypercapnia
   c. Hypoxemia
   d. Acidemia
   e. Pulmonary embolism
   f. Pneumothorax
   g. Positive pressure ventilation
   h. PEEP and CPAP
5. Factors that **decrease** PVR
   a. Improved oxygenation (pulmonary vasodilator)
   b. Alkalemia (hypocapnia)
   c. Vasodilating agents
L. **Measurement of O$_2$ Consumption (Vo$_2$)**
   1. Vo$_2$ is defined as the amount of O$_2$ (in mL) extracted by the peripheral tissues in 1 min. It

is also a measurement of the O$_2$ uptake in the lung.
2. Vo$_2$ may be calculated using the following formula, which is based on the Fick equation

$$Vo_2 = QT \ [C(a-v)o_2] \times 10$$

10 = factor to convert C(a-v)o$_2$ to milliliters of O$_2$ per liter

EXAMPLE:

Given the following data, calculate a patient's O$_2$ consumption (uptake).
   QT   5 L/min
   Cao$_2$ 20 vol %
   Cvo$_2$ 14.5 vol %

$$Vo_2 = 5 \times [20 - 14.5] \times 10$$
$$Vo_2 = 5 \times 5.5 \times 10$$
$$Vo_2 = 275 \ mL/min$$

3. Normal O$_2$ consumption is **150 to 275 mL/min.**
4. Factors that **increase** Vo$_2$
   a. Hyperthermia
   b. Exercise
   c. Seizures
   d. Shivering
5. Factors that **decrease** Vo$_2$
   a. Hypothermia
   b. Cyanide poisoning
   c. Musculoskeletal relaxation

III. **INDIRECT CALORIMETRY**

A. Indirect calorimetry is a method of measuring a patient's Vo$_2$ and Vco$_2$ at the bedside. It is more accurate than using formulas to estimate these values.
B. The data obtained may be used to assess a patient's nutritional needs or response to nutrition therapy, and the patient's overall metabolic state.
C. **Indications for Indirect Calorimetry**
   1. Patients who are difficult to wean from mechanical ventilation.
   2. Patients who are morbidly obese.
   3. Patients who are severely malnourished.
   4. Patients not responding to nutritional support.

D. Indirect calorimetry measures the patient's oxygen consumption, which aids in the evaluation of the hemodynamic status and O_2 cost of breathing of the ventilated patient.

E. Indirect calorimetry may be performed in two ways
   1. The patient exhales into a Douglas bag and the expired air is analyzed for O_2 and CO_2 concentrations. The exhaled volume is measured by a Tissot spirometer.
   2. A metabolic cart is commonly used, which is an automated system in which breath-by-breath analysis can be performed. This method provides for optimal measurement, especially in mechanically ventilated patients.
      a. When using a metabolic cart for a mechanically ventilated patient, a gas sample is taken from the inspiratory limb of the ventilator tubing and the O_2 percentage is analyzed.
      b. The patient's exhaled gas volume is measured as it passes through a flow transducer, where it then enters a mixing chamber where the F_{EO_2} and F_{ECO_2} are measured. This exhaled gas then returns to the ventilator.
      c. After these measurements are obtained, V_{O_2}, V_{CO_2}, and RQ are calculated using the following formulas

$$V_{O_2} = VE \times \frac{1 - F_{EO_2} - F_{ECO_2}}{1 - F_{IO_2}} \times F_{IO_2} - (VE \times F_{EO_2})$$

$$V_{CO_2} = VE \times F_{ECO_2}$$

$$RQ = \frac{V_{CO_2}}{V_{O_2}}$$

F. Problems Associated with Indirect Calorimetry
   1. Errors in calculation: small errors in measurement may result in large errors in the calculated values for V_{O_2}, V_{CO_2}, and energy expenditure. Because of this problem, analyzing equipment must be properly calibrated.
   2. The procedure must be conducted with the patient in a steady-state condition.
   3. Leaks in the ventilator circuit, chest tube, or around the ET-tube cuff render inaccurate results.
   4. The procedure may affect the function of the ventilator.
   5. When conducting indirect calorimetry on a spontaneously breathing patient, the mask or mouthpiece and noseclips used may alter the patient's steady state, rendering inaccurate results.
G. The following should be monitored during indirect calorimetry

1. Patient's steady-state condition
2. Proper equipment function
3. Patient's comfort
4. Patient movement (must lie still during testing)

H. Calculation of resting energy expenditure (REE)
   1. REE estimates the patient's daily energy needs and is calculated from values obtained from indirect calorimetry.
   2. REE is calculated using the following formula

$$REE = [(V_{O_2} \times 3.9) + (V_{CO_2} \times 1.1)] \times 1.44$$

   3. If the REE is within 10% of the predicted value, the patient is **normometabolic.** Patients with REE values of less than 90% of predicted value are considered **hypometabolic,** and patients more than 10% above predicted values are **hypermetabolic.**
   4. REE can be calculated by the following formula if the patient has a pulmonary artery catheter in place

$$REE = QT \times Hb \times (Sa_{O_2} - Sv_{O_2}) \times 95.18$$

   ★ The answer obtained from either of these two equations determines the number of kcal/day needed by the patient.

I. The effects of inadequate nutrition on the patient's respiratory status
   1. Decreased surfactant production: results in a decreased lung compliance.
   2. Decreased response to hypoxia and hypercapnia
   3. Decreased pulmonary clearance mechanisms
   4. Loss of diaphragmatic mass and its ability to contract: results in an increasing difficulty to wean the patient from the ventilator.
   5. Loss of accessory muscle mass and its ability to contract: since patients with severe COPD greatly depend on their accessory muscles during normal ventilation, this may place the patient in acute respiratory failure.

Note

COPD patients have a greater incidence of malnutrition because of their increased energy expenditure, resulting from an increased work of breathing, and because of inadequate caloric intake, resulting from loss of appetite from drug side effects and the dyspnea that they experience during eating.

IV. **ECHOCARDIOGRAPHY**
   A. Doppler techniques and ultrasound echocardiography are useful in the evaluation of intracardiac shunts, valvular disorders, the size of septal defects, and ventricular function.

B. Ultrasonic waves are directed through the heart by a transducer placed on the chest. The ultrasonic waves are reflected backward, or echoed, when they pass from one type of tissue to another (e.g., from cardiac muscle to blood).

C. The transducer then receives the sound waves, which are recorded on a strip chart.

D. An echocardiogram is a graphic display of cardiac movements compiled from the ultrasonic vibrations reflected from the cardiac muscle.

POST-CHAPTER STUDY QUESTIONS

1. List four causes of a "damped" arterial pressure waveform.
2. List five conditions that cause an increased CVP.
3. List four conditions that cause a decreased CVP.
4. What are three drugs used to treat PVCs.
5. What is the treatment for ventricular tachycardia?
6. List three conditions that cause an increased PAP.
7. List two conditions that cause a decreased PAP.
8. PAWP is a measurement of what function?
9. List four conditions that cause an increased PAWP.
10. List two conditions that cause a decreased PAWP.
11. List the normal values for CVP, PAP, and PAWP.
12. Calculate the QT of a patient who has a $\dot{V}O_2$ of 240 mL/min and a $C(a-v)O_2$ of 6 vol%.
13. In a normal, healthy person, what percentage of the cardiac output makes up the intrapulmonary shunt?
14. Calculate the $C(a-v)O_2$, given the following information.

pH	7.43
$PaCO_2$	43 mm Hg
PaO_2	82 mm Hg
SaO_2	95%
PvO_2	37 mm Hg
SvO_2	72%
Hb	14 g/dL

15. List four conditions that increase physiologic shunting.
16. Calculate the percentage of intrapulmonary shunt given the following information.

pH	7.39
$PaCO_2$	40 mm Hg
PaO_2	122 mm Hg
FiO_2	0.50
PB	747 mm Hg

17. List four factors that cause an increased SVR.
18. List three factors that cause a decreased SVR.
19. List five factors that cause an increased PVR.
20. List three factors that cause a decreased PVR.
21. Calculate the oxygen consumption given the following information.

QT	4.5 L/min
CaO_2	19 vol%
CvO_2	14 vol%

22. List four factors that cause an increased O_2 consumption.
23. List three factors that cause a decreased O_2 consumption.

Answers are at the end of the chapter.

REFERENCES

Barnes T: Respiratory care practice, Chicago, 1998, Year-Book Medical Publishers.

Davis D: How to quickly and accurately master ECG interpretation, Philadelphia, 1985, JB Lippincott Co.

Des Jardins T: Cardiopulmonary anatomy and physiology, ed 3, Albany, NY, 1997, Delmar Inc.

Levitzky M: Introduction to respiratory care, Philadelphia, 1990, WB Saunders Co.

Scanlan CL, Wilkins RL, and Stoller JK: Egan's fundamentals of respiratory care, ed 7, St. Louis, 1999, Mosby Inc.

Shapiro B, Kacmarek R, Cane R, et al: Clinical application of respiratory care, ed 4, St. Louis, 1991, Mosby Year-Book.

PRE-TEST ANSWERS

1. D
2. D
3. B
4. C
5. C
6. D

ANSWERS TO POST-CHAPTER STUDY QUESTIONS

1. Clot in catheter, tip of catheter up against vessel wall, clot in transducer, air bubbles in the line
2. Hypervolemia, pulmonary hypertension, right ventricular failure, pulmonary valve stenosis, tricuspid valve stenosis, pulmonary embolism, arterial vasodilation, left-sided heart failure, improper transducer placement, positive pressure ventilator breath, severe flail chest, pneumothorax
3. Hypovolemia, vasodilation, leaks or air in line, improper transducer placement
4. Lidocaine, propranolol, procainamide
5. Defibrillation, chest compressions, lidocaine
6. Pulmonary hypertension, mitral valve stenosis, left ventricular failure
7. Decreased PVR, hypovolemia

8. Left atrial pressure
9. Left ventricular failure, mitral valve stenosis, aortic stenosis, systemic hypertension
10. Hypovolemia, pulmonary embolus (PAWP could also be normal)
11. CVP, less than 8 cm H_2O or less than 6 mm Hg; PAP,
$$\frac{20 - 30 \text{ mm Hg}}{5 - 15 \text{ mm Hg}}$$
or a mean of 10 to 20 mm Hg; PAWP, 4 to 12 mm Hg
12. 4 L/min; $\frac{240 \text{ mL/min}}{6 \times 10} = \frac{240}{60} = 4$ L/min
13. 2% to 5%
14. 4.4 mL/dL; $CaO_2 = (1.34 \times 14 \times .95) + (82 \times .003) = 18$
$CvO_2 = (1.34 \times 14 \times .72) + (37 \times .003) = 13.6$
$18 - 13.6 = 4.4$ mL/dL
15. Pneumonia, pneumothorax, pulmonary edema, atelectasis

16. 11%; $PaO2 = [(747 - 47) \times .50] - 40 \times 1.25 = 300$
$PaO_2 - PaO_2 = 300 - 122 = 178$
$\frac{Q_S}{Q_T} = \frac{178 \times .003}{4.5 + (178 \times .003)} - 11\%$
17. Vasoconstrictors (dopamine, epinephrine), hypovolemia, decreased $PaCO_2$, septic shock (late stages)
18. Vasodilators (nitroprusside sodium, morphine, nitroglycerin), increased $PaCO_2$, septic shock (early stages)
19. Vasoconstrictors, increased $PaCO_2$, hypoxemia, acidemia, pulmonary embolism, pneumothorax, positive pressure ventilation, PEEP, CPAP
20. Vasodilators, hyperoxemia, decreased $PaCO_2$, alkalemia
21. 4.5 [5] $\times$ 10 = 225 mL/min
22. Hyperthermia, exercise, seizures, shivering
23. Hypothermia, cyanide poisoning, musculoskeletal relaxation

Chapter 10

ABG Interpretation

Answer the pre-test questions before studying the chapter. This will help you determine your strong and weak areas regarding the material covered.

1. Which of the following blood gas measurements determines how well a patient is being ventilated?

   A. pH
   B. $Paco_2$
   C. Pao_2
   D. HCO_3^-

2. Which of the following blood gas measurements determines the level of tissue oxygenation?

   A. pH
   B. $Paco_2$
   C. Pao_2
   D. Pvo_2

3. The information below has been obtained from a patient on an aerosol mask at 40% oxygen.

pH	7.42
$Paco_2$	36 mm Hg
Pao_2	122 mm Hg
HCO_3^-	26 mEq/L

   What is this patient's A-a gradient?
   PB = 747 torr

   A. 45 mm Hg
   B. 77 mm Hg
   C. 113 mm Hg
   D. 235 mm Hg

4. Which of the following conditions shifts the HbO_2 dissociation curve to the right?

   A. Hypercapnia
   B. Hypothermia
   C. Alkalemia
   D. HbCO

5. A patient on a 2 L/min nasal cannula has the following ABG results.

pH	7.51
$Paco_2$	27 mm Hg
Pao_2	62 mm Hg
HCO_3^-	23 mEq/L

These results indicate which of the following conditions?

   A. Uncompensated respiratory acidosis
   B. Chronic respiratory alkalosis
   C. Compensated metabolic alkalosis
   D. Acute respiratory alkalosis

6. The respiratory therapist has received an order to obtain ABG levels from a patient, but an Allen's test indicates collateral circulation is not present in the right wrist. At this time the therapist would

   A. Obtain blood from the right radial artery.
   B. Obtain blood from the right brachial artery.
   C. Wait for the physician to evaluate collateral circulation.
   D. Check collateral circulation in the left wrist.

Answers are at the end of the chapter.

REVIEW

I. **ABG ANALYSIS**
   A. Blood gas analysis monitors the following physiologic parameters
      1. Arterial oxygenation: Pao_2
      2. Alveolar ventilation: $Paco_2$
      3. Acid-base status: pH
      4. O_2 delivery to tissues: Pvo_2
   B. Arterial samples are used because the values reflect the patient's total cardiopulmonary status.
   C. Mixed venous blood, obtained from the pulmonary artery via a Swan-Ganz catheter, is used to determine O_2 delivery to the tissues (see chapter on ventilator management).
   D. Blood gases are tested to determine whether to change current therapy or to maintain it.

E. Common sites from which to obtain arterial blood are the radial, femoral, or dorsalis pedis arteries.
   1. Radial artery is the most common site because of the presence of good collateral circulation and easy access.
   2. A modified Allen's test is performed to determine collateral circulation.
      a. Patient is instructed to close hand tightly as practitioner occludes both the radial and ulnar artery.
      b. Patient is instructed to open hand as the practitioner releases the pressure on the ulnar artery while watching for hand to regain normal color.
      c. Color should be restored in 10 to 15 sec. If not restored, the test is considered negative, meaning collateral circulation is not present. Blood must not be obtained from this wrist. Check the other wrist.
F. **ABG Sampling** (via radial artery puncture)
   1. Explain the procedure to the patient.
   2. Perform a modified Allen's test.
   3. Place a folded towel under the patient's wrist to keep the wrist hyperextended.
   4. Clean the puncture site with isopropyl alcohol (70%).
   5. The practitioner must wear gloves for this procedure.
   6. A local anesthetic, such as lidocaine (Xylocaine) may be administered subcutaneously around the puncture site, especially in patients who have been punctured several times. Allow 3 to 5 min for the anesthetic to take effect.
   7. Aspirate 0.5 mL of a 1:1000 solution of heparin into the syringe using a 20- or 23-gauge needle. Pull the plunger of the syringe back and forth so that the entire portion of the syringe is exposed to the heparin. The plunger should then be pushed all the way in to expel the heparin, making sure there are no air bubbles in the syringe. (Most syringes now are previously treated with heparin.)

Note

The heparin lubricates the syringe but is primarily used to prevent the blood from clotting once in the syringe.

   8. With the needle/syringe in one hand, palpate the artery with the other. The needle should enter the skin at a 45° angle with the bevel pointed up. The needle should be advanced until blood is pulsating into the syringe.

Note

Sometimes the needle passes through the artery and only a small amount of blood enters the syringe. If this happens, the needle should be slowly withdrawn until it is in the artery. If the needle needs to be redirected, it should first be withdrawn to the subcutaneous tissue.

   9. After 2 to 4 mL of blood has been obtained, a sterile gauze pad should be applied with pressure over the puncture site for 3 to 5 min or until the bleeding has stopped.
   10. Air bubbles should then be removed from the syringe, since they affect the blood gas levels. Air in the blood causes increased PaO_2 levels and decreased $PaCO_2$ levels.
   11. A cap or rubber stopper should then be placed over the needle, or the needle may be removed and a cap placed over the end of the syringe. This prevents air from entering the syringe.
   12. The practitioner should then roll the syringe back and forth in the hands to ensure proper mixing of the blood and heparin to prevent blood clotting. The syringe is then placed in ice to slow metabolism and keep the ABG levels accurate.
   13. The practitioner should record the following information after the sample is drawn
      a. Patent's name and room number
      b. The patient's FiO_2 level.
      c. If the patient is on ventilator, record
         (1) FiO_2
         (2) V_T
         (3) Respiratory rate
         (4) Mode of ventilation (e.g., CMV, SIMV)
         (5) PEEP level
         (6) Mechanical dead space
      d. Patient's temperature: A fever shifts the HbO_2 curve to the right, indicating that Hb more readily releases O_2 to the tissues but does not pick up the O_2 as easily. This may affect the PaO_2 value, but not usually to a significant degree.

II. **ARTERIAL OXYGENATION**
   A. **PaO_2**
      1. The PaO_2 is the portion of O_2 that is dissolved in the plasma of the blood. It is what is left over after the Hb molecules have been saturated.
      2. For every **1 mm Hg of PaO_2,** there is **0.003 mL of dissolved O_2.**
   B. **PAO_2 (alveolar PO_2)**
      1. It is calculated by the following formula (alveolar air equation)

$$PA_{O_2} = [(PB - 47 \text{ mm Hg})(F_{IO_2})] - (Pa_{CO_2} \times 1.25)^*$$

(47 mm Hg is the level of water vapor pressure at body temperature)

$$PA_{O_2} = [(760 - 47 \text{ mm Hg})(.21)] - 40 \text{ mm Hg} \times 1.25$$
$$PA_{O_2} = (713 \times .21) - 50$$
$$PA_{O_2} = 150 - 50 = \textbf{100 mm Hg}$$

2. This value is often compared to Pa_{O_2} to determine $P(A-a)_{O_2}$ gradient, which refers to the difference between alveolar O_2 tension and arterial O_2 tension. **Normal gradient on room air is 4 to 12 mm Hg.**

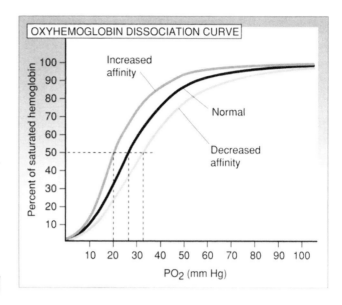

EXAMPLE:

A patient on a 50% Venturi mask has the following ABG levels

pH	7.36
Pa_{CO_2}	45 mm Hg
Pa_{O_2}	94 mm Hg

What is this patient's A-a gradient? (PB = 747 mm Hg)

$$PA_{O_2} = [(747 - 47)(.5)] - 45 \times 1.25$$
$$= 350 - 56$$
$$= 294 \text{ mm Hg}$$

$$P(A-a)_{O_2} = PA_{O_2} - Pa_{O_2}$$
$$= 294 - 94$$
$$= \textbf{200 mm Hg}$$

C. The majority of O_2 carried in the blood is bound to Hb (see chapter on O_2 and medical gas therapy).

D. **HbO_2 Dissociation Curve**
   1. This curve plots the relationship between Pa_{O_2} and Sa_{O_2} and the affinity that Hb has for O_2 at various saturation levels.
   2. This S-shaped curve indicates that at Pa_{O_2} levels of less than 60 mm Hg, small increases in Pa_{O_2} result in fairly large increases in Sa_{O_2}.

EXAMPLES

50% of the Hb molecules would be carrying O_2 at a Pa_{O_2} of only 26 mm Hg. As the Pa_{O_2} increases to 40 mm Hg, the Sa_{O_2} increases substantially, to about 75%. As the Pa_{O_2} continues to rise to 60 mm Hg, the Sa_{O_2} increases to approximately 90%.

---

3. The flat portion of the curve indicates that at Pa_{O_2} levels above 60 mm Hg, saturation rises slowly, with a Pa_{O_2} of 70 mm Hg yielding an Sa_{O_2} of 93% and Pa_{O_2} levels between 80 and 100 mm Hg resulting in Sa_{O_2} levels of 95% to 100%.
4. There are various factors that affect the affinity that Hb has for O_2. These factors shift the HbO_2 dissociation curve to the right or the left.
5. If the curve is **shifted to the right,** it indicates that **hemoglobin's affinity for O_2 has decreased** or Hb will release O_2 to the tissues more readily. **Factors which shift the curve to the right include**
   a. Hypercapnia
   b. Acidosis
   c. Hyperthermia
   d. Increased levels of 2,3 DPG
6. If the curve is **shifted to the left,** it indicates **the affinity of Hb for O_2 has increased,** or Hb will not release O_2 to the tissues as readily. **Factors which shift the curve to the left include:**
   a. Hypocapnia
   b. Alkalosis
   c. Hypothermia
   d. Decreased levels of 2,3 DPG
   e. HbCO
7. As O_2 diffuses from the alveoli to the blood (caused by the pressure gradient), it enters an RBC, where it combines with Hb.
8. As O_2 combines with the Hb, the release of CO_2 is enhanced. This is called the **Haldane effect.**
9. As the RBC travels to the tissue it releases the O_2. This release of O_2 is due to the fact

---

*$(Pa_{CO_2} + 10)$ may be used to simplify the math.

that elevated CO_2 levels, which is present around tissues, decreases hemoglobin's affinity for O_2. This is known as the **Bohr effect.**

10. **Levels of hypoxemia**

60 to 79 mm Hg	Mild hypoxemia
40 to 59 mm Hg	Moderate hypoxemia
< 40 mm Hg	Severe hypoxemia

11. **Normal Pao_2 levels:** Subtract 1 mm Hg from 80 mm Hg for each year over 60 to determine normal Pao_2 by age.

Age (yr)	Pao_2 (mm Hg)
< 60	80–100
60	80
65	75
70	70
75	65
80	60

12. **P-50**
   a. The O_2 tension at which 50% of the Hb is saturated when the blood is 37° C, has a Pco_2 level of 40 mm Hg and a pH level of 7.40.
   b. Normal P-50 is 26.6 mm Hg.
   c. Used to describe affinity of Hb for O_2.
      (1) Increased P-50 indicates decreased affinity
      (2) decreased P-50 indicates increased affinity

13. **Sao_2**
   a. Refers to the quantity of O_2 being carried by the Hb compared with the maximum that may be carried.
   b. **Normal Sao_2 level is 95% to 99%.**

III. CO_2 TRANSPORT AND ALVEOLAR VENTILATION

A. CO_2 makes up approximately 0.03% of inspired air.

B. CO_2 is the by-product of cellular metabolism, and it is by this mechanism that it enters the blood.

C. After CO_2 enters the blood it takes one of two routes.
   1. 5% of the CO_2 dissolves in the plasma.
   2. The remaining 95% enters RBCs.
      a. Approximately 65% of the CO_2 entering the RBC is quickly converted to hydrogen and HCO_3^- ions. (These ions are produced from carbonic acid, which is formed when water and CO_2 dissociate.)
      b. The remaining CO_2 entering the RBC combines with Hb.
      c. Therefore, CO_2 is carried in the blood three ways

   (1) Dissolved in the plasma
   (2) Bound to Hb
   (3) As HCO_3^-

D. **The adequacy of ventilation is determined by the $Paco_2$ level.**
   1. Normal $Paco_2$ range is 35 to 45 mm Hg.
   2. **$Paco_2$ levels < 35 mm Hg** indicate **hypocapnia,** which is excess CO_2 elimination or **hyperventilation.**
   3. **$Paco_2$ levels > 45 mm Hg** indicate **hypercapnia,** which is inadequate CO_2 elimination or **hypoventilation.**

★ E. $Paco_2$ increases when respiratory rate or VT (minute volume) decreases or dead space increases. $Paco_2$ decreases when rate or VT increases or dead space decreases.

IV. ACID-BASE BALANCE (pH)

A. In simple terms, the pH level is determined by the amount of carbonic acid (H_2CO_3) in the blood in relation to the amount of bicarbonate base (HCO_3^-) in the blood.
   1. Henderson Hasselbach equation

$$pH = pK + \log \frac{base}{acid}$$

   pK = dissociation constant = 6.1
   2. Clinically, we may state

$$pH = pK + \log \frac{HCO_3^-}{Pco_2}$$

   3. The important ideas to remember from this equation are
      a. **When HCO_3^- increases** and CO_2 remains unchanged, the **pH increases.**
      b. **When HCO_3^- decreases** and CO_2 remains unchanged, the **pH decreases.**
      c. **When CO_2 increases** and HCO_3^- remains unchanged, the **pH decreases.**
      d. **When CO_2 decreases** and HCO_3^- remains unchanged, the **pH increases.**

> **Note**
>
> For every 20 mm Hg increase in $Paco_2$, the pH will decrease by 0.10. For every 10 mm Hg decrease in $Paco_2$, the pH will increase by 0.10.

B. The ratio of HCO_3^- to H_2CO_3 is 20:1, which is a pH of 7.40.

C. The normal plasma pH range is **7.35 to 7.45.**
   1. A **pH < 7.35** is termed **acidemia** and indicates a higher than normal hydrogen

ion concentration. **Acidemia occurs as a result of**

★ a. Increased P_{CO_2} levels
★ b. Decreased HCO_3^- levels

2. A **pH > 7.45** is termed **alkalemia** and indicates a below-normal hydrogen ion concentration. **Alkalemia occurs as a result of**

★ a. Decreased P_{CO_2} levels
★ b. Increased HCO_3^- levels

D. **Respiratory versus Metabolic Components**
   1. When the initial pH change is the result of a P_{CO_2} change, a respiratory disturbance has occurred.
      a. An **increased P_{CO_2} level (> 45 mm Hg) decreases the pH (< 7.35).** This is **respiratory acidemia,** and if the HCO_3^- level is still within normal limits, it is acute or uncompensated. An example of acute (uncompensated) respiratory acidemia is: pH, 7.25; P_{aCO_2}, 60 mm Hg; HCO_3^-, 25 mEq/L (normal, 22 to 26 mEq/L).
      b. A **decreased P_{CO_2} level (< 35 mm Hg) increases the pH (> 7.45).** This is **respiratory alkalemia,** and if the HCO_3^- level is still within normal limits, it is acute or uncompensated. An example of acute (uncompensated) respiratory alkalemia is: pH, 7.53; P_{aCO_2}, 29 mm Hg; HCO_3^-, 23 mEq/L.
   2. When the initial pH change is the result of a HCO_3^- change, a metabolic disturbance has occurred.
      a. A **decreased HCO_3^- level (< 22 mEq/L) decreases the pH (< 7.35).** This is **metabolic acidemia,** and if the P_{aCO_2} level is within normal limits, it is acute or uncompensated. An example of acute (uncompensated) metabolic acidemia is: pH, 7.24; P_{aCO_2}, 38 mm Hg; HCO_3^-, 13 mEq/L.
      b. An **increased HCO_3^- (> 26 mEq/L) increases the pH (> 7.45).** This is **metabolic alkalemia,** and if the P_{aCO_2} level is within normal limits, it is acute or uncompensated. An example of acute (uncompensated) metabolic alkalemia is: pH, 7.54; P_{aCO_2}, 41 mm Hg; HCO_3^-, 33 mEq/L.

E. **pH Compensation**
   1. The levels of HCO_3^- and CO_2 always change to keep the pH within the normal range. This is called **compensation.**
   2. If the P_{CO_2} initially changes the pH, the HCO_3^- will change accordingly to return the pH to normal.

EXAMPLES

(A) pH 7.27; P_{aCO_2} 58 mm Hg; HCO_3^- 31 mEq/L   (B) pH 7.37; P_{aCO_2} 58 mm Hg; HCO_3^- 35 mEq/L

The (A) example is a **partially compensated respiratory acidemia.** The elevated P_{aCO_2} level caused the initial drop in pH. The HCO_3^- level is increasing to elevate the pH back to normal. Since the pH is approaching normal but is still low, this makes it **partially compensated.**

As the pH returns to normal (B), resulting from the continued increase in the HCO_3^- level, this is called **chronic** or **compensated respiratory acidemia.**

(A) pH 7.53; P_{aCO_2} 26 mm Hg; HCO_3^- 16 mEq/L   (B) pH 7.43; P_{aCO_2} 27 mm Hg; HCO_3^- 12 mEq/L

The (A) example is a **partially compensated respiratory alkalemia.** The decreased P_{aCO_2} level caused the initial increase in pH. The HCO_3^- level is decreasing to drop the pH back to normal. Since the pH is approaching normal but is still high, this makes it **partially compensated.**

As the pH returns to normal (B), resulting from the continuing decreasing HCO_3^- level, this is a **chronic or compensated respiratory alkalemia.**

3. If the HCO_3^- level initially changes the pH, the P_{aCO_2} level will change accordingly to return the pH to normal.

(A) pH 7.21; P_{aCO_2} 22 mm Hg; HCO_3^- 12 mEq/L   (B) pH 7.36; P_{aCO_2} 14 mm Hg; HCO_3^- 13 mEq/L

The (A) example is a **partially compensated metabolic acidemia.** The decreased HCO_3^- level caused the initial drop in pH. The patient is hyperventilating (decreasing P_{aCO_2} levels) to elevate the pH back to normal. Since the pH is approaching normal but is still low, this is **partially compensated.** As the pH returns to normal (B), resulting from the continuing drop in P_{aCO_2}, this is a **compensated metabolic acidemia.**

(A) pH 7.50; P_{aCO_2} 51 mm Hg; HCO_3^- 31 mEq/L   (B) pH 7.44; P_{aCO_2} 59 mm Hg; HCO_3^- 31 mEq/L

The (A) example is a **partially compensated metabolic alkalemia.** The increased HCO_3^- caused the initial increase in pH. The patient is hypoventilating (increasing P_{aCO_2} levels) to drop the pH back to normal. Since the pH is approaching normal but still high, this is **partially compensated.** As the pH returns to normal (B), resulting from the continuing P_{aCO_2} retention, this is a **compensated metabolic alkalemia.**

> **Note**
>
> When interpreting a compensated blood gas: If the compensated pH is 7.35 to 7.40, the pH must be assumed to have been acidotic initially. Decide if the $PaCO_2$ or HCO_3^- caused the initial acidemia. Similarly, if the compensated pH is 7.40 to 7.45, the pH must be assumed to have been alkalotic initially. Decide if the $PaCO_2$ or HCO_3^- caused the initial alkalemia. Metabolic compensation takes several hours to occur, whereas respiratory compensation may occur in minutes.

F. **Mixed Respiratory and Metabolic Component**
- a. When both the $PaCO_2$ and HCO_3^- cause the pH to move in the same direction, this is called a mixed or combined component.
- b. An example of a mixed component is:

pH	7.21
$PaCO_2$	55 mm Hg
HCO_3^-	18 mEq/L

This is an example of **mixed respiratory and metabolic acidemia.** An elevated $PaCO_2$ and decreased HCO_3^- both contribute to acidemia.

V. **ABG INTERPRETATION**
A. **ABG Normal Value Chart Summary**

pH	7.35–7.45
$PaCO_2$	35–45 mm Hg
PaO_2	80–100 mm Hg
HCO_3^-	22–26 mEq/L
Base excess (BE)	−2 to +2

Total base deficit (BD) −2 or total base excess (BE) +2

B. **Basic Steps to ABG Interpretation**
1. Determine the acid-base status by observing the pH.
   - a. Is the pH acidotic (< 7.35)?
   - b. Is the pH alkalotic (> 7.45)?
2. Determine if the pH change is the result of $PaCO_2$ change or a HCO_3^- change.
3. When this is determined, observe for signs of compensation. If the $PaCO_2$ caused the initial pH change, is the HCO_3^- changing to return the pH back to normal?
4. Determine oxygenation status by observing PaO_2.
C. **ABG Example Problems**
1. ABG levels are

pH	7.23
$PaCO_2$	57 mm Hg
PaO_2	81 mm Hg
HCO_3^-	24 mEq/L
BE	−1

- a. Acid/base status: **Acidemia**
- b. Ventilatory status: **Elevated $PaCO_2$; hypoventilation resulting in decreased pH**
- c. Metabolic status: **Normal HCO_3^-; no compensation occurring at this time**
- d. Oxygenation status: **Normal PaO_2**
- e. Interpretation: **Uncompensated (acute) respiratory acidemia**
- f. To correct: **Institute mechanical ventilation** to increase the patient's minute volume, or **increase the ventilator rate or V_T if patient is already on a ventilator.**
2. ABG levels are

pH	7.57
$PaCO_2$	25 mm Hg
PaO_2	98 mm Hg
HCO_3^-	25 mEq/L
BE	0

- a. Acid/base status: **Alkalemia**
- b. Ventilatory status: **Decreased $PaCO_2$; hyperventilation resulting in an increased pH**
- c. Metabolic status: **Normal HCO_3^-; no compensation occurring at this time**
- d. Oxygenation: **Normal PaO_2**
- e. Interpretation: **Uncompensated (acute) respiratory alkalemia**
- f. To correct: **Decrease the ventilator rate or V_T or add mechanical dead space.**
3. ABG levels are

pH	7.45
$PaCO_2$	35 mm Hg
PaO_2	53 mm Hg
HCO_3^-	26 mEq/L
BE	+2

- a. Acid/base status: **Normal pH**
- b. Ventilation status: **Normal $PaCO_2$**
- c. Metabolic status: **Normal HCO_3^-**
- d. Oxygenation status: **Moderate hypoxemia**
- e. Interpretation: **Normal acid/base status with moderate hypoxemia**
- f. To correct: **If patient is on 60% or more O_2 mask, place on CPAP, or add PEEP if ventilator patient is on 60% or more O_2.**

4. ABG levels are

pH	7.38
Pa_{CO_2}	61 mm Hg
Pa_{O_2}	54 mm Hg
HCO_3^-	33 mEq/L
BE	+9

a. Acid/base status: **Normal pH**
b. Ventilatory status: **Increased Pa_{CO_2}; hypoventilation resulting in decreased pH**
c. Metabolic status: **Elevated HCO_3^-; compensating for initial acidemia**
d. Oxygenation status: **Moderate hypoxemia**
e. Interpretation: **Compensated (chronic) respiratory acidemia.** Since the compensated pH is between 7.35 and 7.40, we must assume this was initially an acidemia caused by an elevated Pa_{CO_2}.
f. To correct: **This is a classic example of "normal" ABG levels on a patient with chronic lung disease, therefore no change in present therapy is needed.**

5. ABG levels are

pH	7.29
Pa_{CO_2}	43 mm Hg
Pa_{O_2}	87 mm Hg
HCO_3^-	16 mEq/L
BE	−7

a. Acid/base status: **Acidemia**
b. Ventilatory status: **Normal Pa_{CO_2}**
c. Metabolic status: **Decreased HCO_3^-, resulting in decreased pH**
d. Oxygenation status: **Normal Pa_{O_2}**
e. Interpretation: **Uncompensated metabolic acidemia.** No compensation is occurring, since the Pa_{CO_2} is normal.
f. To correct: **Give $NaHCO_3^-$.** No ventilator parameter changes or oxygenation modifications are necessary at this time.

6. ABG levels are

pH	7.20
Pa_{CO_2}	22 mm Hg
Pa_{O_2}	83 mm Hg
HCO_3^-	15 mEq/L
BE	−10

a. Acid/base status: **Acidemia**
b. Ventilatory status: **Decreased Pa_{CO_2}; hyperventilation compensating for initial acidemia**
c. Metabolic status: **Decreased HCO_3^-; resulting in a decreased pH**
d. Oxygenation status: **Normal Pa_{O_2}**
e. Interpretation: **Partially compensated metabolic acidemia,** This was an initial metabolic acidemia followed by hyperventilation. By removing more CO_2, the pH is returning toward normal. It's not fully compensated, since the pH is not within normal limits at this time. **This is an example of a patient with diabetic acidosis (ketoacidosis).**
f. To correct: **May administer $NaHCO_3^-$.**

VI. **ARTERIAL BLOOD GAS INTERPRETATION CHART**
Key for table: N, normal; I, increased; D, decreased.

	pH	P_{CO_2}	HCO_3^-
Uncompensated (acute)			
Respiratory acidemia	D	I	N
Respiratory alkalemia	I	D	N
Metabolic acidemia	D	N	D
Metabolic alkalemia	I	N	I
Partially compensated			
Respiratory acidemia	D	I	I
Respiratory alkalemia	I	D	D
Metabolic acidemia	D	D	D
Metabolic alkalemia	I	I	I
Fully compensated (chronic)			
Respiratory acidemia	N	I	I
Respiratory alkalemia	N	D	D
Metabolic acidemia	N	D	D
Metabolic alkalemia	N	I	I
Mixed respiratory/metabolic			
Acidemia	D	I	D
Alkalemia	I	D	I

VII. **BLOOD GAS ANALYZERS**
A. Currently, blood gas analyzers have the following capabilities
1. Accurate measurement of pH, P_{CO_2}, and P_{O_2}
2. Self-calibration
3. Accurate measurement of base excess or deficit
4. Accurate measurement of plasma bicarbonate (HCO_3^-)
5. Correction for temperature
6. Self-troubleshooting abilities
7. Automated blood gas interpretation
B. **Blood Gas Electrodes**
1. **Sanz electrode: measures pH** by quantifying the acidity and alkalinity of a solution of blood. This is accomplished by the measurement of the potential difference across a pH-sensitive glass membrane.
2. **Severinghaus electrode: measures P_{CO_2}** by causing the CO_2 gas to produce hydrogen ions by means of a chemical reaction.
3. **Clark electrode: measures P_{O_2}** as a result of a chemical reaction in which electron flow is measured.

POST-CHAPTER STUDY QUESTIONS

1. Interpret the meaning of the following arterial blood gas levels.
   A. pH 7.21, $PaCO_2$ 43 mm Hg, PaO_2 81 mm Hg, HCO_3^- 14 mEq/L
   B. pH 7.36, $PaCO_2$ 62 mm Hg, PaO_2 58 mm Hg, HCO_3^- 36 mEq/L
   C. pH 7.57, $PaCO_2$ 27 mm Hg, PaO_2 89 mm Hg, HCO_3^- 24 mEq/L
   D. pH 7.22, $PaCO_2$ 51 mm Hg, PaO_2 71 mm Hg, HCO_3^- 17 mEq/L
   E. pH 7.44, $PaCO_2$ 28 mm Hg, PaO_2 80 mm Hg, HCO_3^- 18 mEq/L
   F. pH 7.32, $PaCO_2$ 52 mm Hg, PaO_2 84 mm Hg, HCO_3^- 31 mEq/L
2. What do the results of an Allen's test mean?
3. What conditions shift the HbO_2 dissociation curve to the right?
4. When the HbO_2 curve is shifted to the right, how does that affect the affinity of Hb for O_2?
5. Calculate the $P(A-a)O_2$, given the following data.

   PB   747 mm Hg

   ABG levels in patient on 40% O_2

pH	7.42
$PaCO_2$	45 mm Hg
PaO_2	80 mm Hg
HCO_3^-	25 mEq/L

6. Which ABG value best reflects the patient's ability to ventilate?
7. List a set of ABG levels that are typical of a patient with diabetic ketoacidosis.

Answers are at the end of the chapter.

REFERENCES

Barnes TA: Respiratory care practice, Chicago, 1988, Year-Book Medical Publishers.

Eubanks D and Bone R: Comprehensive respiratory care, ed 2, St. Louis, 1990, The CV Mosby Co.

Lane EE: Clinical arterial blood gas analysis, St. Louis, 1987, The CV Mosby Co.

Malley WJ: Clinical blood gases: application and noninvasive alternatives, Philadelphia, 1990, WB Saunders Co.

McPherson SP: Respiratory therapy equipment, ed 5, St. Louis, 1995, The CV Mosby Co.

Shapiro B, Peruzzi W, and Templin R: Clinical application of blood gases, ed 5, St. Louis, 1994, Mosby-Yearbook Inc.

PRE-TEST ANSWERS

1. B
2. D
3. C
4. A
5. D
6. D

ANSWERS TO POST-CHAPTER STUDY QUESTIONS

1. Interpretation is as follows
   A. Uncompensated metabolic acidemia, normal oxygenation
   B. Fully compensated (chronic) respiratory acidemia, moderate hypoxemia
   C. Uncompensated respiratory alkalemia, normal oxygenation
   D. Combined respiratory and metabolic acidemia, mild hypoxemia
   E. Fully compensated respiratory alkalemia, normal oxygenation
   F. Partially compensated respiratory acidemia, normal oxygenation
2. An Allen's test is done before radial artery puncture to determine collateral blood flow to the hand. It is essential to determine if ulnar blood flow is present, in case the radial artery spasms or clots.
3. Hypercapnia, acidosis, hyperthermia, increased 2,3-DPG
4. When the curve shifts to the right, the Hb affinity for O_2 decreases, which makes O_2 binding more difficult, but the O_2 that does bind with Hb will be released more easily to the tissues.
5. 144 mm Hg; $PaO_2 = [(747 - 47) \times 0.40] = (45 \times 1.25)$

   $280 - 56 = 224$
   $PaO_2 - PaO_2 = 224 - 80 = 146$
6. $PaCO_2$
7. pH 7.25, $PaCO_2$ 23 mm Hg, PaO_2 80 mm Hg, HCO_3^- 12 mEq/L; partially compensated metabolic acidemia. The initial problem is metabolic acidemia. The patient responds to this acidemia by hyperventilation to remove CO_2, which begins bringing the pH back up toward normal levels. Your answer should show the levels of pH, $PaCO_2$, and HCO_3^- all decreased.

Chapter 11

Ventilator Management

PRE-TEST QUESTIONS

1. The following information has been obtained from a ventilator patient.

Peak inspiratory pressure	48 cm H_2O
Plateau pressure	27 cm H_2O
V_T	850 mL
PEEP	4 cm H_2O

   Based on this data, the patient's static lung compliance is approximately which of the following?

   A. 18 mL/cm H_2O
   B. 20 mL/cm H_2O
   C. 31 mL/cm H_2O
   D. 37 mL/cm H_2O

2. A volume-cycled ventilator is in the control mode and the I/E ratio alarm is sounding. Which control adjustment would correct this problem?

   A. Decrease the flow rate.
   B. Increase the V_T.
   C. Increase the respiratory rate.
   D. Increase the flow rate.

3. Mechanical ventilation can lead to which of the following complications?

   I. Increased renal output
   II. Barotrauma
   III. Increased cardiac output

   A. I only
   B. II only
   C. I and II only
   D. II and III only

4. Static lung compliance will decrease as a result of which of the following?

   A. Bronchospasm
   B. Mucosal edema
   C. Atelectasis
   D. Bronchial secretions

5. These data have been collected from a ventilator patient in the control mode.

V_T	800 mL	ABG levels: pH	7.50
Rate	15/min	$PaCO_2$	30 mm Hg
FIO_2	0.45	PaO_2	98 mm Hg

   To increase this patient's $PaCO_2$ to 40 mm Hg, the ventilator rate should be adjusted to what level?

   A. 10/min
   B. 11/min
   C. 12/min
   D. 13/min

6. The following data have been collected from a patient on a Bennett 7200 ventilator in the control mode.

V_T	700 mL	ABG levels: pH	7.44
Rate	10/min	$PaCO_2$	42 mm Hg
FIO_2	0.50	PaO_2	58 mm Hg

   Based on this information, the respiratory therapist should recommend which of the following ventilator changes?

   A. Increase FIO_2 to 0.60.
   B. Increase V_T to 800 mL.
   C. Add 5 cm H_2O of PEEP.
   D. Place on CPAP of 4 cm H_2O and an FIO_2 of 0.50.

Answers are at the end of the chapter.

REVIEW

I. **NEGATIVE VS. POSITIVE PRESSURE VENTILATORS**
   A. **Negative Pressure Ventilation**
      1. **Iron lung** (body tank respirator)
         a. Patient is placed in an airtight cylinder up to his or her neck. The head is exposed to ambient conditions.

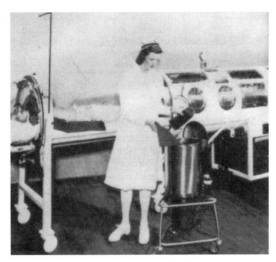

Introduction to Respiratory Care. Philadelphia, 1990, WB Saunders, (Courtesy of JH Emerson Co., Cambridge, Mass.)

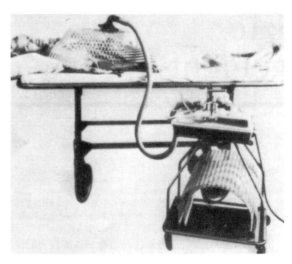

Introduction to Respiratory Care. Philadelphia, 1990, WB Saunders, (Courtesy of JH Emerson Co., Cambridge, Mass.)

b. The underside of the cylinder has a bellows that is powered by an electric motor or by hand.

c. As the bellows descends, it drops the pressure within the airtight chamber to below atmospheric pressure. This sets up a pressure gradient between the inside of the cylinder and the patient's mouth (which is at atmospheric pressure) and air flows into the airways.

d. Gas flow stops as the bellows moves upward and pressures equalize. The patient exhales normally because of the elastic recoil of the lungs. The motor moves the bellows up and down in response to a timing mechanism. Therefore, the iron lung is a **time-cycled ventilator.**

e. The iron lung was used extensively during the polio epidemic of the 1950s. It is not now commonly used to ventilate patients.

f. Negative pressures of up to 15 cm H_2O were commonly used to ventilate the patient.

g. **Disadvantages of the iron lung**
(1) Difficult patient care
(2) Strictly a control ventilator; no means of assisting a breath but may breathe spontaneously between machine breaths.
(3) Difficult to clean
(4) Large and cumbersome
(5) No means of regulating flow
(6) "Tank shock" occurs: pooling of abdominal blood, resulting in decreased venous return

2. **Cuirass** (chest respirator)

a. A plastic shell that covers the chest that was designed to minimize the disadvantages of the iron lung.

b. A flexible hose connects to the shell and is attached to an electric pump, which creates a negative extrathoracic pressure.

c. Since only the thorax receives negative pressure, and not the abdomen, "tank shock" is eliminated. Therefore, venous return is enhanced during inspiration.

d. The cuirass is used to wean patients off the iron lung or for home use on paralyzed patients.

e. **Disadvantages of the cuirass**
(1) Noisy
(2) No means of regulating flow
(3) Difficult to maintain a tight fit
(4) Difficult patient care

f. **Advantages of the cuirass (over the iron lung)**
(1) Patient care is easier
(2) A flow-sensing device may be used to allow patient-triggered breaths.

B. **Positive Pressure Ventilation**
1. Types of positive pressure ventilators
a. Preset volume ventilators (volume-limited or volume-cycled)
b. Preset pressure ventilators (pressure-limited or pressure-cycled)
2. **Volume ventilators**
a. A preset VT is delivered to the patient in each machine breath, and once it is delivered, inspiration ends.
b. The volume-limited ventilator can develop an inspiratory pressure that maintains the preset VT when changes in airway resistance and compliance occur (i.e., volume is constant, pressure is variable).

c. Used for mechanical ventilation of adult patients.

3. **Pressure-cycled ventilators**

a. A preset inspiratory pressure is delivered to the patient, and once it is reached, inspiration ends.

★ b. The delivered V_T is unknown but varies with changes in airway resistance and lung compliance (i.e., volume varies, pressure is constant).

★ c. When lung compliance decreases, delivered V_T decreases. In other words, as the patient's lungs become stiffer and harder to ventilate, the delivered V_T decreases.

d. The pressure control is used like the volume control. When inspiratory pressure is increased, delivered V_T is increased, and vice versa.

e. Used to ventilate infants and postoperative patients and to administer IPPB treatments. Inspiration ends on most infant ventilators when a preset time is reached. The set inspiratory pressure is reached during that time.

f. Recently, **pressure control ventilation (PCV)** has been used as a mode of ventilation, especially for adult patients with ARDS in whom conventional volume ventilation with PEEP has not improved ventilation or oxygenation.

g. Specific indications for PCV vary, but generally the patient should be on the following ventilator parameters before PCV is instituted:
   (1) F_{IO_2}, 1.0
   (2) PEEP > 15 cm H_2O
   (3) PIP > 50 cm H_2O
   (4) Assist/control rate > 16/min

> **Note**
>
> While on these settings, the patient should have decreased lung compliance and hypoxemia.

h. Initial settings for PCV should include
   (1) F_{IO_2}, 1.0
   (2) PIP of about 50% of that on volume ventilation

> **Note**
>
> PIP should be set to obtain a specified exhaled VT. In other words, if the "target" exhaled VT is 600 mL and the actual exhaled VT is 500 mL, the PIP should be increased.

(3) V_T, 6 to 10 mL/kg of ideal body weight
(4) PEEP of about 50% of the volume ventilator setting
(5) I/E, 1:2

> **Note**
>
> PCV is often combined with inverse I/E ratio ventilation. Because this type of ventilation may be uncomfortable, the patient should be sedated and paralyzed.

i. Studies have shown that PCV improves gas exchange, increases oxygenation, reduces PIP, increases mean airway pressure, reduces required PEEP levels, and decreases minute ventilation, especially when it is combined with an inverse I/E ratio. It has also been shown to reduce cardiovascular side effects and barotrauma compared with volume ventilation with PEEP.

j. It is important that exhaled V_T is monitored during PCV. Since inspiration is pressure-limited, the volume will vary with changes in lung compliance and airway resistance.

k. If an inverse I/E ratio of *greater* than 2:1 is used, intrinsic PEEP, also referred to as auto-PEEP, may occur. Auto-PEEP may be detected by monitoring expiratory wave-form curves, which reveals the expiratory flow not returning to zero before the next breath. Auto-PEEP may result in barotrauma, decreased venous return and cardiac output, and increased patient effort to initiate a breath, if the patient is assisting.

l. Extensive monitoring of the patient's cardiovascular and respiratory parameters is vital for patients on PCV.

m. Another type of pressure ventilation is **bilevel positive airway pressure or BiPAP. BiPAP** may be used on intubated or nonintubated patients. Since COPD patients are difficult to wean from mechanical ventilation, BiPAP is being used to ventilate these patients through a nasal mask, avoiding intubation and conventional volume ventilation. BiPAP may buy time for the patient to get past the initial ventilatory crisis and avoid intubation and ventilation. Certainly not always successful, it is becoming a first step in ventilating many COPD patients.

n. BiPAP is also used in home ventilation for patients with neuromuscular dysfunction, obstructive sleep apnea, and other conditions that result in hypoventilation.

o. BiPAP may be time-cycled or patient-cycled. Once inspiration begins, a preset *inspiratory positive airway pressure* (IPAP) is reached. Expiratory positive airway pressure (EPAP) should be preset to avoid CO_2 buildup in the nasal mask. EPAP is the equivalent of PEEP.

p. The initial IPAP setting is usually 10 cm H_2O, and the EPAP setting is 4 cm H_2O. The difference between the IPAP and EPAP settings is the pressure support. In this example, pressure support is 6 cm H_2O. IPAP settings range from 2 to 25 cm H_2O and EPAP ranges from 2 to 20 cm H_2O.

q. A frequency control determines the timed breath rate and is adjustable from 6 to 30 cycles/min. The % IPAP control is set to determine the time spent in inspiration and functions as the I/E ratio control.

r. BiPAP is not a life-support ventilator. The practitioner should use an IPAP that results in an exhaled V_T of 7 to 10 mL/kg of ideal body weight.

s. Criteria for BiPAP mask ventilation include stable hemodynamics, cooperative patient, minimal airway secretions, and no need for airway protection

II. **VENTILATOR CONTROLS**
   A. **Ventilator Modes (Volume Ventilators)**
      1. **Control mode**
         a. Patient cannot initiate inspiration.
         b. Inspiration is initiated by a timing device.

EXAMPLE:

Control rate of 10: the ventilator delivers a breath every 6 seconds (60 ÷ 10). Minute volume remains constant because rate cannot be altered.

      c. Patient should be heavily sedated or paralyzed.
      2. **Assist mode**
         a. The patient initiates inspiration by creating a preset negative pressure, which delivers a machine-controlled V_T.

b. The sensitivity control determines how much negative pressure is required to initiate inspiration. It should be adjusted to **−0.5 to −2.0 cm H_2O.**

c. The patient **must** initiate inspiration. There is no backup rate if the patient becomes apneic. This mode is seldom used.

3. **Assist-control mode**
   a. The patient initiates inspiration by creating a negative pressure, but in case the patient fails to cycle the ventilator into inspiration, a backup rate is set and a machine V_T breath is delivered.
   b. This is a commonly used mode of ventilation.
   c. The patient can receive as many machine breaths as they require above the set rate; therefore, the patient's minute volume is not consistent.

4. **Intermittent Mandatory Ventilation (IMV)**

Exam Note

IMV, using the H-valve assembly, should appear on the RRT examination only.

a. The ventilator delivers a set number of machine breaths, but the patient is able to breathe spontaneously between machine breaths through an **H-valve assembly.**
b. The H valve provides a separate gas source (either a nebulizer or reservoir bag) from which the patient breathes, which is attached to the inspiratory side of the circuit (see diagrams). The sensitivity control is turned off, so that the patient cannot cycle the ventilator into inspiration while breathing spontaneously.
c. **Reservoir bag IMV setup** (see diagram on page 123)
d. **Nebulizer IMV setup** (see diagram on page 123)
e. One way valves (H valves) are incorporated into the setup, so that gas flows only in the direction of the patient from the inspiratory limb of the ventilator circuit.
f. To ensure adequate flow for spontaneous breaths, the reservoir bag should remain one-third to one-half full at all times. If a nebulizer setup is used, mist exiting the H-valve reservoir should be

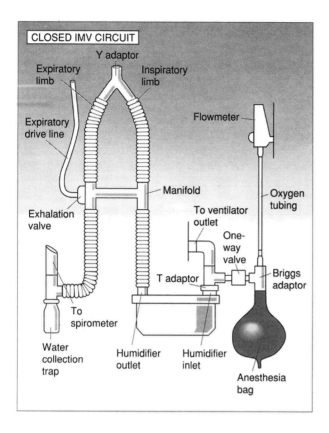

CLOSED IMV CIRCUIT

Y adaptor; Expiratory limb; Inspiratory limb; Flowmeter; Expiratory drive line; Manifold; Oxygen tubing; To ventilator outlet; One-way valve; Exhalation valve; T adaptor; Briggs adaptor; To spirometer; Water collection trap; Humidifier outlet; Humidifier inlet; Anesthesia bag

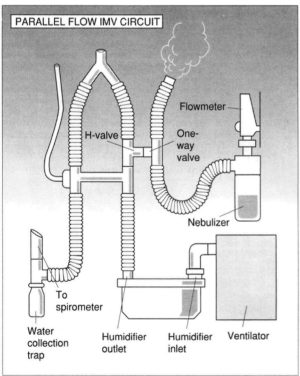

PARALLEL FLOW IMV CIRCUIT

Flowmeter; H-valve; One-way valve; Nebulizer; To spirometer; Water collection trap; Humidifier outlet; Humidifier inlet; Ventilator

visible at all times. If these conditions are not observed, **increase the flow to the H-valve set-up.**

g. The one-way valve must be placed correctly to open **toward** the patient. If

placed backwards, the patient will not be able to open the valve and receive gas flow for spontaneous breathing. This is recognized by observing an increased work of breathing and excessive negative pressure on the ventilator pressure manometer during inspiration.

★ h. During spontaneous inspiration, the manometer needle should be observed deflecting no more than -2 cm H_2O. If it is deflecting more than -2 cm H_2O, make sure the one-way valve is opened towards the patient. If it is, increase the flow. The needle deflecting more than -2 cm H_2O will also occur if inadequate flow to the H-valve assembly is present.

l. IMV was designed to aid in the ventilator weaning process.

★ j. This IMV system allows "breath-stacking" to occur. This means that the ventilator (being time-cycled) will deliver a breath at a specific time, depending on the dialed-in rate. It may come while the patient is breathing spontaneously.

5. **Synchronized Intermittent Mandatory Ventilation (SIMV)**
   a. Allows for spontaneous breathing along with positive pressure ventilator breaths. It is built into the ventilator and senses when the patient is breathing spontaneously, therefore no "breath-stacking" occurs.
   b. It is used as both a weaning technique and for ventilation prior to weaning.
   c. The sensitivity is left on as the patient must open a demand valve to obtain gas flow for spontaneous breathing.

6. **Pressure Support Ventilation (PSV)**
   a. This mode of ventilation is found on the new generation of ventilators that aid in the weaning process from the ventilator.
   b. It is a patient-assisted, pressure-generated, flow-cycled breath, which may be augmented with SIMV or used by itself.
   c. It was designed to make spontaneous breathing through the ET tube during weaning more comfortable by overcoming the high resistance and increased inspiratory work caused by the ET tube (**5 to 10 cm H_2O is all that is required to overcome tubing resistance**).
   d. An inspiratory pressure is set (usually 5 to 10 cm H_2O for weaning purposes). As the patient initiates inspiration, the preset pressure is reached and held constant until a specific inspiratory flow is reached. Then the pressure is terminated.

e. The inspiratory pressure level may be set to achieve a specific VT.

f. PSV may be used for patients who are ventilating well but are intubated to protect their airway or for patients on CPAP with oxygenation deficiencies.

7. **Continuous Positive Airway Pressure (CPAP)**

a. May be achieved with the use of a CPAP mask, nasal prongs, or intubation and a ventilator.

b. A preset pressure is maintained in the airways as the patient breathes totally on his or her own. No positive-pressure breaths are delivered.

c. Patients whose PaO_2 cannot be maintained within normal limits on a **60% or more O_2 mask, and who have normal or low $PaCO_2$ levels, should be placed on CPAP.** Patients with **obstructive sleep apnea benefit from CPAP** to relieve obstruction in the upper airway.

d. CPAP set-ups should always use a **low-pressure alarm** so that leaks in the system will be detected.

e. CPAP separate from the ventilator, such as a CPAP mask, may be accomplished as shown in the diagram.

(1) In this type of setup, the patient's exhaled gas flow enters the expiratory limb of the circuit, where it meets an opposing gas flow entering through a Venturi tube.

(2) This opposing gas flow causes a resistance to exhalation that the patient must overcome.

(3) The pressure the patient must generate to overcome this resistance results in a positive pressure that is read on a manometer placed in the set-up line. This pressure is the CPAP level.

(4) The CPAP level may be increased or decreased by adjusting the opposing gas flow that is passing through the Venturi tube in the expiratory limb.

f. The indications and hazards of CPAP are the same as those listed for PEEP later in this chapter.

B. **VT Control**

1. Determines the delivered VT to the patient in milliliters or liters (varies from 50 mL to 2.2 L)

2. Should be set at **10 to 12 mL/kg of ideal body weight.** Although the old standard of 10 to 15 mL/kg may still be used, current studies advocate using smaller volumes. For children, use 5 to 7 mL/kg of ideal body weight.

a. **Calculating ideal body weight** (in lb)
For males:

$$106 + [6 \times (\text{height in inches} - 60 \text{ in})]$$

For females:

$$105 + [5 \times (\text{height in inches} - 60 \text{ in})]$$

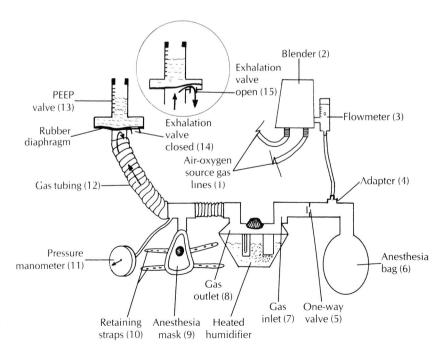

From Eubanks D and Bone R: Comprehensive Respiratory Care, St. Louis, Mosby, 1990.

b. This is very important when you are asked to determine the ventilator V_T for an obese patient.

EXAMPLE:

The physician wants your recommendation for the ventilator V_T setting for a 5 ft 3 in female patient who weighs 150 kg (330 lb).

$$105 + 5 \times (63 - 60)$$
$$105 + (5 \times 3)$$
$$105 + 15 = 120 \text{ lb (ideal body weight)}$$
$$120 \text{ lb} \div 2.2 \text{ lb/kg} = 55 \text{ kg}$$

$$V_T = 12 \text{ mL/kg} \times 55 \text{ kg} = 660 \text{ mL}$$

3. **Increasing the V_T increases alveolar ventilation, while also increasing the minute volume. This decreases the $Paco_2$.**
4. **Decreasing the V_T decreases alveolar ventilation, while also decreasing the minute volume. This increases the $Paco_2$.**

EXAMPLE:

A patient breathing 10/min with a V_T of 600 mL has a minute volume of 6 L. (Minute volume is calculated as respiratory rate $\times$ V_T.) If the patient begins breathing at a respiratory rate of 20/min with a V_T of 300 mL, his or her minute ventilation remains 6 L, but the alveolar ventilation has decreased as a result of the decreased V_T.

5. On volume ventilators:
   a. Increasing the V_T increases the inspiratory time.
   b. Decreasing the V_T decreases the inspiratory time.
6. The preset machine V_T is not the actual volume reaching the patient's lungs.
   a. Volume is "lost" in the ventilator circuit because of airway resistance from gas flow.
   b. Tubing compliance may be calculated to determine how much volume is being lost in the circuit.
   c. With the ventilator set on a specific V_T and the high-pressure limit turned up completely, the machine is cycled into inspiration with the ventilator wye adaptor occluded. Observe the manometer pressure reading.

d. Compliance formula

$$\text{Compliance} = \frac{\text{volume}}{\text{pressure}}$$

EXAMPLE:

Set V_T at 200 mL (0.2 L). Peak pressure reached is 40 cm H_2O.

$$C = \frac{200 \text{ mL}}{40 \text{ cm } H_2O} = 5 \text{ mL/cm } H_2O$$

This means that once the patient is placed on the ventilator, 5 mL of the dialed-in volume will be lost in the tubing for every 1 cm H_2O registering on the manometer.

EXAMPLE:

Tubing compliance, 5 mL/cm H_2O
V_T, 800 mL
Peak inspiratory pressure, 20 cm H_2O

Lost volume = tubing compliance $\times$ peak inspiratory pressure

$$5 \text{ mL/cm } H_2O \times 20 \text{ cm } H_2O = 100 \text{ mL (lost volume)}$$

Dialed-in V_T is 800 mL

$$800 \text{ mL} - 100 \text{ mL (lost volume)} = 700 \text{ mL}$$

e. Lost volume is affected by the water level in the humidifier. Lower water levels allow more compressed volume into the walls of the humidifier, hence more lost volume or less delivered volume to the patient.
f. Volume will also be lost in the patient's conducting airways (e.g., trachea, bronchi) as a result of resistance to gas flow. This part of the patient's airway is called the **anatomic dead space.** It is the part of the airway where no gas exchange occurs, and it is often called "wasted air."

> **Note**
>
> Anatomic dead space is equal to 1 mL/lb of the patient's ideal body weight, but it is reduced by 50% in the intubated patient. Thus, anatomic dead space is equal to about 1 mL/kg.

EXAMPLE:

An intubated 75-kg (165-lb) patient has an anatomic dead space of approximately 75 mL. This means that 75 mL of the patient's VT doesn't reach the alveoli to take part in gas exchange. This may also be subtracted from the ventilator VT setting to obtain a corrected VT.

Note

When using the formula for selecting ventilator VT as 10 to 12 mL/kg of body weight, this lost volume is taken into account, and this is usually an adequate VT. Some ventilators compensate for volume lost in the tubing by delivering a higher VT automatically.

7. Exhaled VT is measured with a bellows spirometer, with the MA-1 ventilator, or by a digital readout. Exhaled VT is most accurately measured with a respirometer placed between the ET tube and ventilator wye adaptor or at the exhalation valve. To most accurately measure **the VT delivered by the ventilator, a respirometer should be placed on the ventilator outlet.**

★ 8. Volume may be lost from other causes.
   a. Loose humidifier jar or tubing connections will register a low exhaled VT reading on spirometer.
   b. Leak around ET-tube cuff results in low exhaled VT reading

★ 9. If the bellows spirometer on the MA-1 ventilator rises during inspiration (it should drop), the most likely cause is a leak in the exhalation valve or a disconnected exhalation valve drive line.

★ 10. If the bellows spirometer (MA-1) fails to empty during inspiration, check the dump valve or reconnect dump-valve tubing.

Exam Note

Although the MA-1 ventilator is not as commonly used as in the past, questions may still be asked on the examination.

C. **Respiratory Rate Control**
   1. **Normal initial setup is 8 to 12 breaths/min.**
   2. **Adjusting the rate control alters the expiratory time, therefore altering the I/E ratio.**
      a. Increasing the rate decreases expiratory time.
      b. Decreasing the rate increases expiratory time.
   3. **Adjusting the rate alters the minute volume.**
      a. Increasing the rate increases minute volume.
      b. Decreasing the rate decreases minute volume.
   4. **Adjusting the rate affects the PaCO$_2$ level.**
      a. Increasing the rate decreases PaCO$_2$.
      b. Decreasing the rate increases PaCO$_2$.

Note

Adjusting the rate to alter the patient's PaCO$_2$ level is more beneficial for patients on controlled ventilation or on SIMV or IMV. On assist/control, the patient may obtain as many machine breaths as needed, no matter what rate is set so the PaCO$_2$ is most effectively altered by adjusting the VT control.

   5. Adjustable on most ventilators from 0.5/min to 60/min.
D. **Inspiratory Flow Control**
   1. Normal setting: 40 to 60 L/min.
   2. Adjusting the flow rate alters the inspiratory time, therefore altering the I/E ratio.
      a. Increasing the flow rate decreases inspiratory time.
      b. Decreasing the flow rate increases inspiratory time.
   3. Adjustable on most ventilators from 20 to 120 L/min.
E. **I/E Ratio**
   1. A comparison of the inspiratory time with the expiratory time.
   2. **Normal I/E ratio for the adult is 1:2.** This means that expiration should be twice as long as inspiration.
   3. Normal I/E ratio for the infant is 1:1.
   4. The I/E ratio is established by the use of **three** ventilator controls on the volume ventilator.
      a. **VT control**
         (1) Increasing the **VT** increases inspiratory time (makes inspiratory time longer).
         (2) Decreasing the **VT** decreases inspiratory time (makes inspiratory time shorter).
      b. **Flow rate control**
         (1) Increasing the flow rate decreases inspiratory time.
         (2) Decreasing the flow rate increases inspiratory time.
      c. **Respiratory rate control**

(1) Increasing the respiratory rate decreases expiratory time.
(2) Decreasing the respiratory rate increases expiratory time.
5. Calculate I/E ratio with following formula

$$I/E = \frac{\text{inspiratory flow rate (L/min)}}{\text{minute volume (L/min)}} - 1 \text{ (for inspiration)}$$

EXAMPLE:

VT	800 mL (.8 L)
Rate	12/min
Flow rate	40 L/min

$$\text{I/E ratio} = \frac{40 \text{ L/min}}{(.8 \text{ L} \times 12)} = \frac{40 \text{ L/min}}{9.6 \text{ L/min}} = 4.2 - 1 = 1:3.2$$

6. **Calculation of inspiratory time**

$$\text{I time} = \frac{\text{total cycle time}}{\text{sum of I/E ratio parts}}$$

EXAMPLE:

Calculate the inspiratory time if the I/E ratio is 1:2 and the ventilator rate is 10/min.

$$\text{Total cycle time} = \frac{60}{10 \text{ (rate)}} = 6 \text{ sec}$$

$$\text{I time} = \frac{6 \text{ sec}}{3 \text{ (I/E parts)}} = 2 \text{ sec}$$

7. Inspiratory time should not exceed expiratory time, except in specific situations. This is referred to as an **inverse I/E ratio.** It may greatly compromise venous blood return to the heart and increase intrathoracic pressure.
   a. If the I/E ratio alarm is sounding on the ventilator, indicating an inverse I:E ratio, three controls may be altered to correct it.
      (1) Rate: decrease to lengthen expiratory time
      (2) Volume: decrease to shorten inspiratory time
      ★ (3) Flow: increase to shorten inspiratory time

Note

Increasing flow is the most common adjustment to correct for an inverse I/E ratio.

F. **O₂ Percentage Control**
   1. Adjustable from 21% to 100% to maintain normal PaO₂ levels.
   ★ 2. O₂ percentage should be increased to a maximum of 60% to maintain normal PaO₂ levels. Once 60% is reached, PEEP should be added or increased.
   ★ 3. O₂ percentage should be reduced first to a level of 60% before decreasing PEEP levels in hyperoxygenated patients.
G. **Sensitivity Control**
   1. This determines the amount of patient effort required to cycle the ventilator into inspiration.
   2. Should be set so that the patient generates **−0.5 to −2.0 cm H₂O pressure.**
   3. If the ventilator self-cycles, the sensitivity is too high. Decrease the sensitivity.
   4. **If it takes more than −2.0 cm H₂O pressure to cycle the ventilator into inspiration, increase the sensitivity.**
   5. In the control mode of ventilation, the sensitivity is turned off and does not allow the patient to trigger a machine breath.
   6. The sensitivity is also turned off on the MA-1 ventilator when using an external gas source (H-valve setup) for the IMV mode.
   ★ 7. On the MA-1, when PEEP is added or increased, the sensitivity must be increased accordingly, and it must be decreased if PEEP is decreased to maintain the patient effort at −2 cm H₂O for triggering a machine breath.
H. **Sigh controls**
   1. Sigh rate should be set at 6 to 12 sighs/hour.
   2. Sigh volume should be set 1.5 to 2.0 times the VT.
   3. Sighs aid in preventing atelectasis.
   4. Usually not functional in the SIMV mode

Exam Note

Although sighs are not commonly used in practice in many areas, the examination may still offer questions on the subject.

I. **Inflation Hold Control**
   1. Adjustable from 0 to 2 sec.
   2. Mechanism keeps the exhalation valve closed, causing the ventilator V_T to be held in the lungs for a preset time.
   3. Used to improve oxygenation by reducing atelectasis and shunting and increasing the diffusion of gases.
   4. Using an inspiratory hold causes an increased intrathoracic pressure.
   5. Used to obtain a plateau pressure to calculate static lung compliance.

J. **Expiratory Retard**
   1. Used to prevent premature airway collapse during expiration (on MA-1 ventilator).
   2. Increases the expiratory time, therefore altering the I/E ratio and increasing intrathoracic pressure.

K. **Positive End-Expiratory Pressure (PEEP)**
   1. Used to maintain positive pressure in the airway after a ventilator breath.
   2. **Indications for PEEP**
      a. Atelectasis
    ★ b. Hypoxemia on 60% or more O_2
      c. Decreased functional residual capacity (FRC)
      d. Lowering O_2 percentage to safe levels (less than 60%)
      e. Decreased lung compliance
      f. Pulmonary edema
   3. **Hazards of PEEP**
      a. Barotrauma
      b. Decreased venous return
      c. Decreased cardiac output
      d. Decreased urinary output
   4. Excessive PEEP levels may lead to decreases in PaO_2 and lung compliance by overdistending already open alveoli and shunting blood to collapsed alveoli.
   5. A decreased cardiac output caused by PEEP is evidenced by a drop in blood pressure and PvO_2 values.
   6. **Optimal PEEP: the level of PEEP that improves lung compliance without decreasing the cardiac output.**
   7. A mixed venous PO_2 (PvO_2) level may be obtained from the pulmonary artery by means of a Swan-Ganz catheter.
      a. **Normal PvO_2 is 35 to 45 mm Hg.**
      b. **A PvO_2 of less than 35 mm Hg indicates a possible decrease in cardiac output. If the PvO_2 drops after initiation of PEEP, it is an indicator of reduced venous return and cardiac output caused by PEEP.**
      c. The PvO_2 value indicates the adequacy of tissue oxygenation.
      d. **Use the PEEP level that provides the best lung compliance and PvO_2 value.**

EXAMPLES:

Determining optimal PEEP
Which of the following represents optimal PEEP?

PEEP (cm H_2O)	PaO_2 (mm Hg)	PvO_2 (mm Hg)
4	68	34
6	74	37
8	78	33
10	82	32

Notice how the PvO_2 decreased after the increase in PEEP from 6 cm H_2O to 8 cm H_2O. This indicates a drop in cardiac output with this PEEP change. Therefore, return to the PEEP level that maintains the highest PvO_2. In this example, the optimal PEEP level is 6 cm H_2O.

Remember that the PaO_2 does not determine optimal PEEP level. Even though the PaO_2 in this example continued to increase at increasing PEEP levels, it did so at the expense of a decreasing cardiac output. This indicates a worsening oxygenation status.

III. **VENTILATOR ALARMS AND MONITORING**
   A. **Low-Pressure Alarm**
      1. Should be set 5 to 10 cm H_2O below peak inspiratory pressure.
    ★ 2. This alarm is activated by leaks in the ventilator circuit or by patient disconnection.
   B. **High-Pressure Alarm**
      1. Should be set 5 to 15 cm H_2O above peak inspiratory pressure.
      2. When this pressure is reached on a volume ventilator, inspiration ends prematurely, decreasing delivered V_T.
    ★ 3. This alarm may be activated by
      a. Decreasing lung compliance
      b. Increasing airway resistance caused by
         (1) Airway secretions
         (2) Bronchospasm
         (3) Water in the ventilator tubing
         (4) Kink in the ventilator tubing
         (5) Patient coughing
   C. **Low PEEP/CPAP Alarm**
      1. Should be set 2 to 4 cm H_2O below the baseline level.
      2. This alarm is activated by leaks in the ventilator circuit or by patient disconnection.

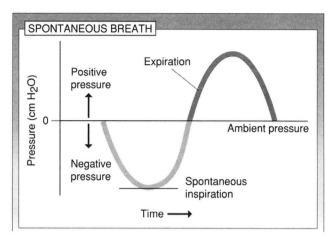

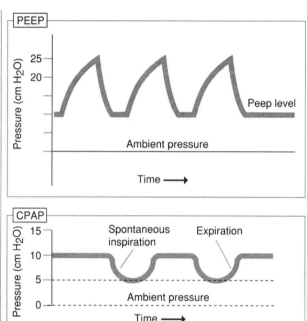

PEEP pressure curves compared with other curves.

f. PEEP level

g. Pressure waveform

h. I/E ratio

3. $\bar{P}aw$ is commonly measured by a digital reading on a $\bar{P}aw$ monitor, or it may be calculated using the following equation.

$$\bar{P}aw = 0.5 + [PIP - PEEP \times \frac{(\text{inspiratory time})}{\text{total respiratory cycle}}$$

4. Optimal $\bar{P}aw$ is the level that improves oxygenation and ventilation without resulting in cardiovascular embarrassment and barotrauma.

5. Studies have shown that $\bar{P}aw$ levels above 12 cm H_2O result in an increased risk of barotrauma.

6. Providing that there has been no change in dynamic compliance or ventilator parameters, if $\bar{P}aw$ decreases, it indicates less pressure required to ventilate the patient's lungs or an increased static lung compliance. An increased $\bar{P}aw$ indicates higher pressure required to ventilate or a decreased static lung compliance.

F. **End-Tidal CO_2 Monitoring (Capnography)**

1. Capnography is a technique by which exhaled CO_2 is measured. This measurement is obtained by the use of a mass spectrometer. (End-tidal CO_2 is abbreviated $PETCO_2$.)

2. Normal $PETCO_2$ is approximately the same as alveolar CO_2, which is equal to arterial PCO_2. $PETCO_2$, therefore, is a noninvasive technique to obtain the patient's $PaCO_2$.

3. $PETCO_2$ may be expressed as partial pressure or a percentage. Normal $PETCO_2$ is 35 to 45 mm Hg **or 4.5% to 5.5%.**

4. There is a difference of approximately 2-5 mm Hg between normal $PaCO_2$ and $PETCO_2$.

5. $PETCO_2$ readings may decrease as a result of any of the following

a. Hyperventilation

b. Apnea (reading falls to zero)

c. Total airway obstruction (reading falls to zero)

d. Conditions in which perfusion is decreased (hypotension, pulmonary embolism, decreased cardiac output). Low reading results from decreased perfusion to the pulmonary capillaries, rendering an inaccurate $PETCO_2$ reading. $PaCO_2$ may be increasing.

6. $PETCO_2$ readings may increase as a result of the following

D. **Apnea Alarm**

1. Set according to the patient's respiratory rate.

2. This alarm is activated after a preset time passes with no inspiratory flow through the tubing.

3. Important alarm for patients on the ventilator in the CPAP mode or low SIMV rates.

E. **Mean Airway Pressure ($\bar{P}aw$) Monitoring**

1. $\bar{P}aw$ is the average pressure applied to the airway over a specific time.

2. $\bar{P}aw$ is directly affected by

a. Ventilator rate

b. Peak inspiratory pressure

c. Inspiratory time

d. Inspiratory hold

e. Expiratory retard

a. Hypoventilation
b. Hyperthermia (increased CO_2 production)

7. Continuous $PETCO_2$ monitoring with tracings is becoming an important technique in monitoring critically ill patients. The tracing records CO_2 readings during inspiration (which should be zero, since little CO_2 is in inspired air) and during expiration, when CO_2 begins to increase.

8. An $PETCO_2$ measurement by itself should not be used to predict $PaCO_2$ in patients with left ventricular failure (decreased cardiac output), pulmonary embolism, or COPD because of inaccurate readings under these conditions.

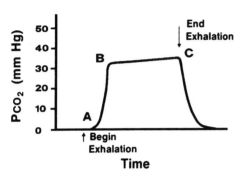

From Eubanks D and Bone R: Comprehensive respiratory care, ed 2, St. Louis, 1990, Mosby, Inc.

IV. **INDICATIONS FOR MECHANICAL VENTILATION**

A. **Apnea**
B. **Acute Ventilatory Failure**
1. $PaCO_2$ of greater than 50 mm Hg indicates ventilatory failure and a need for mechanical assistance.
2. To determine ventilatory failure on a COPD patient who chronically retains CO_2, note whether the pH is below 7.30. If so, there may be a need for ventilator assistance.

C. **Impending Acute Ventilatory Failure**
1. Sometimes normal ABG levels can be deceiving. A patient may have normal ABG levels but the respiratory rate may be 30/min to 40/min to achieve this normal PCO_2 level. This indicates pending ventilatory failure. The patient is likely to tire soon, resulting in an increasing $PaCO_2$ level and ventilatory failure.
2. A patient with a neuromuscular disease, such as Guillain-Barré syndrome, must be monitored closely for lung muscle involvement. **Measurement of the patient's negative inspiratory force and vital capacity best determines the lung status.**

D. **Oxygenation**
1. Patient may be ventilating adequately but oxygenating poorly.
2. Mechanical ventilation is indicated if O_2 deficiency is directly related to an abnormal ventilatory pattern or an increased work of breathing.
3. A patient on an O_2 mask at **60% or more** who is ventilating well (normal or low $PaCO_2$) but is not oxygenating adequately (low PaO_2) is probably exhibiting a large intrapulmonary shunt. This may be corrected with CPAP. Mechanical ventilation may not be necessary initially.

V. **COMMON CRITERIA FOR INITIATION OF MECHANICAL VENTILATION**

A. Vital capacity (VC) of less than 15 mL/kg; normal is 65 to 75 mL/kg.
B. $P(A-a)O_2$ of greater than 450 mm Hg on 100% O_2; normal is 25 to 65 mm Hg.
1. When the PaO_2 is low and the $P(A-a)O_2$ is normal for ambient conditions and the patient's age, hypoxemia is most likely the result of hypoventilation.
2. When the PaO_2 is low and the $P(A-a)O_2$ is high, hypoxemia is most likely the result of either a V/Q mismatch, diffusion defect, or shunting. In this situation, the patient may be hyperventilating to compensate for the hypoxemia.
C. VD/VT ratio of greater than 60%; normal is 25 to 35%.

$$\frac{VD}{VT} = \frac{PaCO_2 - PECO_2}{PaCO_2}$$

D. Unable to obtain a MIP of at least -20 cm H_2O; normal is -50 to -100 cm H_2O.
E. PEP of less than 40 cm H_2O; normal is 100 cm H_2O.

F. Respiratory rate of greater than 35/min; normal is 10/min to 20/min.

VI. GOALS OF MECHANICAL VENTILATION
A. Increased minute ventilation
B. Decreased work of breathing
C. Increased alveolar ventilation
D. ABG levels maintained within normal range
E. Improved distribution of inspired gases. It has been shown that positive pressure breaths on 21% O_2 increase the PaO_2 slightly.

VII. COMPLICATIONS OF MECHANICAL VENTILATION
A. **Barotrauma**
   1. Pneumothorax: may be characterized by **subcutaneous emphysema** (air in the subcutaneous tissues)
   2. Pneumomediastinum
   3. Pneumopericardium
B. **Pulmonary Infection**
   1. Debilitated patients have lower resistance
   2. Contaminated equipment
   3. Improper airway care (e.g., tracheostomy care, suctioning)
   4. Retained secretions as a result of ET tube and poor cough
   5. Ciliary dysfunction caused by ET tube

> **Note**
>
> The most cost-effective method of preventing cross-contamination of patients and equipment is proper handwashing techniques.

C. **Atelectasis**
   1. Using a minimum V_T of 10 mL/kg of body weight prevents this.
   2. Instituting a sigh breath periodically reduces risk.
D. **Pulmonary O_2 Toxicity**
   1. May result in ARDS.
   2. Results from using high O_2 concentrations for prolonged periods.
   3. It is characterized by
      a. Impaired surfactant production
      b. Capillary congestion
      c. Edema
      d. Fibrosis
      e. Thickening of alveolar membranes
      f. Decreased lung compliance, resulting in high peak pressures being required to ventilate the patient. (See chapter on disorders of the respiratory system.)
E. **Tracheal Damage**
   Usually at the cuff site

F. **Decreased Venous Blood Return to the Heart**
   Results from *the positive airway pressures* being transferred onto the large veins returning blood to the heart, resulting in decreased pulmonary blood flow, decreased cardiac output, and decreased blood pressure.
G. **Decreased Urinary Output**
   1. Results from decreased renal blood flow (caused by decreased cardiac output)
   2. Also results from an increased production of *antidiuretic hormone* (ADH).
      a. ADH production increases because of baroreceptors in the atria of the heart, which sense the decreased venous return.
      b. These receptors send a message to the hypothalamus, which stimulates the pituitary gland to secrete more ADH, thereby inhibiting urine excretion.
H. **Lack of Nutrition**
   1. Malnutrition may lead to
      a. Difficulty weaning from the ventilator as a result of weakened respiratory muscles
      b. Reduced response to hypoxia and hypercarbia
      c. Impaired wound healing
      d. Decreased surfactant production
      e. Infection
      f. Pulmonary edema from decreased serum albumin levels
   2. Since oral feeding is not possible, nasogastric feedings should be implemented. Other feeding routes include an intravenous line or enteral feedings through a catheter in the stomach.
   3. High-protein, high-carbohydrate diets are recommended.

VIII. DEAD SPACE (V_D)
A. V_D is that portion of the V_T that does not take part in gas exchange.
B. **Types of deadspace (V_D)**
   1. **Anatomic V_D** (discussed earlier) consists of the conducting airways from the nose and mouth to the terminal bronchioles, i.e., air that doesn't reach the alveolar epithelium where gas exchange occurs.
      a. Anatomic V_D = 1 mL/lb body weight.
      b. **A tracheostomy decreases the anatomic V_{DS} by 50%** by bypassing the upper airway.
   2. **Alveolar V_D**
      a. Air reaching the alveoli but not taking part in gas exchange
      b. Results from lack of perfusion to air-filled alveoli

c. May result from hyperinflated alveoli where blood is not able to use all the air

3. **Physiologic V$_D$**
   a. The sum of anatomic and alveolar V$_D$s
   b. The most accurate measurement of V$_D$
4. **Mechanical V$_D$**
   a. Ventilator circuits have a certain amount of V$_D$, ranging from 75 to 150 mL.
   b. Since anatomic V$_D$s decreases when a patient has an ET tube or tracheostomy tube, the V$_D$ created by the circuit is balanced out.
   c. Additional mechanical deadspace (V$_D$) may be added to the ventilator circuit **between the ventilator wye adaptor and the ET tube adaptor to increase Pa$_{CO_2}$ levels.**
      (1) For every 100 mL of dead space added, the Pa$_{CO_2}$ increases approximately 5 mm Hg.
      (2) Mechanical deadspace (V$_D$) may be added to the circuits of patients on control or assist/control modes only. **Never add deadspace if the patient is on SIMV, IMV or CPAP.**

IX. LUNG COMPLIANCE (C$_L$)

A. Lung compliance is defined as the ease with which the lung expands. It varies inversely with the pressure required to move a specific volume of air.

$$C_L = \frac{V}{P}$$

1. The higher the compliance, the easier it is to ventilate the lung. (The lung requires less pressure to ventilate.)
2. The lower the compliance, the stiffer the lung is and the harder it is to ventilate. (The lung requires more pressure to ventilate.)
3. **Normal total lung compliance** (sum of the compliance of lung tissue and thoracic cage) is **0.1 L/cm H$_2$O.**

B. **Calculation of Lung Compliance**
   1. **Dynamic compliance**
      a. Formula

$$\text{Dynamic } C_L = \frac{V_T}{PIP - PEEP}$$

Given the following data, calculate the patient's dynamic lung compliance.

V$_T$	600 mL
PIP	35 cm H$_2$O
PEEP	5 cm H$_2$O

$$\text{Dynamic } C_L = \frac{600 \text{ mL}}{30 \text{ cm H}_2\text{O}} = 20 \text{ mL/cm H}_2\text{O}$$

   b. Dynamic compliance is measured as air is flowing through the circuit and airways, therefore is actually a measurement of airway resistance (abbreviated Raw).
   ★ c. Dynamic compliance changes with changes in Raw caused by:
      (1) Water in the ventilator tubing
      (2) Bronchospasm
      (3) Secretions
      (4) Mucosal edema
   d. Dynamic compliance is not an accurate measurement of how compliant the lungs are.

2. **Static compliance**
   a. Is a more accurate measurement of lung compliance, or how easily the lung is expanded, since it is measured with no air flowing through the circuit and airways (i.e., under static conditions).
   b. Air flow may be stopped with the volume remaining in the lungs by adjusting a 1- to 2-sec inspiratory hold or by pinching off the expiratory drive line after inspiration has begun.
   c. Once the flow has stopped, a **plateau pressure** occurs after peak pressure has been reached. The drop from peak to plateau pressure represents the pressure change from when gas flow is occurring to when it stops.
   d. Static compliance is calculated as follows

$$\text{Static } C_L = \frac{V_T}{\text{Plateau presssure} - \text{PEEP}}$$

EXAMPLE:

V$_T$	800 mL
Plateau pressure	25 cm H$_2$O
PEEP	5 cm H$_2$O
Peak pressure	45 cm H$_2$O

Calculate the static lung compliance.

$$\text{Static } C_L = \frac{800 \text{ mL}}{20 \text{ cm H}_2\text{O}} = 40 \text{ mL/cm H}_2\text{O}$$

C. Important Points Concerning Lung Compliance

★ 1. Increasing plateau pressures indicate the lung compliance is decreasing, or the lungs are harder to ventilate.
★ 2. If the peak pressures are increasing, but the plateau pressure remains the same, then lung compliance is not decreasing. An increased Raw is occurring from bronchospasm, secretions, coughing and tubing obstructions, etc.

EXAMPLE:

Time	Peak Pressure	Plateau Pressure
6:00 AM	28 cm H_2O	10 cm H_2O
7:00 AM	34 cm H_2O	10 cm H_2O
8:00 AM	42 cm H_2O	10 cm H_2O

In this example, the peak pressures are increasing, while the plateau pressures are remaining stable. This indicates an increase in Raw and not a decreasing lung compliance.

EXAMPLE:

Time	Peak Pressure	Plateau Pressure
1:00 PM	34 cm H_2O	16 cm H_2O
2:00 PM	40 cm H_2O	22 cm H_2O
3:00 PM	44 cm H_2O	26 cm H_2O

In this example, the plateau pressures are increasing along with the peak pressures. This indicates a decreasing lung compliance.

3. Decreasing static lung compliance results from
   a. Pneumonia
   b. Pulmonary edema
   c. Consolidation
   d. Atelectasis
   e. Air-trapping
   f. Pleural effusion
   g. Pneumothorax
   h. ARDS
4. Normal static lung compliance on the ventilated patient is 60 to 70 mL/cm H_2O.

Note

Calculation of lung compliance is also important in determining optimal PEEP level.

EXAMPLE:

Optimal PEEP is represented by which of the following

PEEP (cm H_2O)	Peak pressure (cm H_2O)	Plateau pressure (cm H_2O)	VT (mL)
4	36	20	500
6	39	22	500
8	42	23	500
10	45	27	500

Remember that optimal PEEP is the level of PEEP that produces the highest static lung compliance. There is no need to calculate the compliance for all four PEEP levels in this problem. Since the VT is the same at all PEEP levels, simply subtract the PEEP level from the plateau pressure. The lowest number you get after doing this will be the optimal PEEP level, since the lower the number divided into the VT, the better the results in lung compliance. In other words, a PEEP of 4 resulted in a plateau pressure of 20, a difference of 16. A PEEP of 6 also resulted in difference of 16; a PEEP of 8, a difference of 15; a PEEP of 10, a difference of 17. The lower the number divided into the VT, the higher the compliance result, therefore the optimal PEEP level in this example is 8 cm H_2O.

C. Calculation of Airway Resistance (Raw)

On an intubated ventilator patient, the amount of pressure being delivered to the airways and how much is going to the alveoli must be known. The difference between these two is the amount of pressure lost as a result of Raw. We can determine this loss by subtracting the plateau pressure from the peak inspiratory pressure (PIP). The closer the plateau pressure is to the peak pressure, the lower the pressure loss caused by Raw, and vice versa. When this pressure difference is divided by the inspiratory flow, we can measure Raw.

$$Raw = \frac{(PIP - Plateau\ pressure)}{Flow\ rate}$$

Note

Since Raw is measured in cm H_2O/L/sec, flow rate must be converted from L/min to L/sec by dividing flow by 60.

EXAMPLE:

The following data have been collected from a patient on a volume ventilator.

Peak inspiratory pressure	35 cm H_2O
Plateau pressure	20 cm H_2O
Flow rate	60 L/min = 1 L/sec

$$Raw = \frac{35 \text{ cm } H_2O - 20 \text{ cm } H_2O}{1 \text{ L/sec}}$$

$$= \frac{15 \text{ cm } H_2O}{1 \text{ L/sec}} = 15 \text{ cm } H_2O/\text{L/sec}$$

Since normal Raw in an intubated patient is around 5 cm H_2O/L/sec, this example reflects a high Raw.

★ Normal Raw in nonintubated individuals is 0.6 to 2.4 cm H_2O/L/sec, based on a flow rate of 30 L/min or 0.5 L/sec.

X. VENTILATION OF THE PATIENT WITH HEAD TRAUMA

A. Higher than normal flow rates should be used to make inspiratory time shorter, lessening the time of positive pressure in the airways. The longer the time of positive pressure in the airways, the more impedance of blood flow from the head which increases intracranial pressure (ICP).

B. Maintain the **$Paco_2$ between 25 and 30 mm Hg,** since this reduces ICP by vasoconstriction of cerebral vessels. **ICP should be maintained below 15 mm Hg; normal ICP is < 10 mm Hg.**

> **Exam Note**
>
> Although the exam may still advocate using hyperventilation in patients with head trauma, recent studies have shown this should not be used because of inadequate perfusion to healthy brain tissue.

C. If the ICP begins to increase, the patient should be hyperventilated (preferably with a resuscitation bag) to reduce the cerebral blood flow, thus lowering ICP.

D. Caution must be exercised when suctioning, since this tends to increase ICP as a result of hypoxemia.

XI. WEANING FROM MECHANICAL VENTILATION

A. Criteria For Weaning

1. V_T equal to 3 times the body weight in kg
2. VC of greater than 15 mL/kg, or twice the V_T
3. Able to achieve a MIP of at least −20 cm H_2O
4. V_D/V_T of less than 0.60
5. P(A-a)O_2 less than 350 mm Hg on 100% O_2
6. Respiratory rate of less than 25/min

7. Patient should be alert and able to follow commands.
8. Patient should be off any medications that may hinder spontaneous ventilation.
9. Life-threatening situations, such as shock or hypotension, should not be present.
10. Anemia, fever or electrolyte imbalances should not be present.

B. Weaning Techniques

1. Using SIMV or IMV to decrease the number of mechanical ventilator breaths, while allowing for more spontaneous breathing.
   a. Patient should be on 40% O_2 or less before extubation.
   b. Patient should be on SIMV or IMV rate of 4/min or less before removal from the ventilator.
   c. Postoperative patients may be weaned as they begin waking up. Provided patients have normal blood gas levels and are beginning to awaken, the SIMV or IMV rate can begin to be decreased.

2. **Time On-Time Off Method**
   a. Patient is taken off the ventilator periodically and placed on flow-by for a specific length of time, then placed back on the ventilator.
   b. The time off the ventilator is gradually increased, until the patient is spending more time off the ventilator than on.
   c. Patient is often returned to the ventilator while asleep.
   d. Patient must be monitored closely (e.g., blood pressure, V_T, heart rate, respiratory rate, ABG levels, Sao_2) while on flow-by.
   e. Often, the O_2 percentage is increased 10% while on flow-by.

XII. HIGH-FREQUENCY VENTILATION (HFV)

> **Exam Note**
>
> HFV will appear on the RRT examination only.

A. HFV refers to breathing rates that are four times the normal rate (60/min in the adult). Smaller than normal V_T is used, sometimes less than anatomic V_D. HFV has been shown to improve gas exchange without the barotrauma and cardiovascular problems associated with conventional volume-limited and pressure-limited ventilation in both infants and adults.

B. **Three Classifications of HFV**
   1. **High-frequency positive pressure ventilation (HFPPV)**

a. Gas delivery to the patient occurs with the use of a time-cycled or pressure- or volume-limited device through ventilator tubing that has a low compressible volume. This ensures that little volume is lost in the tubing.

b. Gas is directed through an insufflation catheter that is placed through the ET tube, and the rapid opening and closing of the exhalation valve determines gas flow into and out of the lungs.

c. The exhalation valve opens and closes in response to a pneumatic or electric source. Some pneumatic units incorporate fluidic gates to accomplish the opening and closing of the exhalation valve.

d. **Ventilatory rates with HFPPV are between 60/min and 100/min with a small VT of 3 to 5 mL/kg of body weight. I:E ratios of 1:3 or less are normally used.**

★ e. Delivery of a small VT results in lower peak inspiratory pressure and lower mean airway pressure, at a much higher rate than conventional ventilation, and an improved distribution of gas.

f. PEEP may also be used with HFPPV to improve oxygenation with less cardiovascular side effects than conventional positive pressure ventilation and PEEP.

g. HFPPV has also been used during thoracic surgery, such as lobectomy or pneumonectomy, in which conventional ventilation may not be effective.

2. **High-frequency jet ventilation (HFJV)**

a. A high-pressure gas source injects short, rapid bursts of gas through a jet catheter, usually incorporated into a special ET tube. Air is entrained through a separate channel during inspiration, increasing flow to the patient.

b. Frequency rates vary from about 100 to 600 cycles per minute at I:E ratios of 1:1 to 1:4. Peak inspiratory pressures are usually about 8 to 10 cm H_2O above baseline. VT is usually a little larger than anatomic VD.

★ c. A low-pressure alarm set 2 to 3 cm H_2O below peak inspiratory pressure should be incorporated to determine power loss or system leaks.

★ d. A high-pressure alarm should be set 5 to 10 cm H_2O above peak inspiratory pressure. This alarm may be activated by a plugged ET tube, air-trapping (resulting from short exhalation time at high rates), pneumothorax, or airway secretions requiring suctioning.

e. The gas is most effectively humidified with the use of a heat exchanger that is designed to withstand high pressure. Water and the jet gas mix and then pass through the exchanger. This warms the gas and also humidifies it.

f. An infusion pump may also be used to humidify the inspired gas. The pump places water in front of the jet nozzle and, as the gas passes through the jet, it combines with the water just outside the jet, humidifying the gas.

g. Because a low VT is delivered with HFV, resulting in an increased potential for atelectasis, PEEP should be employed to reduce the incidence of this.

3. **High-frequency oscillation (HFO)**

a. HFO requires an oscillating device that forces small impulses of gas into and out of the patient's airway.

b. Three types of oscillating devices are used.

(1) Piston: As the piston moves inward, a small volume of gas is delivered to the patient. As the piston withdraws, the same amount of gas is drawn away from the patient (exhalation). A sine-type flow wave is usually produced.

(2) Diaphragm: Audio loudspeakers have been used to accomplish HFO. As the diaphragm vibrates, the rapid movement, both forward and backward, moves a volume of gas into and out of the patient's lungs.

(3) Flow interruptor: As flow is being delivered to the patient's airways, it passes through a rotating bar with a hole in it. Gas flow periodically passes through the hole and is delivered in small bursts to the patient. Exhalation occurs by normal passive recoil of the lung.

c. Oscillations occur at a rate of 60 to 3600/min at a VT of less than anatomic deadspace.

d. HFO may be beneficial in treating patients with large degrees of intrapulmonary shunting. It is being used currently to ventilate infants with respiratory distress syndrome.

C. **Potential Advantages of HFV over Conventional Ventilation**

1. Reduced risk of barotrauma

2. Reduced risk of cardiac side effects (decreased venous return and decreased cardiac output)
3. Less fluctuation in ICP
4. Improvement of mucociliary clearance

XIII. INDEPENDENT LUNG VENTILATION (ILV)

> **Exam Note**
>
> ILV will appear on the RRT examination only.

A. In the case of unilateral lung disease or conditions such as unilateral bronchopleural fistula or massive hemoptysis, the diseased lung may be ventilated independently from the healthy lung. If conventional ventilation is used, generally the healthy lung gets ventilated more effectively than the diseased lung.
B. Single-lung transplant patients may also be more effectively ventilated with ILV.

XIV. ESTIMATING DESIRED VENTILATOR PARAMETER CHANGES
A. Making Changes in the FIO₂

$$\text{Desired } F_{IO_2} = \frac{Pa_{O_2} \text{ (desired)} \times F_{IO_2} \text{ (current)}}{Pa_{O_2} \text{ (current)}}$$

EXAMPLE:

The data below are from a patient on a volume ventilator.

Mode	Control	ABGs:	pH	7.43
Vт	750 mL		Paco₂	42 mm Hg
Rate	12/min		Pao₂	53 mm Hg
Fio₂	0.40			

To increase this patient's Pao₂ to 80 mm Hg, to what level must the Fio₂ be changed?

$$\text{Desired } F_{IO_2} = \frac{80 \times .4}{53} = \frac{32}{53} = .60$$

B. Making Changes in the Ventilator Rate

$$\text{Desired rate} = \frac{\text{Rate (current)} \times Pa_{CO_2} \text{ (current)}}{Pa_{CO_2} \text{ (desired)}}$$

EXAMPLE:

Data collected from a patient in the control mode on a volume ventilator.

Vт	800 mL	ABGs:	pH	7.51
Fio₂	0.35		Paco₂	26 mm Hg
Rate	16/min		Pao₂	94 mm Hg

To raise the patient's Paco₂ to 35 mm Hg, the ventilator rate should be adjusted to what level?

$$\text{Desired rate} = \frac{16 \times 26}{35} = \frac{416}{35} = 11.8 \text{ or } 12/min$$

C. Making Changes in Minute Volume (V̇E)

Formula: V̇E = respiratory rate × Vт

$$\text{Desired } (\dot{V}_E) = \frac{\dot{V}_E \text{ (current)} \times Pa_{CO_2} \text{ (current)}}{Pa_{CO_2} \text{ (desired)}}$$

EXAMPLE:

Below is data collected from a patient on a volume ventilator in the control mode.

Vт	700 mL (.7 L)	ABGs:	pH	7.28
Rate	10/min		Paco₂	54 mm Hg
Fio₂	0.45		Pao₂	74 mm Hg

Which of the following ventilator settings would decrease the patient's Paco₂ to 45 mm Hg?

Vт	650 mL	Rate	10/min
Vт	700 mL	Rate	12/min
Vт	700 mL	Rate	14/min
Vт	750 mL	Rate	10/min

In this question, we use the equation above to derive the necessary V̇E to decrease the Paco₂ to the desired level. Then choose the answer with the appropriate V̇E that has been calculated.

$$\text{Desired } \dot{V}_E = \frac{7 \times 54}{45} = \frac{378}{45} = 8.4 \text{ L}$$

The V̇E required to decrease the Paco₂ to 45 mm Hg is 8.4 L. In the example, the second choice gives a minute volume of 8.4 L (700 mL × 12/min).

D. Making Changes in Alveolar Ventilation (V̇A)

Formula: V̇A = (Vт − anatomic Vd) × respiratory rate

$$\text{Desired } \dot{V}_A = \frac{\dot{V}_A \text{ (current)} \times Pa_{CO_2} \text{ (current)}}{Pa_{CO_2} \text{ (desired)}}$$

EXAMPLE:

Below are data recorded on a patient who is on a volume ventilator in the control mode.

V_T	800 mL (.8 L)	ABGs: pH	7.30
Rate	12/min	Pa_{CO_2}	50 mm Hg
FiO_2	0.40	Pa_{O_2}	76 mm Hg
Anatomic V_D	150 mL		

Which of the following ventilator settings would decrease the patient's Pa_{CO_2} to 40 mm Hg?

V_T	700 mL	Rate	15/min
V_T	800 mL	Rate	18/min
V_T	800 mL	Rate	15/min
V_T	850 mL	Rate	12/min

In this question, we use the equation above to derive the alveolar ventilation necessary to bring the Pa_{CO_2} down to 40 mm Hg. It is the same equation that we used in the previous problem, except that we correct for anatomic V_D, in this case, 150 mL, which is subtracted from the V_T. This value is then multiplied by the respiratory rate to determine the V_A.

$$(800 - 150 = 650 \text{ mL or .65 L}) \ .65 \times 12 = 7.8 \text{ L}$$

$$\text{Desired } \dot{V}_A = \frac{7.8 \times 50}{40} = \frac{390}{40} = 9.75 \text{ L}$$

Therefore, an alveolar volume of 9.75 L is required to decrease the Pa_{CO_2} to 40 mm Hg. You now choose the appropriate choice from the table above, in this case, the third one.

XV. PRACTICE VENTILATOR PROBLEMS

A. A 75-kg male patient is placed in the control mode on a volume ventilator. Appropriate data from his chart are

V_T	700 mL	ABGs: pH	7.28
Rate	12/min	Pa_{CO_2}	54 mm Hg
FiO_2	0.50	Pa_{O_2}	74 mm Hg
PEEP	5 cm H_2O	HCO_3^-	23 mEq/L

Based on this information, the RCP should recommend which of the following ventilator changes?

1. Increase PEEP to 10 cm H_2O.
2. Add 100 mL of mechanical V_D.
3. Increase the FiO_2 to 0.60.
4. Increase the V_T to 800 mL.

Answer: The fourth choice. The patient is hypoventilating as a result of an inadequate V_T. The patient weighs 75 kg, and using 10 to 12 mL/kg of ideal body weight to determine adequate V_T, the ventilator should be set on a V_T between 750 and 900 mL.

B. A patient on the Bennett 7200 ventilator is placed on the control mode of ventilation. Pertinent data are

V_T	800 mL	ABGs: pH	7.41
Rate	12/min	Pa_{CO_2}	37 mm Hg
FiO_2	0.60	Pa_{O_2}	137 mm Hg
PEEP	8 cm H_2O	HCO_3^-	26 mEq/L

What is the most appropriate ventilator change to recommend at this time?

1. Decrease the FiO_2 to 0.50.
2. Increase the V_T to 900 mL.
3. Decrease the rate to 10/min.
4. Decrease the PEEP to 6 cm H_2O.

Answer: The fourth choice. Patient is ventilating well but is hyperoxygenating on 60% O_2. Since the O_2 percentage is at a relatively safe level, we may reduce the Pa_{O_2} by decreasing the level of PEEP.

C. A 46-year-old, 80-kg (176-lb) man is being mechanically ventilated on a volume ventilator in the assist/control mode. Data include

FiO_2	0.30	ABGs: pH	7.48
Rate	12	Pa_{CO_2}	32 mm Hg
V_T	800 mL	Pa_{O_2}	53 mm Hg

What is the most appropriate recommendation at this time?

1. Decrease the rate to 8/min.
2. Decrease V_T to 750 mL.
3. Increase the FiO_2 to 0.50.
4. Place patient on 8 cm H_2O of PEEP.

Answer: The third choice. This patient is slightly hyperventilating as a result of hypoxemia. As the Pa_{O_2} increases, hyperventilation should subside. Increasing the FiO_2 or adding PEEP both will elevate the Pa_{O_2}, but since the FiO_2 is 0.30, we can safely increase it to as high as 0.60 before adding PEEP.

D. A patient is in the control mode of ventilation on the following settings.

V_T	800 mL
Rate	10/min
FiO_2	0.35

ABG values:

pH	7.50
Pa_{CO_2}	29 mm Hg
Pa_{O_2}	97 mm Hg
HCO_3^-	25 mEq/L

What would be the most appropriate ventilator change to make at this time?

1. Increase the inspiratory flow.
2. Add 5 cm H$_2$O PEEP.
3. Increase the FIO$_2$ to 0.50.
4. Decrease VT to 700 mL.

Answer: The fourth choice. This patient is hyperventilating resulting in a low PaCO$_2$. Since the PaO$_2$ is normal, hypoxemia is not the cause of the hyperventilation. Minute ventilation is too high and can be reduced by decreasing VT, thereby increasing PaCO$_2$.

E. A 60-kg (132-lb) female patient is on a volume ventilator in the control mode set on the following settings.

VT	800 mL	ABGs: pH	7.52
Rate	12/min	PaCO$_2$	28 mm Hg
FIO$_2$	0.40	PaO$_2$	92 mm Hg

What is the appropriate ventilator change at this time?

1. Increase the FIO$_2$ to 0.50.
2. Add PEEP of 5 cm H$_2$O.
3. Decrease rate to 6/min.
4. Decrease VT to 600 mL.

Answer: The fourth choice. The VT setting is more than 12 mL/kg, resulting in the patient being hyperventilated. Decreasing the VT will increase the PaCO$_2$. Decreasing the rate will also increase the PaCO$_2$, but a rate of 6/min (third choice) in the control mode is too low.

XVI. **VENTILATOR FLOW, VOLUME, AND PRESSURE WAVE FORMS**
   A. **Flow Wave Forms**

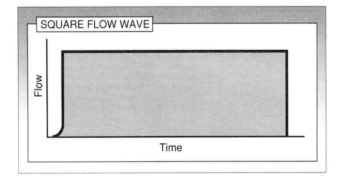

1. **Square wave (constant flow)**
   a. With this flow pattern, the flow remains constant throughout inspiration.
   b. Changes in Raw and compliance won't change the flow pattern under normal circumstances.
   c. This type of flow pattern is beneficial to patients with increased respiratory rates.

2. **Sine (sinusoidal) wave**

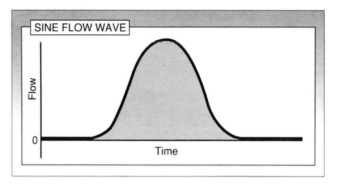

   a. Flow gradually accelerates from the beginning of inspiration, then decelerates toward the end of inspiration.
   b. This flow pattern benefits patients with increased Raw by decreasing airway turbulence produced by this flow.

3. **Decelerating ramp wave**

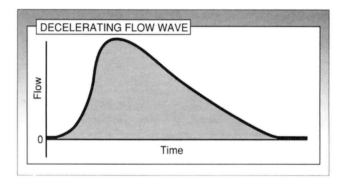

   a. Initial flow is high and begins decelerating as inspiration continues.
   b. Flow never decreases more than 50% to 55% of initial flow.
   c. Benefits patients with low compliance, since this pattern allows ventilation to occur at a decreased pressure.

4. **Accelerating ramp wave**

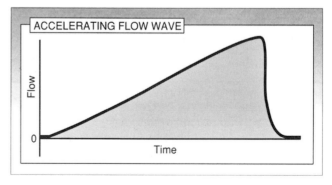

a. Flow is initially slow and accelerates to a peak flow by the end of inspiration.

b. This pattern creates less turbulence of flow in the beginning of inspiration, therefore more volume may be delivered through narrowed or obstructed airways.

B. **Volume Wave Form**

1. This is a typical volume wave form showing volume in milliliters on the vertical axis and time in seconds on the horizontal axis. Notice how the waveform returns to zero (baseline) during exhalation.

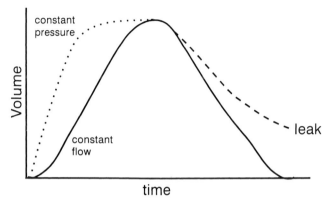

From Branson, Hess, Chatburn: Respiratory Care Equipment. Lippincott. 1995.

2. If the volume tracing does not return to baseline at the end of exhalation, it is an indication of leaks in the ventilator circuit or around the ET-tube cuff or chest tube or it may result from air trapping.

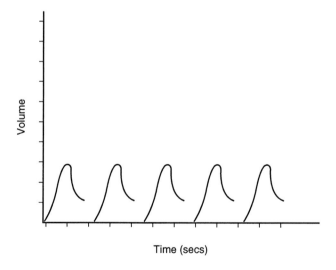

3. If the volume tracing goes below the baseline, this is an indication of auto-PEEP or the patient may be coughing or agitated.

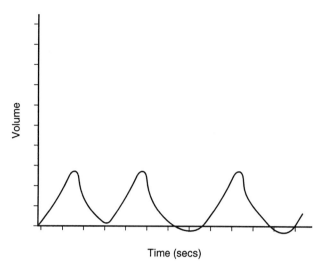

4. Obstructive lung disease causes the tracing to be flat during exhalation as a result of decreased expiratory flows.

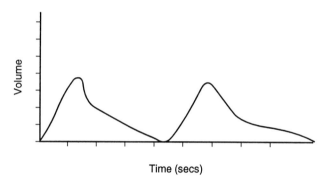

C. **Pressure Wave Form**

1. This is a typical pressure wave form that is shown during volume ventilation; pressure is shown on the vertical axis, time on the horizontal axis. (When using pressure ventilation, the pressure wave form is almost square in nature.)

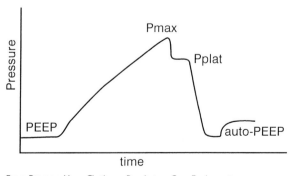

From Branson, Hess, Chatburn: Respiratory Care Equipment. Lippincott. 1995.

2. Peak pressure rises during inspiration and is determined by V_T, Raw, lung compliance, and inspiratory flow.

3. The difference between peak pressure and plateau pressure is Raw.
4. If the wave form does not return to baseline during exhalation, the patient is on PEEP, or auto-PEEP is occurring.

XVII. SUMMARY OF VENTILATOR ADJUSTMENTS ACCORDING TO ABG RESULTS

ABG Abnormality	Ventilator Adjustment
Decreased pH Increased $PaCO_2$ Decreased or normal PaO_2	Increase V_T (Maintain 10 to 12 mL/kg) Increase rate
Increased pH Decreased $PaCO_2$ Normal or increased PaO_2	Decrease V_T Decrease rate Add mechanical V_D
Normal pH Increased $PaCO_2$ PaO_2 of 50 to 65 mm Hg Increased HCO_3^-	No adjustment needed; this is a COPD patient. May begin weaning if other weaning criteria are met.
Normal or increased pH Normal or decreased $PaCO_2$ Decreased PaO_2	Increase FIO_2 if <0.60. Add or increase PEEP if FIO_2 is 0.60 or more.
Normal pH Normal $PaCO_2$ Increased PaO_2	Decrease FIO_2 if it is higher than 0.60; decrease PEEP if FIO_2 is 0.60 or lower.
Decreased pH Normal $PaCO_2$ Decreased HCO_3^-	No ventilator changes are necessary; administer HCO_3^-.

XVIII. MAINTENANCE OF THE VENTILATOR CIRCUIT

A. While routine ventilator circuit changes vary from hospital to hospital, the circuit should be changed at least once per week. Bacterial culturing of the circuits will determine whether more frequent circuit changes are necessary.
B. When changing the ventilator circuit, the patient should be hyperoxgenated before removal of the circuit. In some cases, when the patient may not tolerate even the shortest time off the ventilator during the circuit change, the patient should be manually ventilated by a practitioner or nurse, while another practitioner changes the circuit.

POST-CHAPTER STUDY QUESTIONS

1. Pressure control ventilation is most commonly used on adults with what lung condition?
2. What effect does decreasing lung compliance have on delivered V_T on a neonate on a pressure-limited ventilator?
3. How can you determine adequate flow is available to the patient through an external circuit used in the IMV mode?
4. As the oxygenation status of a patient worsens on an O_2 mask, at what point should CPAP be employed?
5. How is minute ventilation calculated?
6. How is alveolar minute ventilation calculated?
7. Calculate the ventilator tubing compliance when the volume is set at 200 mL (.2 L), generating an inspiratory pressure of 50 cm H_2O.
8. Using the tubing compliance in question #7, calculate the corrected V_T when the patient is on a V_T of 700 mL with a peak inspiratory pressure of 20 cm H_2O.
9. On the initial ventilator setup, at what range should the ventilator rate be set?
10. How should the appropriate ventilator V_T be determined?
11. List six indications for the use of PEEP.
12. List four hazards of PEEP.
13. Define optimal PEEP.
14. After increasing the PEEP level, how can it be determined that cardiac output has been adversely affected?
15. How may the ventilator low-pressure alarm be activated?
16. List ways that the ventilator high-pressure alarm may be activated.
17. How should the high-pressure alarm be set?
18. List some factors that affect airway resistance (Raw).
19. What is normal $PETCO_2$?
20. List four conditions that result in a decreased $PETCO_2$ reading.
21. List two conditions that result in an increased $PETCO_2$ reading.
22. List six criteria that indicate mechanical ventilatory assistance is necessary.
23. List eight complications of mechanical ventilation.
24. Calculate the static lung compliance if the V_T is 750 mL, PIP is 46 cm H_2O, PEEP is 8 cm H_2O, and plateau pressure is 28 cm H_2O.
25. List some conditions that result in decreased lung compliance.
26. What is indicated if peak inspiratory pressures are increasing with no increase in plateau pressure?
27. List the criteria that patients should meet before beginning to wean them from the ventilator.
28. What respiratory rates are used with HFJV?
29. List four advantages of high-frequency ventilation over conventional ventilation.
30. A ventilator patient on an FIO_2 of 0.30 has a PaO_2 of 60 mm Hg. To increase the PaO_2 to 80 mm Hg, what change to the FIO_2 must be made?
31. A ventilator patient in the control mode is on a ventilator rate of 8/min and has a $PaCO_2$ of 55 mm Hg. To decrease the $PaCO_2$ to 40 mm Hg, what change must be made to the ventilator rate?

32. A 36-year-old woman is on assist/control mode, rate of 10/min, V_T of 650 mL, and an FIO_2 of 0.40. ABG results: pH 7.27, $PaCO_2$ 54 mm Hg, PaO_2 75 mm Hg, HCO_3^- 26 mEq/L. What ventilator alteration should be made?

33. A ventilator patient on a FIO_2 of 0.70 and a PEEP of 8 cm H_2O has a PaO_2 of 147 mm Hg. What ventilator adjustment should be made to reduce the PaO_2?

34. In what conditions is ILV used?

35. On a volume wave form, if the tracing does not return to baseline, what does this indicate?

Answers are at end of the chapter.

REFERENCES

Chang D: Clinical application of mechanical ventilation, ed 1, Albany, NY, 1997, Delmar Publishers.

Dupuis YG: Ventilators: theory and clinical application, St. Louis, 1986, The CV Mosby Co.

Eubanks D and Bone R: Comprehensive respiratory care, ed 2, St. Louis, 1990, The CV Mosby C.

McPherson SP: Respiratory therapy equipment, ed 5, St. Louis, 1995, Mosby-Yearbook, Inc.

Pilbeam SP: Mechanical ventilation: physiological and clinical applications, ed 2, St. Louis, 1998, Mosby, Inc.

Scanlan C, Wilkins R, and Stoller J: Egan's fundamentals of respiratory care, ed 7, St. Louis, 1999, Mosby, Inc.

PRE-TEST ANSWERS

1. D
2. D
3. B
4. C
5. B
6. A

ANSWERS TO POST-CHAPTER STUDY QUESTIONS

1. ARDS
2. Decreases V_T
3. If there is inadequate flow, the reservoir bag totally deflates or mist totally disappears from reservoir tube during inspiration; manometer pulls past -2 cm H_2O during inspiration.
4. If 60% O_2 still results in hypoxemia (and $PaCO_2$ is normal or low)
5. $V_T \times RR$
6. $(V_T - V_D) \times RR$
7. 4 mL/cm H_2O; volume/pressure = 200 mL/50 cm H_2O = 4 mL/cm H_2O
8. 620 mL; lost volume = PIP × tubing compliance = 20 × 4 = 700 − 80 = 620 mL.
9. 8/min to 12/min
10. 10 to 12 mL/kg of ideal body weight
11. Atelectasis, hypoxemia on 60% O_2 or more, decreased FRC, to prevent using more than 60% O_2 to maintain normal PaO_2 level, decreased lung compliance, pulmonary edema
12. Barotrauma, decreased venous return, decreased cardiac output, decreased urinary output
13. The level of PEEP that improves lung compliance without decreasing cardiac output.
14. Decreasing PvO_2 levels and drop in blood pressure
15. Leaks in the circuit, patient disconnection
16. Decreasing lung compliance, airway secretions, bronchospasm, water in ventilator tubing, kink in ventilator tubing, coughing
17. 5 to 15 cm H_2O above average peak inspiratory pressure
18. Bronchospasm, water in ventilator tubing, mucosa edema, secretions
19. 35 to 45 mm Hg, or 4.5% to 5.5%
20. Hyperventilation, apnea, total airway obstruction, hypotension, pulmonary embolism, decreased cardiac output
21. Hypoventilation, hyperthermia
22. VC < 15 mL/kg, $P(A-a)O_2$ > 450 mm Hg on 100% O_2, VD/VT > 60%, unable to obtain a MIP of at least -20 cm H_2O, PEP < 40 cm H_2O, respiratory rate > 35/min
23. Barotrauma, pulmonary infection, atelectasis, tracheal damage, decreased venous return, decreased urinary output, lack of nutrition, pulmonary O_2 toxicity
24. 37.5 mL/cm H_2O; 750 mL/20 cm H_2O = 37.5 mL/cm H_2O
25. Pneumonia, pulmonary edema, consolidation, atelectasis, air-trapping, pleural effusion, pneumothorax, ARDS
26. Raw is increasing
27. VC > 15 mL/kg, V_T three times body weight (kg), able to obtain a MIP of at least -20 cm H_2O, VD/VT <60%, $P(A-a)O_2$ < 350 mm Hg on 100% O_2, respiratory rate < 25/min; and life-threatening conditions, anemia, fever, or electrolyte imbalances not present
28. 100 to 600 cycles/min
29. Reduced risk of barotrauma, reduced risk of cardiac side effects, less fluctuation in ICP, improvement in mucociliary clearance
30. Increase the FIO_2 to 0.40; 80 × .3 ÷ 60 = 0.40
31. Increase ventilator rate to 11/min; 8 × 55 ÷ 40 = 11
32. Increase the V_T or ventilator rate (to decrease $PaCO_2$)
33. Decrease the FIO_2 to 0.60
34. Single lung transplantation, bronchopleural fistula, massive hemoptysis
35. Leaks in the tubing or around the ET tube or chest tube; air-trapping

Chapter 12

Disorders of the Respiratory System

Answer the pre-test questions before studying the chapter. This will help you determine your strong and weak areas regarding the material covered.

1. Pursed lip breathing would be most beneficial in which of the following lung disorders?

   A. Emphysema
   B. Pulmonary edema
   C. Pneumonia
   D. Pleural effusion

2. On assessing a patient's laboratory results, you notice a sputum culture that reveals a high eosinophil count. This is characteristic of which of the following pulmonary conditions?

   A. TB
   B. Asthma
   C. Pneumonia
   D. Pulmonary embolism

3. Which lung condition is characterized by consolidation on chest films?

   A. Pulmonary edema
   B. Emphysema
   C. Pneumonia
   D. Pleural effusion

4. A 17-year-old asthmatic girl enters the emergency department in moderate respiratory distress. She states that the attack began about 1 hour before she came to the emergency department. You would expect her ABG results to reveal

   A. Acute respiratory acidosis with hypoxemia.
   B. Metabolic acidosis with hypoxemia.
   C. Acute respiratory alkalosis with hypoxemia.
   D. Chronic metabolic alkalosis.

5. Which of the following causative organisms for pneumonia is characteristically seen in patients with AIDS?

   A. Pneumocystis carinii
   B. Klebsiella species
   C. Pseudomonas species
   D. Haemophilus influenzae

6. The drug streptokinase is used to treat which of the following lung disorders?

   A. Pneumonia
   B. Pleural effusion
   C. Pneumothorax
   D. Pulmonary embolism

Answers are at end of the chapter.

I. **CHRONIC OBSTRUCTIVE PULMONARY DISEASE (COPD)**

> **Note**
>
> COPD is a condition that means there is a chronic obstruction to air flow within the lungs. The following diseases are classified as COPD and are discussed in the outline.

Emphysema
Chronic bronchitis
Asthma
Cystic fibrosis
Bronchiectasis

A. **Emphysema**
   1. **Definition:** A permanent abnormal enlargement of the air spaces distal to the terminal bronchioles, associated with destructive changes of the alveolar walls.
      a. Panlobular (panacinar) type
         (1) An acinus is the anatomic gas exchange unit of the lung, made up of the respiratory bronchiole, alveolar duct, alveolar sacs, and the alveoli.
         (2) The entire acinus is involved in this emphysema.

(3) There is significant loss of lung parenchyma.

(4) Alveoli are destroyed.

(5) Bullae are present.

(6) Usually associated with emphysema resulting from α_1-antitrypsin deficiency.

b. Centrilobular (centriacinar)

(1) Lesion is in the center of the lobules, which results in enlargement and destruction of the respiratory bronchioles.

(2) Usually involves the upper lung fields and is most commonly associated with chronic bronchitis.

c. Bullous emphysema

(1) Emphysematous changes are isolated and accompanied by the development of bullae, which are weak air spaces and prone to rupture.

(2) **Bullae** are defined as air spaces in their distended state, more than 1 cm in diameter.

(3) **Blebs** are defined as air spaces adjacent to the pleura, usually less than 1 cm in diameter in their distended state.

2. **Causes**

a. Smoking

b. α_1-antitrypsin deficiency (hereditary)

3. **Pathophysiology**

★ a. Elastic recoil of the lung is diminished, resulting in premature airway closure.

★ b. Inspiratory flow rates are normal, while expiratory flow rates are reduced.

★ c. Air-trapping leads to chronic hyperinflation of the lungs and an increased FRC.

d. **Lung compliance is increased** as a result of the destruction of elastic lung tissue.

e. Emphysema diminishes the area over which gas exchange occurs and is accompanied by regional differences in ventilation and perfusion. This accounts for increased physiologic deadspace and the abnormal ABG results observed in emphysema patients.

4. **Clinical signs and symptoms**

a. Dyspnea: initially occurs on exertion, then progressively worsens.

b. Digital clubbing: results from **chronic hypoxemia**

★ c. Increased AP chest diameter (barrel chest)

★ d. Use of accessory muscles during normal breathing

★ e. Elevated hemoglobin level, hematocrit, and RBC count

★ f. ABGs reveal chronic CO_2 retention and hypoxemia (advanced stages of the disease)

g. Reduced breath sounds and hyperresonance to percussion

h. Cyanosis

i. **Right-sided heart failure (cor pulmonale)** in advanced stages

(1) Cor pulmonale results from an increased workload on the right ventricle as it attempts to deliver blood through constricted pulmonary blood vessels.

(2) These vessels are constricted (causing pulmonary hypertension) as a result of arterial hypoxemia and hypercarbia.

(3) Chronic pulmonary hypertension results in right ventricular hypertrophy and, eventually, right-sided heart failure.

(4) **Cor pulmonale results in peripheral edema, such as pedal (ankle) edema, distended neck (jugular) veins, and an enlarged liver.**

(5) **O_2 therapy is essential in the prevention or treatment of cor pulmonale in patients with chronic respiratory failure.** O_2 is a pulmonary vasodilator that decreases pulmonary hypertension.

(6) Diuretic and digitalis therapy are indicated when right ventricular failure supervenes the underlying respiratory problems.

5. **Characteristics on chest x-ray films**

★ a. Flattened diaphragm

★ b. Hyperinflation

c. Reduced vascular markings

d. Bullous lesions

6. **Characteristics on pulmonary function studies**

★ a. Increased RV and FRC

b. Decreased diffusion capacity

c. Decreased VC

★ d. Decreased FEV_1

★ e. Decreased FEV_1/FVC

f. Prolonged nitrogen washout

7. **Treatment**

a. Smoking cessation program

(1) Group counseling

(2) Nicotine replacement therapy

(3) Frequent reminders from health care providers about the need to stop smoking to improve quality of life

(4) Discussions with RCP or other health care provider to help the patient understand the effects that smoking has on the cardiopulmonary system

b. Adequate hydration

c. Postural drainage

d. Bronchodilators

e. Prevention of infections by immunizations
f. Exercise (walking)
★ g. Breathing exercise training
  ★ (1) Diaphragmatic breathing exercises
  (2) **Pursed-lip breathing:** prevents premature airway closure by producing a back pressure into the airways on exhalation
★ h. Care must be taken when administering oxygen to emphysema patients who chronically retain CO_2 and are chronically hypoxemic. PaO_2 levels should be maintained between 50 and 65 mm Hg to avoid knocking out the patient's "hypoxic drive."

Note

If, after placing a patient with severe COPD on O_2, the PaO_2 increases above 70 mm Hg and the $PaCO_2$ begins increasing, this should be recognized as knocking out the patient's "hypoxic drive" and the oxygen percentage should be decreased. Remember to maintain the PaO_2 level at 50 to 65 mm Hg.

Note

If given a choice of O_2 delivery devices, such as a nasal cannula or air entrainment mask at approximately the same percentage, choose the air entrainment mask for a COPD patient.

B. **Chronic Bronchitis**
1. **Definition:** Chronic excessive mucus production, resulting from an increase in the number and size of mucus glands and goblet cells. Symptoms are a cough and increased mucus production for at least 3 months of the year for more than 2 consecutive years. Males are most commonly affected.
2. **Cause**
Smoking
3. **Pathophysiology**
a. Increase in the size of mucus glands
b. Increase in the number of goblet cells
c. Inflammation of bronchial walls
d. Mucus plugs in peripheral airways
e. Loss of cilia
f. Emphysematous changes in advanced stages of disease
g. Narrowing airways, leading to air flow obstruction
4. **Clinical signs and symptoms**
a. Cough with sputum production

b. Dyspnea on exertion, progressing to dyspnea with less effort
c. CO_2 retention and hypoxemia in advanced stages
d. Increased pulmonary vascular resistance in advanced stages
e. Increased hemoglobin level, hematocrit, and RBC count in advanced stages
f. Right-sided heart failure (cor pulmonale) in advanced stages
5. **Characteristics on chest x-ray films**
a. Not significant in early disease
b. Hyperinflation (in advanced stages)
6. **Characteristics on pulmonary function studies**
a. None in early disease
b. Increased RV
c. Decreased FEV_1
d. Decreased inspiratory flow rates in obstructive bronchitis
7. **Treatment**
Same as for emphysema
C. **Asthma**
1. **Definition:** A disease characterized by increased reactivity of the trachea and bronchi to various stimuli, resulting in bronchoconstriction (bronchospasm), increased mucus production, and swelling of mucosal tissue.
2. **Causes**
a. **Extrinsic asthma (allergic asthma)**
  (1) Begins early in life
  (2) Caused by inhalation of airborne antigens (e.g., dust, pollen)
  (3) Exercise often precipitates bronchospasm
b. **Intrinsic asthma (nonallergic asthma)**
  (1) A nonseasonal, nonallergic form of asthma that occurs later in life
  (2) Caused by inhalation of pollutants (e.g., dust, fumes, smoke), infections, and emotional crises
  (3) Usually is a chronic form of asthma that is persistent in nature as opposed to the episodic nature of extrinsic asthma
3. **Pathophysiology**
a. Mast cells in the bronchial tree are stimulated, causing the release of
  (1) Histamine
  (2) Leukotrienes
  (3) Slow-reacting substance of anaphylaxis (SRS-A)
  (4) Eosinophilic chemotactic factor of anaphylaxis (ECF-A)
  (5) Prostaglandins
b. The release of these substances results in

(1) Bronchoconstriction
(2) Mucosal edema
(3) Increased mucus production
(4) Accumulation of eosinophils in the blood and sputum
(5) Vasodilation

4. **Clinical signs and symptoms**
   a. Mild wheezing and cough initially, which may progress to severe dyspnea if the attack isn't arrested
   b. Cough is initially nonproductive, progressing to productive cough by the end of the episode.
   ★ c. Secretions contain high levels of eosinophils.
   d. Intercostal and supraclavicular retractions
   e. Use of accessory muscles to breathe (in a severe attack)
   ★ f. Paradoxical pulse: Systolic blood pressure is 10 mm Hg higher on expiration than on inspiration.
   g. Tachycardia and tachypnea
   ★ h. ABG levels initially reveal hypoxemia and low $PaCO_2$. $PaCO_2$ increases as attack worsens and patient begins to tire.
   I. Cyanosis

5. **Characteristics on chest x-ray films**
   a. Hyperinflation (hyperlucency of lung fields)
   b. Atelectasis
   c. Infiltrates

6. **Characteristics on pulmonary function studies**
   ★ a. Decreased FEV_1
   ★ b. Decreased FVC
   ★ c. Decreased FEV_1/FVC
   ★ d. Increased RV

7. **Treatment (preventive)**
   a. Prevention (avoid known allergens or causative factors)
   b. Medications
      (1) Bronchodilators
      (2) Cromolyn sodium: **prevents attacks by stabilizing the mast cell. Not used during an attack.**
      (3) Corticosteroids

8. **Treatment (during an attack)**
   a. Bronchodilators
   b. IV fluids
   c. O_2 therapy
   d. IV aminophylline (theophylline ethylenediamide)

9. **Status asthmaticus:** severe asthmatic attack not responding to treatment with an adequate amount of routine medications within a few hours.
   a. Patient should be hospitalized immediately.

b. IV aminophylline
c. Hydration
d. IV corticosteroids
e. Supplemental oxygen
f. Close monitoring of ABG levels and pulse oximetry (SpO_2)
g. Bronchodilating agents
h. Chest physical therapy (if tolerated) to remove mucus plugs and secretions
I. If not controlled by previous measures, intubate and institute mechanical ventilation.

D. **Cystic Fibrosis**
Covered in detail in chapter on neonatal and pediatric lung disease.

E. **Bronchiectasis**
1. **Definition:** A dilation of the bronchi and bronchioles, chronic in nature, that results in inflammation and damage to the walls of these airways.
2. **Causes**
   a. Chronic respiratory infections
   b. TB lesion
   c. Secondary to patients with cystic fibrosis
   d. Bronchial obstruction
3. **Pathophysiology**
   a. It is not clear whether the chronic dilation is a result of destructive changes in the bronchial walls caused by inflammation and infection or, possibly, a congenital defect of the airways.
   b. Bronchial obstruction may render the mucociliary transport system ineffective, leading to an accumulation of thick secretions.
   c. The bronchial wall is destroyed, with a resultant atrophy of the mucosal layer.
   d. Because of the decreased values in both flows and volumes this disease may be either obstructive or restrictive in nature (see characteristics on pulmonary function studies).
4. **Clinical signs and symptoms**
   ★ a. Productive cough with large amounts of thick, purulent secretions, which may be foul-smelling. Often, a layering of the sputum occurs.
   b. Tachypnea and tachycardia
   c. Hemoptysis
   d. Recurrent pulmonary infections
   e. Digital clubbing
   f. Cyanosis
   g. Respiratory alkalosis with hypoxemia (in the early stage)
   h. Chronic respiratory acidosis with hypoxemia (in the late stage)
   i. Barrel chest

5. **Characteristics on chest x-ray films**
   a. Increased lung markings
   b. Flattened diaphragm
   c. Segmental atelectasis
6. **Characteristics on pulmonary function studies**
   a. Decreased FVC
   b. Decreased FRC
   c. Decreased FEV_1
   d. Decreased $FEF_{25\%-75\%}$
7. **Treatment**
   a. Chest physical therapy
   b. Aerosol therapy
   c. Bronchodilator therapy
   d. Mucolytics, e.g., acetylcysteine (Mucomyst)
   e. Antibiotics
   f. O_2 therapy
   g. Expectorants

II. **LOWER RESPIRATORY TRACT INFECTIONS**
A. **Pneumonia**
   1. **Definition:** acute inflammation of the gas exchange units of the lungs.
   2. **Cause**
      a. A variety of organisms (discussed later)
      b. Decreased airway defense mechanisms caused by
         (1) Ineffective cough
         (2) Obtunded airway reflexes
         (3) Impaired mucociliary transport system
         (4) Obstructed airways
      c. Various conditions result in a predisposition to pneumonia
         (1) COPD
         (2) Alcoholism
         (3) Malnutrition
         (4) Seizure disorders
         (5) Chronic debilitating illnesses
         (6) Major surgical procedures
         (7) Old age
   3. **Pathophysiology**
      a. Pathogenic microorganisms that reach the gas exchange areas of the lung cause an intense tissue reaction, resulting in production of inflammatory exudates and cells.
      b. The WBCs phagocytize the invading organisms, leading to further inflammation.
      c. As the lungs begin filling with the inflammatory exudates and cells, they become **consolidated.**
      d. If tissue necrosis is not present, the lung heals and returns to normal function.
      e. If tissue necrosis occurs, healing is slow, with production of fibrous scar tissue resulting in pulmonary fibrosis and loss of normal lung function.

4. **Clinical signs and symptoms**
   a. Infection
   b. Malaise
   c. Fever
   d. Chest pain
   e. Dyspnea and tachycardia
   f. Inspiratory crackles on auscultation
5. **Characteristics on chest x-ray films**
   ★ a. Consolidation
   b. Air bronchogram
6. **Types of pneumonia**
   a. Bacterial
      (1) Causative organism is **Streptococcus pneumoniae:** called pneumococcal pneumonia; **most common bacterial pneumonia**
      (2) *Haemophilus influenzae*
      (3) *Klebsiella pneumoniae*
      (4) *Legionella pneumoniae*
      (5) *Pseudomonas aeruginosa*
   b. *Mycoplasma pneumoniae:* smaller than bacteria; disease is more common in children
   c. Viral
      (1) Influenza viruses
      (2) Adenoviruses
      (3) Chickenpox (varicella-zoster virus)
   d. Protozoan
      (1) ***Pneumocystis carinii pneumonia (PCP)***
      (2) This type of pneumonia is seen in 60% of AIDS cases. Definitive diagnosis is made from cultures of lung secretions and tissue.
      (3) *P. carinii* pneumonia is commonly treated with the antiprotozoal drug **pentamidine** via aerosolization.
7. **Treatment** (for pneumonia in general)
   a. Antibiotics
   b. Supplemental O_2
   c. Chest physical therapy
   d. Adequate hydration
   e. Adequate nutrition
   f. Tracheal suctioning (if there has been poor removal of secretions because of ineffective cough)
B. **Lung Abscess**
   1. **Definition:** An infection of the lung that is characterized by a localized accumulation of pus with destruction of the surrounding tissue.
   2. **Causes**
      a. The most common causative organisms are anaerobic bacteria.
      b. Aerobic bacteria, including staphylococci, streptococci, and some gram-negative bacteria may be less common causes.
      c. May occur after aspiration

d. Seen in conjunction with lung cancer

3. **Pathophysiology**
   a. In the acute phase, it looks much like pneumonia.
   b. As progression occurs, necrosis is evident, which may spread to adjacent lung tissue.

4. **Clinical signs and symptoms**
   a. Fever
   b. Cough, initially nonproductive (or minimal production), followed by production of **purulent, foul-smelling secretions.**
   c. Chest pain
   d. Weight loss
   e. Hemoptysis
   f. Digital clubbing
   g. Tachycardia
   h. Tachypnea

5. **Characteristics on chest x-ray films**
   a. Localized area of consolidation
   b. Most common sites are the superior segments of the lower lobes and posterior segments of upper lobes (as a result of position during an aspiration event).

6. **Characteristic laboratory findings**
   a. Increased WBC count
   b. Anemia (decreased RBC count)
   c. Sputum culture reveals purulence and necrosis

7. **Treatment**
   a. Antibiotics
   b. Postural drainage
   c. Adequate nutrition

> **Note**
>
> If an abscess ruptures into the pleura, pus accumulates in the pleural space. This is called empyema, and it should be drained before chest physical therapy.

C. **Tuberculosis (TB)**
   1. **Definition:** A granulomatous bacterial infection, chronic in nature, affecting the lungs and other organs of the body.
   2. **Cause:** The inhalation or ingestion of the bacterium, *Mycobacterium tuberculosis.* Infection is usually spread through coughing and sneezing. Diagnosis is based on skin tests, chest films, and sputum culture showing bacilli that are acid-fast, which means not readily decolorized by acid after staining, a specific characteristic of this bacteria.
   3. **Pathophysiology**
      a. After the bacillus is inhaled, it enters the alveoli, resulting in an inflammatory reaction similar to that seen in pneumonia.
      b. Macrophages enter the infected area and engulf the bacilli without fully killing them.
      c. The lung tissue surrounding this area encapsulates the bacilli, providing a protective covering. This is called a granuloma, or tubercle.
      d. The granuloma fills with necrotic material and is referred to as a caseous (cheese-like) granuloma.
      e. If the patient's immunologic system controls this process or if antituberculosis drugs are given, the lung tissue becomes fibrotic and calcifies as healing occurs. This may result in stiffness or decreased lung compliance in the affected area.
      f. In most cases, the patient's own immunologic mechanisms keep the bacilli in check, but the bacillus remains dormant in the lungs for many years, resulting in a positive result on TB skin tests. These encapsulated bacilli can escape in later years, causing infection.
      g. Chronic dilation of the bronchi (bronchiectasis) may result during the healing process of TB.
      h. In uncontrolled cases, the tubercles increase in size and combine to form larger tubercles, which may rupture and permit air and the infected material to enter the pleural space, bronchi, and bronchioles.

4. **Clinical signs and symptoms**

> **Note**
>
> Most individuals infected with TB have few, if any, symptoms. The primary TB lesion heals completely, possibly leaving a small scar, which could calcify later in life.

   a. Cough
★ b. Sputum production that tests positive for acid-fast bacilli
   c. Tachycardia
   d. Increased cardiac output
   e. Chest pain
   f. Hemoptysis
   g. Dull percussion note
   h. Crackles and rhonchi with chest auscultation
   i. Hyperventilation and hypoxemia (in early stages)
   j. Chronic respiratory acidosis with hypoxemia (in late stages)
   k. Cyanosis (in severe cases)

5. **Characteristics on chest x-ray films**
   a. Enlarged lymph nodes in hilar region (lymphadenopathy)
   b. Pleural effusion
   c. Cavitation
   d. Ghon's complex (lung lesion and lymph node involvement)
   e. Fibrosis
   f. Infiltrates
6. **Characteristics on pulmonary function studies**
   a. Decreased VC
   b. Decreased FRC
   c. Decreased RV
   d. Decreased TLC

> **Note**
>
> These findings are characteristic of the restrictive lung processes that occur in TB.

7. **Treatment**
   a. Supplemental O_2
   b. Antituberculosis drugs: These drugs are used in combination for 2 to 4 months.
      (1) Rifampin
      (2) Isoniazid (INH)
      (3) Ethambutol
      (4) Streptomycin
   c. Placement in respiratory isolation
   d. Routine airway maintenance

III. **OTHER LUNG DISORDERS**
   A. **Pulmonary Edema (Cardiogenic)**
      1. **Definition:** An excessive amount of fluid in the lung tissues or alveoli, caused by an increase in pulmonary capillary pressure resulting from hydrostatic left-sided abnormal heart function.
      2. **Causes**
         a. Left-sided heart failure
         b. Aortic stenosis
         c. Mitral valve stenosis
         d. Systemic hypertension

> **Note**
>
> These four mechanisms cause back up of fluid from the heart into the pulmonary capillaries until they become engorged, leading to pulmonary edema, and are evidenced by increased PCWP levels.

      e. Alveolar capillary membrane leak caused by injury, such as seen in ARDS (noncardiogenic pulmonary edema). **PCWP is normal in this instance.**
      3. **Pathophysiology**
         a. Fluid balance is maintained within the capillaries by two forces.
            (1) **Plasma oncotic pressure** (pressure trying to keep fluid in the capillaries)
            (2) **Capillary hydrostatic pressure** (pressure trying to push fluid out of the capillaries)
         b. Oncotic pressure is normally much higher than capillary hydrostatic pressure, keeping fluid in the capillaries.
         c. As blood from the heart backs up into the pulmonary circulation, capillary hydrostatic pressure increases above plasma oncotic pressure, and fluid from the blood leaks out into the interstitial spaces.
         d. Excess fluid overwhelms the lymphatic system (which normally drains the interstitial spaces) and the fluid drains into the alveoli, resulting in **decreased lung compliance.**
         e. Raw increases because of the excess fluid.
         f. A-a gradient widens as a result of intrapulmonary shunting and V/Q mismatch results.
      4. **Clinical signs and symptoms**
         a. Dyspnea
            (1) **Orthopnea:** dyspnea while lying down (relieved by sitting upright in semi-Fowler's or Fowler's position)
            (2) **Paroxysmal nocturnal dyspnea:** severe attack of dyspnea that occurs during sleep and awakens the patient (relieved by sitting up in semi-Fowler's position).
         ★ b. Productive cough with thin, pink frothy secretions
         ★ c. Crackles may be auscultated in bases of lung (or in all lung fields in severe edema)
         d. Tachypnea
         e. Cyanosis
         ★ f. Diaphoresis (sweating)
         g. Distended neck veins
         h. Tachycardia or other arrhythmias
      5. **Characteristics on chest x-ray films**
         a. Increased vascular markings
         b. Interstitial edema
         c. Enlarged heart shadow
      6. **Treatment**
         a. O_2 administration (percentage based on PaO_2)
         b. Cardiac glycosides
         c. Ventilatory support with PEEP (if condition is severe)

d. Maintain adequate airway
e. Morphine
f. IPPB with ethyl alcohol (40% to 50% dilution)
g. Diuretics such as furosemide (Lasix)

B. **Pulmonary Embolism (PE)**
1. **Definition:** Obstruction of the pulmonary artery or one of its branches by a blood clot. **Embolus:** A clot that travels through the bloodstream from its vessel of origin to lodge in a smaller vessel, obstructing blood flow.
2. **Causes**
   a. The blood clot usually originates in deep veins of the legs or pelvic area, dislodges, travels back to the heart through the venous system, and lodges in the pulmonary artery.
   b. Clot originally forms because of stagnation or venous stasis from prolonged bed rest, immobility from the pain of trauma or surgery, or paralysis.
   c. Seen in COPD patients because of venous stasis, resulting from the increased viscosity of their blood.
3. **Pathophysiology**
   a. Blood flow is obstructed to areas of the involved lung, contributing to dead-space ventilation (ventilation without perfusion).
   b. Lung compliance decreases as atelectasis occurs in the region of the decreased perfusion. This is the lung's response to inadequate perfusion to try and maintain normal V/Q matching.
   c. Widened A-a gradient results from intrapulmonary shunting and V/Q mismatch.
4. **Clinical signs and symptoms**
   a. Dyspnea
   b. Chest pain
   c. Tachypnea
   d. Cough
   e. Pleuritic pain
   f. Hemoptysis
   g. Tenderness and swelling in lower extremities due to thrombophlebitis
   h. Tachycardia
   i. Cyanosis
   j. Decreased breath sounds over the affected area. Wheezing and crackles may be heard.
5. **Characteristics on chest x-ray films**
   a. May be normal
   b. Decreased lung volume
   c. Linear densities of atelectasis
   d. Pleural effusion
   e. Elevated hemidiaphragm caused by atelectasis
6. **Diagnostic procedures**
   A valuable procedure for the diagnosis of PE is a V/Q lung scan. Normal results on a perfusion scan should rule out PE. **Pulmonary angiography** is another procedure that is sometimes performed for definitive diagnosis of PE.
   (a) **V/Q scan:** The patient inhales a harmless radioactive substance, which is distributed throughout the alveoli. A small amount of radioactive imaging material is injected into a vein, and it too travels to the lung and outlines the blood supply or perfusion to the lung. Areas with inadequate perfusion appear dark on the scan because the radioactive particles are unable to pass to an area of obstruction.
   (b) **Pulmonary angiography** is the most accurate method for detection of pulmonary emboli. A dye that is visible on x-ray film is injected into an artery and travels to the pulmonary arteries, where the obstruction is outlined and can be viewed.
7. **Treatment**
   a. Prevention
      (1) Elastic stockings
      (2) Leg elevation
      (3) Ambulation
      (4) Small doses of heparin (an anticoagulant)
   b. Anticoagulation therapy
      (1) Heparin
      (2) Warfarin sodium (Coumadin)
      (3) Streptokinase or urokinase in cases of massive embolus
   c. Supplemental O_2
   d. If hypotension present:
      (1) Vasopressors
      (2) Fluids

C. Acute Respiratory Distress Syndrome **(ARDS)**
1. **Definition:** A group of symptoms causing acute, catastrophic respiratory failure, resulting from pulmonary injury. For the lung condition to be considered ARDS, three criteria must be met.
   a. Infiltrates on chest x-ray confirm that fluid is leaking into the interstitial spaces.
   b. Normal heart function as evidenced by normal PCWP.
   c. PO_2/FIO_2 ratio of less than 200
2. **Causes**
   a. Diffuse lung injury
      (1) Sepsis

(2) Aspiration

(3) Near-drowning

(4) O_2 toxicity

(5) Shock

(6) Thoracic trauma

(7) Extensive burns

(8) Inhalation of toxic gases (e.g., smoke inhalation)

(9) Fluid overload

(10) Fat embolism

(11) Narcotic overdose

  b. Most patients have no previous pulmonary problems.

3. **Pathophysiology**

  a. Lung injury occurs and is followed by an inflammatory process.

  b. Alveolar capillary membrane begins to leak, causing noncardiogenic pulmonary edema.

  c. Fluid builds up in the interstitial spaces, alveoli, and distal airways.

  d. Surfactant production decreases, resulting in atelectasis, while excessive fluid fills the alveoli and airways.

★ e. Because of inflammatory cells, fibrin, and cellular debris that result from the inflammatory process, the lungs become stiff and lung compliance decreases.

  f. In severe cases, the lungs may become almost entirely atelectatic, leading to massive intrapulmonary shunting.

4. **Clinical signs and symptoms**

★ a. Hypoxemia: In severe cases, it is refractory (not responsive) to O_2 therapy.

  b. Cyanosis

  c. Severe dyspnea and cough

★ d. Decreased lung compliance

  e. Suprasternal and intercostal retractions

  f. Widened A-a gradient on 100% O_2 (severe cases)

  g. Tachypnea

5. **Characteristics on chest x-ray films**

  a. Interstitial edema

  b. Alveolar edema (fluffy infiltration)

6. **Treatment**

  a. Patients are usually not managed well on high O_2 concentrations alone because of decreased lung compliance.

  b. Mechanical ventilation with **PEEP**

★ (1) Because the lungs are noncompliant, peak inspiratory pressures are quite elevated.

★ (2) Add PEEP if PaO_2 is below normal when the patient is on an FIO_2 of 0.60 or more.

Note

To prevent further lung tissue damage caused by high inspiratory pressures, lower tidal volumes are being used. This results in elevated $PaCO_2$ levels. This type of ventilator management, referred to as "permissive hypercapnia," is decreasing the mortality rate in ARDS patients according to recent studies.

---

  c. Monitor heart pressures (PAP, PCWP) with Swan-Ganz catheter

  d. Diuretics

  e. Routine airway maintenance

D. **Pneumothorax**

1. **Definition:** The presence of air in the pleural space.

2. **Causes**

  a. Spontaneous pneumothorax

    (1) Develops without previous trauma

    (2) Seen most commonly in tall, thin young males as a result of bleb rupture

    (3) Seen in COPD patients as a result of bullous disease and bleb rupture

  b. Traumatic pneumothorax

    (1) Broken ribs

    (2) Puncture wound

    (3) Chest or neck surgery

3. **Pathophysiology**

  a. When air enters the pleural space, the negative pressure in the pleural space becomes atmospheric resulting in the "negative" pull on the lung to be lost. The lung begins to collapse because of its natural recoil properties diminishing ventilation to the lung.

  b. A **tension pneumothorax** occurs if the opening to the pleural space in the lung acts as a one-way valve, permitting air to enter the space but not allowing the air to exit.

    (1) Ventilation of the affected lung diminishes.

★ (2) The trapped air increases pressure on the affected side, pushing the trachea and mediastinum to the unaffected side. Pressure compresses the heart resulting in a decreased cardiac output. This is a life-threatening condition.

    (3) The **immediate action** to take is to relieve the pressure in the pleural space by inserting a needle in the second or third intercostal space.

  c. The volume of the unaffected lung will increase and more blood will perfuse it, which helps to prevent severe hypoxemia.

4. **Clinical signs and symptoms**
   a. Chest pain
   b. Dyspnea
   c. Decreased breath sounds over affected lung
   d. Hyperresonant percussion note over affected lung
   e. Asymmetric chest excursion
   f. Tachypnea (in severe cases)
   g. Cyanosis (in severe cases)
5. **Characteristics on chest x-ray films**
   ★ a. Hyperlucency
   ★ b. Deviation of heart, trachea, and mediastinum to the opposite (unaffected) side, if tension pneumothorax is present.
6. **Diagnostic procedures**
   a. Although chest x-ray films enable a definitive diagnosis of pneumothorax in patients of all ages, transillumination with a fiberoptic probe has been successful in diagnosis of pneumothorax in infants. The transilluminator has a light on its distal tip, and when placed over areas of free air in the pleural space, transillumination is greater than in other areas.
7. **Treatment**
   a. Needle aspiration: **immediately in tension pneumothorax**
   b. Placement of chest tube
   c. Supplemental O_2 as needed (monitor SpO_2 and/or ABG levels)
E. **Pleural Effusion**
   1. **Definition:** Excessive fluid in the pleural space.
      a. Transudate: fluid caused by an imbalance between transcapillary pressure and plasma oncotic pressure.
      b. Exudate: fluid caused by increased capillary permeability, as in inflammation.
   2. **Causes**
      a. Causes of transudative pleural effusion
         ★ (1) CHF (most common cause)
         (2) Cirrhosis of the liver
         (3) Kidney disease
      b. Causes of exudative pleural effusion
         (1) Infections
         (2) Trauma
         (3) Surgery
         (4) Tumors
         (5) Pulmonary embolism (PE)
   3. **Pathophysiology**
      a. Fluid accumulates in the pleural space as a result of an imbalance between the formation of the fluid and how much is absorbed.

b. Increased fluid formation may cause pleural effusion.
c. Decreased absorption may cause pleural effusion.
4. **Clinical signs and symptoms**
   a. Chest pain
   b. Dyspnea
   c. Dullness to percussion
   d. Absent breath sounds over the fluid
5. **Characteristics on chest x-ray films**
   a. Blunting of costophrenic angle
   b. Homogeneous density in dependent part of the hemithorax

> **Note**
>
> A radiograph taken in the lateral decubitus position (patient lying on side) should confirm the effusion. The fluid moves with gravity as the patient lies on the side.

6. **Treatment**
   a. Drain fluid by thoracentesis
   b. Chest tube drainage may be necessary in chronic cases
   c. Supplemental O_2 as needed (monitor ABG levels and/or SpO_2)
F. **Atelectasis**
   1. **Definition:** Partial or complete collapse of alveoli. It may involve small localized areas of the lung, a lobe, or the entire lung.
   2. **Causes**
      a. Obstructed airways: This may result from secretions, tumors, mucus plugs, or foreign body aspiration. These obstructions to gas flow prevent air from reaching the alveoli for gas exchange. This is referred to as **absorption atelectasis.** Another example of absorption atelectasis occurs when high levels of O_2 are delivered to the lung. This "washes out" the nitrogen in the lung, resulting in collapsed alveoli.
      b. Loss of negative pleural pressure: There is subatmospheric pressure present in the pleural space, which creates a pull on the lung that helps to keep it from collapsing. Any condition that results in loss of this subatmospheric (negative) pressure, causes the lung to collapse. Pneumothorax and pleural effusion are both causes of the loss of negative intrapleural pressure.
      c. Right mainstem bronchus intubation: If the right mainstem bronchus is inadvertently intubated, no gas flow enters the left lung. This results in atelectasis of the left lung.

The same holds true, obviously, for a left mainstem bronchus intubation, but the incidence is much less common, since the angle of the left mainstem bronchus is 45° to 55°; the right mainstem bronchus angles off the trachea at about 25°, making right bronchus intubation more likely.

d. Deficiency or loss of surfactant: Surfactant is present in the fluid that lines the alveolar wall and reduces surface tension, so that alveoli do not collapse during exhalation. Conditions resulting in reduced surfactant include: O_2 toxicity, in which high O_2 levels damage the alveolar type II cells that produce surfactant, which leads to ARDS; near-drowning, which results in loss of surfactant from the aspiration of certain substances; and in premature birth, surfactant is immature, resulting in atelectasis (see chapter on neonatal and pediatric lung disease).

e. Hypoventilation: Decreased VT from any condition eventually results in atelectasis. Examples include: chest or abdominal pain, phrenic nerve paralysis, abdominal or thoracic surgery, high-level spinal cord injury, inadequate ventilator VT settings, unconsciousness.

f. Decreased pulmonary blood flow: If a PE is blocking blood flow to the alveoli, the lungs compensate by reducing volume to the specific alveoli (resulting in atelectasis) in which there is deficient perfusion, so blood will more likely perfuse open alveoli.

3. **Pathophysiology**

a. As a result of the conditions resulting in atelectasis mentioned in the previous section, FRC and VC decrease.

b. Intrapulmonary shunting occurs as capillary blood passes by collapsed alveoli, preventing gas exchange from taking place normally and resulting in hypoxemia.

4. **Clincial signs and symptoms**

a. Asymptomatic in mild atelectasis

b. Hypoxemia

c. Dyspnea

d. Cough

e. Dullness to percussion

f. Elevated diaphragm

g. Crackles in lung bases

h. Diminished or absent breath sounds

i. Tracheal deviation toward the atelectatic lung

5. **Characteristics on chest x-ray films**

a. Increased density (white)

b. Elevated diaphragm

c. Displaced interlobar fissures

d. Mediastinal shift

e. Altered bronchial and carinal angles

6. **Treatment**

a. Prevention of postoperative atelectasis by administration of incentive spirometry or IPPB

b. Adequate pulmonary hydration to prevent mucus plugs and mobilization of secretions

c. Treatment of underlying atelectasis with deep-breathing exercises, such as incentive spirometry or IPPB

d. Placement on CPAP if patient is hypoxemic on 60% O_2 or more

e. Placement on PEEP if patient is on ventilator

IV. **SLEEP APNEA**

A. Sleep apnea is present in patients who have at least 30 episodes of apnea over a 6-hr period of sleep.

B. The apneic period may last from 20 sec to more than 90 sec.

C. **Types of Sleep Apnea**

1. **Obstructive sleep apnea**

a. Apnea caused by upper airway anatomic obstruction.

b. During the apneic period, the patient exhibits **strong and often intense respiratory effort.**

c. Although sleep posture (sleeping on side rather than supine) has some benefits, **the use of CPAP or BiPAP while sleeping is the most effective method for treating obstructive sleep apnea.**

d. Obstructive sleep apnea may be associated with
(1) Obesity
(2) Excessive pharyngeal tissue
(3) Deviated nasal septum
(4) Laryngeal web
(5) Laryngeal stenosis
(6) Enlarged adenoids or tonsils

e. **Symptoms of obstructive sleep apnea**
(1) Loud snoring
(2) Hypersomnolence (excessive sleeping during the day)
(3) Morning headache
(4) Nausea
(5) Personality changes

2. **Central sleep apnea**

a. Apnea occurs because of the failure of the central respiratory centers (in the medulla) to send signals to the respiratory muscles.

b. **It is characterized by the absence of inspiratory effort with no diaphragmatic movement (unlike obstructive sleep apnea).**

c. This type of sleep apnea is associated with CNS disorders.

d. Central sleep apnea may be associated with
   (1) Hypoventilation syndrome
   (2) Encephalitis
   (3) Spinal surgery
   (4) Brainstem disorders

e. **Symptoms of central sleep apnea**
   (1) Insomnia
   (2) Mild snoring
   (3) Depression
   (4) Fatigue during the day

Note

Some patients may have a combination of both obstructive and central sleep apnea, which is defined as mixed sleep apnea.

D. **Diagnostic Sleep Studies**
   1. Sleep studies are a very effective method for the diagnosis of sleep apnea and other breathing disorders such as sudden infant death syndrome (SIDS).
   2. Sleep studies are also valuable in determining the cause, severity, and pathophysiologic effects of the breathing disorder during sleep.
   3. **Polysomnography** refers to events that are recorded graphically while the individual is sleeping.
   4. Continuous recordings on graph paper **(polysomnogram)** during the sleep study include
      a. Eye movement (electrooculogram)
      b. Brain wave activity (EEG)
      c. ECG
      d. Absence of air flow (apnea) is determined with the use of a CO_2 analyzer, thermistor, tracheal sound recorder, or a pneumotachograph
      e. Chest and abdominal movement
      f. O_2 saturation using an ear oximeter

POST-CHAPTER STUDY QUESTIONS

1. List the five diseases classified as COPD.
2. List the common findings on an emphysema patient's chest films.

3. What PaO_2 level should be maintained on a COPD patient who is chronically hypoxemic?
4. List the clinical signs and symptoms of cor pulmonale.
5. How does O_2 therapy help prevent or treat cor pulmonale?
6. The count of which type of WBC is characteristically elevated in the sputum and blood of an asthmatic?
7. What aerosolized medication is used to treat *Pneumocystis carinii* pneumonia?
8. List four causes of cardiogenic pulmonary edema.
9. List the signs and symptoms of pulmonary edema.
10. List the treatment modalities for pulmonary edema.
11. List the various causes of ARDS.
12. List the signs and symptoms of ARDS.
13. List treatment modalities for ARDS.
14. Define pneumothorax.
15. What is the immediate treatment for a tension pneumothorax?
16. What is the most effective method for treating obstructive sleep apnea?
17. List six parameters that are measured during a sleep study.

Answers are at the end of the chapter.

REFERENCES

Des Jardins T: Clinical manifestations of respiratory disease, ed 2, Chicago, 1990, Year-Book Medical Publishers.

Farzan S: A concise handbook of respiratory diseases, ed 4, Stamford, CT, 1997, Appleton & Lange Co.

The Merck Manual of Medical Information, 1997, Merck and Co.

PRE-TEST ANSWERS

1. A
2. B
3. C
4. C
5. A
6. D

ANSWERS TO POST-CHAPTER STUDY QUESTIONS

1. Emphysema, chronic bronchitis, asthma, bronchiectasis, cystic fibrosis
2. Flattened diaphragm, increased lung markings (hyperinflation), reduced vascular markings, bullae or bleb formation
3. 50 to 65 mm Hg

4. Pedal edema, distended jugular (neck) veins, enlarged liver
5. By causing pulmonary vasodilation of pulmonary vessels thereby decreasing pulmonary hypertension
6. Eosinophils
7. Pentamidine
8. Left ventricular failure, mitral valve stenosis, aortic stenosis, systemic hypertension
9. Dyspnea; pink, frothy secretions; crackles; tachypnea; cyanosis; diaphoresis; distended neck veins; arrhythmias
10. Supplemental O_2, cardiac medications, ventilatory support, maintain airway, morphine, IPPB with ethyl alcohol, diuretics

11. Sepsis, aspiration, near-drowning, O_2 toxicity, shock, thoracic trauma, extensive burns, toxic gas inhalation, fluid overload, fat embolism, narcotic overdose
12. Hypoxemia (often not responsive to O_2), cyanosis, severe dyspnea, decreased lung compliance, retractions, widened $P(A-a)O_2$ gradient, tachypnea
13. Mechanical ventilation with PEEP, diuretics, airway maintenance, monitor cardiac pressures
14. Air in the pleural space
15. Needle aspiration in the second or third intercostal space
16. CPAP or BiPAP
17. Eye movement, EEG, ECG, apnea, chest or abdominal movement, SpO_2

Chapter 13

Neonatal and Pediatric Respiratory Care

PRE-TEST QUESTIONS

Answer the pre-test questions before studying the chapter. This will help you determine your strong and weak areas regarding the material covered.

1. An APGAR score of 5 is determined 5 min after delivery of a term infant. Which of the following should be done at this time?

   A. Stimulate and deliver low-to-moderate O_2 concentrations.
   B. Intubate and place on mechanical ventilation.
   C. Intubate and place on CPAP and 80% O_2.
   D. Place on nasal CPAP and 100% O_2.

2. The foramen ovale and ductus arteriosis remain patent in infants with persistent fetal circulation as a direct result of which of the following?

   A. Hypocarbia
   B. Pulmonary hypertension
   C. Hyperoxia
   D. Arterial hypotension

3. Which of the following is not an indication for nasal CPAP in an infant?

   A. To increase static lung compliance.
   B. To decrease FRC.
   C. To decrease PVR.
   D. To decrease intrapulmonary shunting.

4. Which of the following are complications of an umbilical artery catheter (UAC)?

   I. Pneumothorax
   II. Thromboembolism
   III. Infection

   A. I only
   B. II only
   C. I and III only
   D. II and III only

5. Which of the following may occur as a result of cold stress to an infant?

   I. Hypoxemia
   II. Metabolic acidemia
   III. Hypoglycemia
   IV. Decreased O_2 consumption

   A. I and III only
   B. II and IV only
   C. I, II, and III only
   D. I, II and IV only

6. An elevation in the levels of chloride in sweat is diagnostic for which of the following lung conditions?

   A. Bronchiolitis
   B. Cystic fibrosis
   C. Hyaline membrane disease
   D. Epiglottitis

Answers are at end of the chapter.

REVIEW

I. NEONATAL RESPIRATORY CARE
A. The "High-Risk Infant"
   1. The term "high-risk infant" describes an infant who is at greater risk of death or who has a higher probability of a permanent disability.
   2. Maternal factors involved with high risk infants
      a. Maternal age (less than 16 or more than 35 years)
      b. Diabetes
      c. Drug, alcohol, or tobacco abuse
      d. Maternal infections
      e. Previous cesarean section
      f. High blood pressure
      g. Previous history of infant with respiratory problems or anomalies
      h. Lack of adequate prenatal care
   3. Other factors that characterize high-risk infants
      a. premature rupture of membranes (PROM)—increases the risk for fetal infection, especially pneumonia

b. Premature delivery (at less than 38 weeks gestation)
c. Postmature delivery (at more than 42 weeks gestation)
d. Meconium in amniotic fluid
e. Prolapsed cord
f. Prolonged labor
g. Abnormal fetal presentation (i.e., breech presentation)

B. **Assessment of the Neonate**
1. Assessing gestational age
   a. The **Dubowitz** scoring system is one of the most accurate means of estimating the baby's gestational age.
   b. The Dubowitz system scores the infant on 11 neuromuscular signs and 10 external characteristics.
   c. Each specific sign is worth a given number of points and the infant is given all or part of those points, depending on the assessment of that particular sign or characteristic.
   d. Points from each assessed area are totaled and plotted on a graph, which determines the infant's gestational age.
   e. Areas assessed include skin thickness, color and transparency of skin, amount of vernix present on the infant, plantar creases, posture, and muscle tone.
   f. Normal gestational age is 38 to 42 weeks.
   g. The calculated gestational age can then be plotted on a graph, along with the infant's birth weight, to determine if the infant is appropriate for gestational age (AGA), small for gestational age (SGA), or large for gestational age (LGA).

2. **Apgar scoring system**
   a. This system evaluates the infant's general condition within 5 min after birth.
   b. The five areas of assessment and the 0- to 2-point scoring system for each area are listed in the following table.

	SCORE		
Assessed sign	**0**	**1**	**2**
Heart rate	Absent	< 100 beats/min	> 100 beats/min
Respiratory effort	Absent	Slow, irregular	Strong cry
Color	Pale, blue	Body pink, extremities blue	Totally pink
Reflex irritability	No response	Grimace	Sneeze or cough
Muscle tone	Limp	Some flexion	Active flexion

c. The Apgar assessment is done at 1 min after delivery to determine if immediate intervention is required and again at 5 min after birth.
d. Apgar results at 1 min and corresponding intervention.
   (1) **Score of 7 to 10** is normal; requires routine observation, suction upper airway with bulb syringe, dry the infant, and place under a warmer.
   (2) **Score of 4 to 6** indicates moderate asphyxia; requires stimulation and O_2 administration.
   (3) **Score of 0 to 3** indicates severe asphyxia; requires immediate resuscitation with ventilatory assistance.
e. The 5-min Apgar score is useful in determining the infant's response to intervention; a score of less than 6 is associated with major complications and treatment in an intensive care nursery.
f. The five assessed signs in the Apgar scoring system may be more easily remembered by using the following mnemonic.

"A" for appearance (color)
"P" for pulse (heart rate)
"G" for grimace (reflex irritability)
"A" for activity (muscle tone)
"R" for respiration (respiratory effort)

Note

Acrocyanosis, or cyanosis in the hands and feet, is normal after birth, but cyanosis observed in the mucous membranes or lips indicates that O_2 therapy must be administered immediately.

3. **Silverman scoring system**
   a. This system helps determine the severity of respiratory distress.
   b. The infant is assessed in five areas:
      (1) Intercostal retractions
      (2) Xiphoid retractions
      (3) Chest lag or paradoxical breathing
      (4) Nasal flaring: often the first or only sign of respiratory distress
      (5) Grunting: An audible expiratory grunt, caused by the infant partially closing the glottis during exhalation to prevent alveolar collapse, is a common sign of respiratory distress in infants.
   c. Each assessed area is worth from 0 to 2 points, with the *lowest* score indicating minimal distress (as opposed to the *highest*

score being the best on the Apgar scoring system).

4. **Other clinical assessments**
   a. Respiratory rate: normally 40/min to 60/min
   b. Heart rate: 130 to 150 beats/min
   c. Blood pressure: normal systolic = 60 to 90 mm Hg; normal diastolic = 30 to 60 mm Hg.
   d. Normal ABG levels on room air.

pH	7.35 to 7.45 (no less than 7.25 at birth)
$Paco_2$	35 to 45 mm Hg
Pao_2	50 to 70 mm Hg
HCO_3^-	20 to 26 mEq/L
BE	−5 to +5

C. **O_2 Delivery Devices for Neonates**
   1. **Incubators**

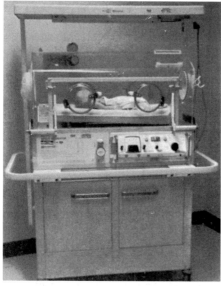

From Scanlan C, Spearman C, Sheldon R: Egan's fundamentals of respiratory care, ed 5, St. Louis, 1990, The CV Mosby Co.

   a. Inlet nipples on the incubator allow for attachment of O_2 tubing that supplies the flow of O_2 to the inside of the incubator.
   b. Low levels (21% to 40%) and high levels (40% to 100%) are obtainable on most models by adjusting a lever that alters the amount of room air entrainment. Most units have a red lever that identifies low or high levels of O_2 use. If the lever is in a vertical position, the O_2 percentage is

above 40%. If the lever is in a horizontal position, it indicates that O_2 percentages of less than 40% are being delivered.
   c. O_2 may also be delivered into the incubator via aerosol tubing from a nebulizer set on a specific percentage. The tubing is placed through one of the portholes of the incubator.
   d. The disadvantage of using an incubator for an infant on supplemental O_2 is that inconsistent O_2 percentage delivery results from leaks in the incubator when it is opened to administer care to the infant.

2. **O_2 hood**

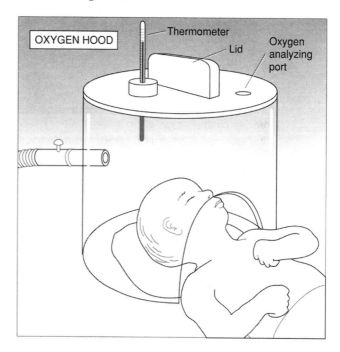

   a. The O_2 hood is the recommended method for delivering O_2 in the range of 21% to 100% to the infant.
   b. A heated nebulizer connected to an O_2 blender is the most common method of O_2 delivery. The aerosol tubing connects into the back of the hood. If a blender is used to regulate the O_2 percentage, the nebulizer must be set on 100% so that no air entrainment occurs, which would alter the blender percentage.
   c. A heated humidifier (Cascade or pass-over) is often used rather than a nebulizer to prevent overhydration of the infant.
   d. The percentage of O_2 should be analyzed continuously with an O_2 analyzer. A port in the top of the hood makes analyzing possible. **It should be noted that the O_2 percentage should be analyzed as close to the infant's airway as**

possible, since the percentage of O$_2$ is somewhat higher at the bottom of the hood as opposed to the top.

  e. A heated nebulizer or humidifier should be used because cold gas blowing on the infant's face may induce apnea and colder temperatures in the hood may increase the infant's O$_2$ consumption.

  f. Flows into the hood should be at least 5 L/min to prevent CO$_2$ build up in the hood.

  g. Temperatures inside the hood should be closely monitored through a port in the top of the hood to avoid overheating or underheating the infant.

  h. Noise levels inside the hood have been proven to be a source of hearing loss to the infant. To keep noise levels to a minimum, nebulizers that entrain air should not be used because they produce increased noise levels.

3. **Nasal catheter or cannula**

  a. Nasal catheters and cannulas are available in infant sizes and are most commonly used for long-term O$_2$ therapy in the treatment of bronchopulmonary dysplasia (BPD) and other chronic diseases.

  b. The flowmeters used to deliver O$_2$ through the catheter or cannula should be calibrated so that increments of 0.25 and 0.50 L/min can be used.

4. **Nasal CPAP**

  a. CPAP is most commonly administered to infants with nasal prongs.

  b. CPAP may also be administered with a mask, ET tube, or nasopharyngeal tube.

  c. **Indications for nasal CPAP**

    (1) To improve oxygenation

> **Note**
>
> In order to prevent pulmonary tissue damage (such as BPD) from high FIO_2 levels, CPAP should be administered. FIO_2 should be no higher than 0.60 to maintain normal PaO_2 levels, if possible. If PaO_2 is less than normal, on 0.60 institute CPAP, do not increase the FIO_2.

    (2) To increase static lung compliance
    (3) To increase FRC
    (4) To decrease the work of breathing
    (5) To decrease intrapulmonary shunting
    (6) To decrease PVR

  d. **Complications of nasal CPAP**

    (1) Barotrauma (pneumothorax)

    (2) Decreased venous return, resulting in decreased cardiac output

> **Note**
>
> Decreased venous return is less likely to occur if the infant has decreased static lung compliance caused by RDS. Infants with normal lungs would be more prone to this complication because the lungs are more compliant and the airway pressure is more easily transferred to the superior and inferior vena cavae.

    (3) Air-trapping
    (4) Pressure necrosis
    (5) Loss of CPAP from crying or displacement

  e. ABGs must be drawn frequently if CPAP is used to monitor PaCO_2 levels. Should PaCO_2 begin to rise, mechanical ventilation is necessary.

  f. The use of nasal CPAP on infants is based on the fact that infants are obligate nose breathers. If the baby cries, CPAP is lost.

D. **Hazards of O$_2$ Therapy in the Neonate**

  1. **Retrolental fibroplasia (RLF)**

    a. This condition is also called neonatal retinopathy and retinopathy of prematurity (ROP).

    b. RLF is caused by high levels of O$_2$ in the blood **(PaO_2 of more than 100 mm Hg).**

    c. RLF occurs primarily in premature infants who have very fragile retinal blood vessels.

    d. Initially, the high arterial O$_2$ levels cause constriction of the retinal vessels. As the vessels remain constricted, new vessels form in an attempt to oxygenate the retina.

    e. This growth of new vessels leads to hemorrhaging within the retina, retinal detachment, and blindness.

    f. The degree of blindness varies in each situation and infants exposed to supplemental O$_2$ should have an eye examination before discharge.

    g. ABG samples should be frequently obtained while the infant is on O$_2$ to determine the O$_2$ level in the blood. **If the infant has a ductal shunt (discussed later in this chapter), the blood must be drawn from the right radial, brachial, or temporal artery to measure the PaO_2 of the blood going to the head.** If no shunt exists, blood may be drawn from the umbilical artery catheter or any peripheral artery.

  2. Bronchopulmonary dysplasia (BPD)

a. BPD is caused by long-term supplemental O_2 therapy and mechanical ventilation.

b. Damage occurs in the alveolar epithelium, causing destruction of pulmonary tissues.

c. **BPD is discussed in detail later in this chapter.**

E. **Sites for Obtaining Arterial Blood**
   1. **Umbilical artery**
      a. An umbilical artery catheter (UAC) is normally placed in critically ill infants who require frequent ABG analysis.
      b. The catheter is inserted into one of the two umbilical arteries. After insertion, the position of the catheter should be determined by radiograph.
      c. The tip of the catheter should rest in the **descending aorta** at either one of the following vertebral levels as seen on radiographic image.
         (1) T6 to T10 (thoracic aorta)
         (2) L3 to L4 (lumbar aorta)
      d. The catheter may be secured in place with umbilical tape or sutures attached to the umbilical stump, and the catheter is then taped to the abdomen.
      e. **Advantages of the UAC**
         (1) Frequent ABG samples are easily obtained
         (2) Prevents frequent peripheral arterial punctures
         (3) Allows continuous monitoring of blood pressure
         (4) Allows the infusion of drugs and fluids
      f. **Complications of the UAC**
         (1) Infection
         (2) Thromboembolism (To help prevent this, flush line with heparin after a blood sample is drawn.)
         (3) Air embolism
         (4) Hemorrhage
      g. UACs should be left in place for no longer than **7 to 10 days** to help avoid these complications.
      h. Generally, no more than 0.5 mL of blood is necessary for ABG analysis.
      i. If there is inadequate perfusion to the lower extremities, blanching or cyanosis of the legs or feet will be evident. The catheter should be withdrawn or replaced.
   2. **Peripheral artery puncture**
      a. Arterial blood may be drawn from one of several arteries in the neonate, including the radial, brachial, temporal, and posterior tibial arteries.
      b. The radial artery is the most common site because of its easy accessibility, good collat-

eral circulation, and lack of immediately adjacent nerves or veins.

   c. A 25- or 26-gauge needle is generally used to puncture the artery at a 35° to 45° angle to the artery. The bevel of the needle should be facing up when radial puncture is performed.
   d. Location of the radial artery is determined by a radial pulse or by placing a **transilluminator** under the back of the wrist. This lighted device aids in the location of the artery.
   e. Since the radial artery in a neonate is very small, it is not uncommon to insert the needle completely through the artery. If, after advancing the needle, there is no blood obtained, withdraw the needle slightly until blood enters the needle.
   f. When an adequate amount of blood has been obtained, the needle is withdrawn, and pressure should be applied to the puncture site for approximately 5 minutes.
   g. Any air bubbles in the sample should be removed before analysis. If this is not done, the blood gas analysis will come back with erroneous values, indicating a high Pa_{O_2} and low Pa_{CO_2}.

   3. **Arterialized capillary blood sampling**
      a. Arterialized capillary blood is normally obtained from the heel of the neonate by using a lancet to puncture the capillary.
      b. The infant's foot should be warmed for several minutes (usually by wrapping a warm moist diaper around the foot) to cause peripheral vasodilation, which improves capillary perfusion and arterializes the capillary blood.
      c. The heel should then be cleaned with alcohol and the capillary punctured, using a lancet. The blood is contained in a heparinized glass capillary tube.
      d. Care should be taken not to squeeze the heel, because this may cause damage to the foot and contaminate the sample with venous blood and interstitial fluid.
      e. The capillary tube should be as close to the puncture site as possible to avoid contaminating the sample with room air.
      f. Once the sample is obtained, pressure should be applied to the heel until the bleeding stops, and then an adhesive bandage should be applied.
      g. Capillary blood samples offer fairly reliable correlations for arterial pH and PCO_2, but are unreliable for PO_2 values. While the capillary PO_2 (Pc_{O_2}) may be low, the Pa_{O_2}

may actually be high, which increases the risk of RLF or BPD. It is also possible to have a high PcO_2 when the PaO_2 is low, risking hypoxic damage. **Arterial PO_2 levels must be monitored periodically to prevent this potential hazard. Normal $PaCO_2$ is 40 to 50 mm Hg.**

F. **Transcutaneous $Paco_2$ and PaO_2 Monitoring**
   1. By applying blood gas electrodes over the skin, the neonate's PaO_2 and $Paco_2$ may be monitored continuously without having to perform arterial sticks as frequently.
   2. The probe is attached to the skin, which warms the skin, resulting in vasodilation and increased perfusion to the dermal layer of the skin. O_2 and CO_2 diffuse through the skin in concentrations similar to those in arterial blood.
   3. **Disadvantages of transcutaneous monitoring**
      a. The heated probe (42–44° C) may burn the skin. The location of the probe should be changed every **3 to 4 hours** to prevent this. In the more premature infant with very fragile skin, the probe position should be changed every **2 hours.**
      ★ b. The infant must have adequate perfusion to the area of the skin where the probe is attached to provide accurate readings.
      ★ c. Inaccurate readings occur if the probe is inadequately heated, the monitor is not calibrated properly, or the probe becomes loose and air comes between the probe and the skin.
   4. The monitor requires calibrating during the initial setup and after probe position changes. This is done with the sensor off the infant and is calculated by (PB − 47 mm Hg) × 0.21. After calibration, the monitor takes 20 to 30 min to equilibrate before accurate readings are displayed.

G. **Oximetry**
   1. Monitoring arterial O_2 saturation with a pulse oximeter (SpO_2) is becoming a popular method to determine the oxygenation status of infants.
   2. Oximetry uses photometrics (a light beam shining through the skin or nailbed) to determine SaO_2, therefore burning of the skin that is possible with transcutaneous monitoring is not a factor.

Note

For more detailed information on oximetry, see the chapter on ABG interpretation.

H. **Thermoregulation of the Infant**

Exam Note

Incubators and radiant warmers appear on the RRT examination only.

   1. It is very important that infants are kept in a **thermal neutral environment,** which is an environment that keeps the infant's body temperature normal, resulting in a normal level of O_2 consumption.
   2. Neonates are unable to shiver if they are exposed to a cold environmental temperature. The infant becomes cold-stressed. For neonates to generate heat, they begin to break down brown fat that is stored mainly in the neck and thorax. This is called "nonshivering thermogenesis."
   ★ 3. As brown fat is metabolized, O_2 consumption increases, which may result in hypoxemia. This leads to lactic acidosis (metabolic acidosis). Cold stress also results in apnea and hypoglycemia.
   4. Incubators are common devices used to maintain a thermal neutral environment.
   5. **Radiant warmers** are also used as a way of controlling temperature. These devices deliver warm air from above the infant in an open bed. The infant is therefore more easily accessible than in an incubator.
   ★ 6. A skin probe is applied to the right upper abdomen of the infant. The probe measures the infant's temperature, which should be maintained around 36.5° C. Should the infant's body temperature increase or decrease, a servo control adjusts the amount of heat needed to maintain the temperature that is set on the control (usually 36.5° C).

II. **NEONATAL CARDIOPULMONARY DISORDERS**
A. Respiratory distress syndrome (RDS)
   1. **Definition:** A syndrome affecting premature infants that is caused by inadequate amounts of pulmonary surfactant, which leads to massive atelectasis and hypoxemia. (Also known as hyaline membrane disease or HMD.)
   2. **Causes**
      a. Immature lungs with surfactant deficiency
      b. **Lecithin-sphingomyelin (L:S) ratio of less than 2:1**. These lipid levels may be obtained from amniotic fluid to determine the maturity of the surfactant. A ratio of more than 2:1 indicates mature surfactant.
      c. Infants born before 35 weeks of gestation are at risk for RDS.

3. **Pathophysiology**
   a. Surfactant lines the inner surface of alveoli, decreasing the surface tension and thereby reducing their tendency to collapse.
   b. Immature surfactant or decreased surfactant production, as seen in RDS, leads to alveolar collapse, decreased lung compliance, hypoxemia, and metabolic acidosis.
   c. Alveolar surface tension increases from lack of surfactant, resulting in fluid being pulled into the alveoli. Because of damage to the capillary endothelial cells by acidosis and hypoxemia, the fluid entering the alveoli contains protein and the blood-clotting component fibrin. This makes the alveoli very stiff (noncompliant) and causes the hyaline membrane formation.
4. **Clinical manifestations**
   a. Nasal flaring
   b. Grunting
   c. Retractions
   d. Tachypnea
   e. Cyanosis
   f. ABG levels reveal hypercapnia and hypoxemia with a mixed respiratory and metabolic acidosis.
5. **Chest X-ray findings**
   a. "Ground glass" appearance
   b. Diffuse atelectasis
   c. Air bronchograms
6. **Treatment**
   a. O_2 therapy to maintain PaO_2 above 50 mm Hg
   b. Nasal CPAP or ET-tube CPAP if infant's PaO_2 remains below 50 mm Hg on 60% O_2
   c. Positive pressure ventilation with PEEP if $PaCO_2$ is increasing with a pH of less than 7.25
   d. Surfactant replacement
   e. Thermoregulation
   f. Adequate fluids to prevent dehydration
   g. Packed RBCs are given to prevent anemia and blood loss from frequent ABG samples
B. Bronchopulmonary dysplasia (BPD)
   1. **Definition:** A form of chronic lung disease seen in infants with severe RDS after prolonged positive pressure ventilation and supplemental O_2. Dysplasia refers to abnormal development; in this case, of the bronchi and lungs.
   2. **Causes**
      a. Although the cause of BPD is widely debated, it is thought to be caused by prolonged (more than 7 days) exposure to high concentrations of O_2 with positive pressure ventilation.

   b. A major cause of BPD is thought to be high inspiratory pressures associated with mechanical ventilation, leading to barotrauma.
   c. It occurs more frequently in infants weighing less than 1500 g.
3. **Pathophysiology**
   a. There are four stages of BPD
      (1) **Stage 1** occurs 2 to 4 days after birth and consists of
         (a) Hyaline membrane formation
         (b) Atelectasis
         (c) Necrosis of bronchiolar mucosa
         (d) Bronchiolar metaplasia
      (2) **Stage 2** occurs 4 to 10 days after birth and includes necrosis, repair of alveolar and bronchial epithelium, and emphysematous changes.
      (3) **Stage 3** occurs 10 to 20 days after birth and includes
         (a) Interstitial fibrosis
         (b) Atelectasis
         (c) Continuation of bronchiolar metaplasia
         (d) Increased mucus production
         (e) Bullae formation
      (4) **Stage 4** occurs 30 days after birth and includes
         (a) Formation of emphysematous alveoli
         (b) Atelectasis
         (c) Continuation of interstitial fibrosis
   b. Large amounts of mucus production occur, leading to air-trapping with resultant atelectasis.
4. **Clinical manifestations**
   a. Increased airway resistance
   b. Normal or increased static lung compliance
   c. V/Q mismatch
   d. Hypoxemia on room air
   e. Hypercapnia
   f. Tachypnea
   g. Barrel chest
   h. Retractions
5. **Chest X-ray findings**
   a. "Ground glass" appearance
   b. Opacification
   c. Atelectasis
   d. Hyperlucency
   e. Presence of bullae
6. **Treatment**
   a. O_2 therapy to maintain PaO_2 between 50 and 70 mm Hg (helps prevent pulmonary hypertension resulting from hypoxemia)
   b. Pressure-limited, time-cycled ventilator may be required to maintain normal ABG levels
   c. Adequate humidification to prevent mucus plugging in the airways or ET tube

d. Chest physical therapy and suctioning
e. Adequate nutrition
f. Maintenance of fluid balance or diuretic administration to minimize the infant's increased risk of cor pulmonale, pulmonary edema, and CHF.
g. Bronchodilator therapy

C. **Meconium aspiration**
1. **Definition:** Aspiration of meconium is most commonly associated with full-term or post-term infants. Meconium is discharged in the first fetal bowel movement and is composed of mucus, vernix, epithelial cells, and amniotic fluid.
2. **Causes**
    a. If, while *in utero,* the infant becomes hypoxic, meconium is passed into the amniotic fluid.
    b. Infants, *in utero,* breathe in a shallow manner, moving amniotic fluid into and out of the oropharynx. But if the infant is stressed or asphyxiated, the breaths are much deeper and meconium may be aspirated through the vocal cords and into the lungs.
    c. The **post-term** infant is at greater risk for meconium aspiration because less amniotic fluid is present; therefore, there is less dilution of the meconium.
    d. Even if the meconium is present only in the mouth or the glottic area, aspiration may occur with the infant's first few breaths.
3. **Pathophysiology**
    a. The substances that make up meconium make it very thick, and therefore, if aspirated, it will plug airways, leading to atelectasis and increased airway resistance.
    b. Generally, air flow passes through the obstruction during inspiration but gets trapped during expiration as the airway diameter decreases, resulting in hyperinflation.
    c. This air-trapping often leads to pneumothorax.
    d. Infants with this condition often present with patent ductus arteriosis (discussed later) caused by the intrauterine hypoxia. Hypoxia causes pulmonary vasoconstriction, which prevents the ductus arteriosis and foramen ovale from closing, resulting in a right to left shunt.
4. **Clinical manifestations**
    a. Long fingernails and peeling skin (signs of post-maturity)
    b. Hypoxemia
    c. Hypercarbia
    d. Tachypnea
    e. Retractions, nasal flaring, grunting

f. Barrel chest (from air-trapping)
g. Cyanosis
h. Crackles and rhonchi on chest auscultation
5. **Chest X-ray findings**
    a. Patchy infiltrates
    b. Atelectasis
    c. Consolidation
    d. Pneumothorax (commonly observed)
    e. Hyperinflation
6. **Treatment**
    a. If meconium is observed during delivery, the infant's oral and nasal pharynx should be suctioned once the head is delivered and before the first cry, to prevent aspiration of the meconium.
    b. Immediately after delivery, the infant should be intubated and suctioned to remove meconium from the lower airway.
    c. Positive pressure ventilation should not be started until all meconium is cleared, since this would push it farther into the airways.
    d. O_2 therapy or mechanical ventilation, depending on severity of the condition
    e. Chest physical therapy
    f. Frequent suctioning

D. Persistent fetal circulation (PFC)
1. **Definition:** A condition in which fetal blood circulation through the heart persists after birth. PFC is also referred to as persistent pulmonary hypertension of the neonate (PPHN)
    a. **Normal fetal circulation:** Blood flow through the heart of the infant *in utero* differs from the pathway the blood takes after birth. Only about 10% of blood returning to the right side of the infant's heart flows on into the pulmonary circulation. The other 90% or so of the blood volume in the right side of the heart shunts over to the left side via two pathways. One is through the foramen ovale, a pathway that allows blood to flow from the right atrium into the left atrium. The second area where shunting occurs is through the ductus arteriosus, which is a communication between the pulmonary artery and the descending aorta.
    b. These two communications between the right and left heart are kept open *in utero* because of the high pressure in the pulmonary vasculature. After the infant is delivered and begins breathing O_2 from the air, pulmonary vasodilation occurs, reducing the pulmonary hypertension and allowing the foramen ovale and ductus arteriosus to gradually close.
    c. If closure of these two pathways does not occur, blood will bypass the lungs and be

shunted directly into the left side of the heart and out to the body without oxygenation. **PaO_2 levels do not increase as FIO_2 is increased.**

2. **Causes**
   a. The condition is most common in full-term or post-term infants because the pulmonary vessels are more reactive to hypoxia, leading to pulmonary vasoconstriction
   b. Conditions often accompanied by PFC
      (1) Perinatal asphyxia
      (2) Meconium aspiration
      (3) Pneumonia
      (4) Sepsis
      (5) Congenital heart defects
      (6) Diaphragmatic hernia
      (7) Hypoplastic lungs
      (8) Hypoglycemia

> **Note**
>
> Any condition that results in increased pulmonary vascular resistance (PVR) can cause PFC.

3. **Pathophysiology**
   a. The foramen ovale and ductus arteriosus remain patent as a result of pulmonary hypertension.
   ★ b. This results in right-to-left shunting that causes hypoxemia that is not responsive to O_2 therapy.

4. **Clinical manifestations**
   a. Tachypnea
   b. Hypoxemia
   c. Cyanosis (not in all cases)
   ★ d. More than a 15-mm Hg difference in the PaO_2 between preductal blood (radial or temporal artery) and postductal blood (umbilical artery) on 100% O_2 (i.e., preductal PaO_2 is higher than postductal PaO_2)

> **Note**
>
> Even though this is characteristically diagnostic of a right-to-left shunt, PFC should not be ruled out if this is not observed, because it may still be present. A PDA can be positively identified using ultrasonography. Transcutaneous PO_2 monitors may also be used in place of arterial sticks to determine right-to-left shunting. One $TcPO_2$ probe is placed on the right arm (preductal) and one placed on the abdomen or lower extremities (postductal) and the difference is monitored.

   e. Significant increase in PaO_2 (more than 100 mm Hg) when $PaCO_2$ is maintained at 20 to 25 mm Hg

> **Note**
>
> Maintaining low $PaCO_2$ levels results in pulmonary vasodilation, which should allow less blood flow through the ductus arteriosus and foramen ovale. If shunting is occurring, PaO_2 levels would increase during this test.

5. **Chest X-ray findings**
   a. May be normal
   b. Decreased pulmonary vasculature

6. **Treatment**
   a. Mechanical hyperventilation to maintain $PaCO_2$ levels at 20 to 25 mm Hg with an alkaline pH
   b. Maintenance of PaO_2 levels at more than 100 mm Hg

> **Note**
>
> Maintaining $PaCO_2$ and PaO_2 levels as mentioned above should be done only for the first few days of therapy.

   c. Drug therapy
      (1) Tolazoline (Priscoline), a vasodilator
      (2) Nitroprusside sodium (Nipride), a vasodilator
      (3) Sodium bicarbonate to produce alkalemia
      (4) Dopamine, which increases systemic vascular resistance and thus reduces the right-to-left pressure gradient, which decreases shunting
   d. Weaning from mechanical ventilation should be done slowly because small decreases in ventilator respiratory rates, peak inspiratory pressure, and FIO_2 may result in a return to shunting, which will require even higher ventilator parameters (respiratory rate, PIP, FIO_2) than before.

> **Note**
>
> A PDA may also produce a left-to-right shunt. This occurs in premature infants in whom aortic pressures exceed pulmonary artery pressures; blood flows from the aorta to the pulmonary artery; and the blood is recirculated through the lungs. This may lead to CHF and pulmonary edema. Chest films reveal increased pulmonary vascularity and cardiomegaly.

e. Furosemide (Lasix) is indicated for treatment of the edema, and indomethacin is often used to help constrict the ductus so that blood can't flow through it.

III. **EXTRACORPOREAL MEMBRANE OXYGENATION (ECMO)**
A. Infants who do not respond to conventional mechanical ventilation may be placed on ECMO.
B. In this procedure, venous blood is removed from the right atrium via an indwelling catheter and pumped through a membrane where the blood is oxygenated. The blood is then returned to the infant via the right jugular vein.
C. Neonatal conditions that may warrant this procedure are
   1. meconium aspiration syndrome
   2. RDS
   3. PPHN
   4. sepsis
   5. perinatal asphyxia
   6. congenital diaphragmatic hernia
D. To be placed on ECMO, an infant must meet the following criteria:
   1. A gestational age of more than 35 weeks
   2. Reversible lung disease
   3. No pre-existing head bleeds
   4. Significant shunting
   5. Reversible anatomic shunting
   6. Reversible pulmonary hypertension

IV. **AIRWAY DISORDERS OF THE PEDIATRIC PATIENT**
A. **Epiglottitis**
   1. **Definition:** A bacterial infection of the epiglottis, most commonly affecting children 3 to 7 years old, that results in inflammation and edema of the supraglottic area.
   2. **Causes**
      a. Bacterial infection
      b. Bacterial pathogens responsible for epiglottis:
         (1) *Haemophilus influenzae,* the most common cause
         (2) *Streptococcus* species
         (3) *Staphylococcus aureus*
         (4) *Pneumococcus* species
   3. **Pathophysiology**
      a. Bacterial infection leads to inflammation of the epiglottis, glottis, and hypopharynx
      b. Inflammation leads to swelling of the supraglottic area, resulting in a sudden onset of severe respiratory distress and often precipitating a life-threatening situation.
   4. **Clinical manifestations**
      a. High fever
      b. Drooling

c. Sore throat
d. Dyspnea
e. Tachycardia
f. Inspiratory stridor
g. Intercostal and sternal retractions
h. Use of accessory muscles during inspiration
i. Hoarseness
j. As swelling progresses, child sits up and leans forward to maintain the airway
k. Epiglottis is swollen and red upon direct visualization, which may result in complete upper airway obstruction; so, if attempted, intubation and tracheostomy equipment must be readily available. Avoid direct visualization if possible.
l. Initial ABG levels reveal hypoxemia and respiratory alkalosis, progressing to respiratory acidosis if hypoxemia not reversed
   5. **X-ray findings**
   Lateral neck x-ray film reveals swollen epiglottis, known as the **"thumb sign"** because it resembles the distal end of a thumb.
   6. **Treatment**
      a. Tracheal intubation
         (1) Tracheotomy performed if nasal or oral intubation is impossible
         (2) Usually the patient may be extubated in 36 to 48 hr
      b. O$_2$ therapy in uncomplicated cases
      c. Antibiotics (for *H. influenzae*)
      d. Mechanical ventilation is rarely necessary
B. **Laryngotracheobronchitis (Croup)**
   1. **Definition:** Upper airway obstruction resulting from inflammation of the larynx and subglottic area; most commonly seen in children 8 months to 4 years old.
   2. **Causes**
      a. Primarily parainfluenza virus infection
      b. May result from adenovirus or respiratory syncytial virus (RSV) infection (discussed later in this chapter)
   3. **Pathophysiology**
      a. Swelling and edema of the laryngeal and subglottic area results from inflammation that leads to a narrowing airway lumen.
      b. The subglottic area is the narrowest portion of the infant's or child's airway, so a small degree of edema causes a significant reduction in the cross-sectional area.
      c. The inflammation results in increased mucus production from the mucus glands.
   4. **Clinical manifestations**
      a. Tachypnea
      b. Tachycardia
      c. Cyanosis
      d. Inspiratory stridor

e. Intercostal and sternal retractions

f. Use of accessory muscles for breathing

g. Barking cough

h. Fever

I. Initial ABG levels reveal hypoxemia and respiratory alkalosis, progressing to respiratory acidosis if hypoxemia is not reversed.

5. **X-ray findings**

Lateral neck x-ray film indicates haziness in the subglottic region.

6. **Treatment**

a. O_2 therapy

b. Cool aerosol to reduce swelling

c. Aerosolized racemic epinephrine to reduce swelling

d. Adequate hydration

C. **Foreign Body Aspiration**

1. **Definition:** Inhalation of a foreign body into the tracheobronchial tree

2. **Causes**

a. Young children often place objects in their mouths and, in some instances, aspirate the object into the respiratory tract.

b. The most commonly aspirated objects are seeds, peanuts, and coins.

3. **Pathophysiology**

a. The aspirated object usually lodges in the right mainstem bronchus, because of its angle of bifurcation from the trachea.

b. Certain objects (especially peanuts) may result in a chemical bronchitis that causes mucosal swelling and edema.

c. Commonly, infection distal to the obstruction occurs, resulting in abscess, pneumonia, or bronchiectasis.

4. **Clinical manifestations**

a. Choking or coughing, depending on severity

b. Dyspnea

c. Cyanosis

d. Wheezing (normally unresponsive to bronchodilator therapy)

e. Hemoptysis (uncommon)

5. **Chest X-ray findings**

a. Chest films may indicate hyperinflation of the affected lung.

b. Mediastinal shift away from the side of the aspiration during expiration, as the affected lung becomes hyperinflated.

> **Note**
>
> Inspiratory and expiratory chest films should be taken to determine if mediastinal shift is present.

6. **Treatment**

a. Abdominal thrusts (severe cases of obstruction)

b. Bronchoscopy to remove foreign object

c. Bronchodilator therapy followed by postural drainage and percussion is often successful in removing the object before bronchoscopy.

D. **Bronchiolitis**

1. **Definition:** An inflammation of the bronchioles that is most commonly seen in children during the first 2 years.

2. **Causes**

a. Most commonly results from **RSV** infection

b. Adenovirus and influenza virus infection (less commonly)

3. **Pathophysiology**

a. The viral infection causes inflammation of the bronchioles, mucosal edema, and spasm of the bronchiolar smooth muscle.

b. In severe cases, mucus and fibrin may accumulate in the lumen of the affected bronchioles.

c. Inspiratory and expiratory flows become obstructed, increasing FRC.

d. Atelectasis may result from the inflammation in severe cases.

4. **Clinical manifestations**

a. Recent upper respiratory tract infection

b. Fever

c. Cough

d. Tachypnea

e. Dyspnea

f. Crackles and wheezing on chest auscultation

g. Apnea (in infants)

h. Sternal and intercostal retractions

i. Hypoxemia

4. **Chest x-ray findings**

a. Marked hyperradiolucency

b. Infiltrates

5. **Treatment**

a. Mild cases do not require hospitalization

b. **Severe cases**

(1) O_2 therapy (via hood or tent, depending on age of the child)

(2) CPAP to treat severe hypoxemia

★ (3) Ribavirin (antiviral drug), administered via a SPAG nebulizer for 12 to 18 hr daily through an O_2 hood for 3 to 7 days

(4) Mechanical ventilation, if ribavirin treatment is unsuccessful

(5) Adequate hydration

E. **Cystic Fibrosis**

1. **Definition:** A hereditary disease affecting the exocrine glands of the body that results in the

production of thick mucus from these glands. The glands most commonly affected are located in the pancreas, the sweat glands, and the lungs. The disease is classified as COPD.

2. **Causes**
   a. Genetic transmission
   b. The mother and father both must be carriers of this recessive gene. Each child of the couple has a one-in-four chance of having the disease.

3. **Pathophysiology**
   a. Large amounts of thick mucus are produced as a result of the abnormally large numbers of bronchial glands and goblet cells located in the tracheobronchial tree.
   b. Thick mucus stagnates in the airways, leading to airway obstruction and facilitation of bacterial growth.
   c. Mucus plugging results in atelectasis, hyperinflation, and pneumonia.
   d. Abnormalities in the pancreatic ducts and glands result in inadequate absorption and digestion of food, causing malnutrition if not properly treated.

4. **Clinical manifestations**
   a. Tachypnea
   b. Tachycardia
   c. Cough with thick mucus production
   d. Increased AP chest diameter
   e. Digital clubbing
   ★ f. Elevated chloride levels in sweat (diagnostic of this disease)
   g. Use of accessory muscles during normal breathing
   h. Early in disease process, ABG levels indicate hypoxemia with respiratory alkalosis.
   i. In late stages of disease, ABG levels reveal chronic ventilatory failure with hypoxemia.
   j. Cyanosis
   k. Cor pulmonale, in late stages
   l. Pulmonary function studies reveal decreases in expiratory flow values and increased FRC values

5. **Chest x-ray findings**
   a. Hyperinflation
   b. Flattened diaphragm
   c. Increased lung markings
   d. Cardiomegaly

6. **Treatment**
   ★ a. Aerosolized bronchodilator therapy with mucolytic, such as acetylcysteine (Mucomyst), followed by chest physical therapy.
   b. O_2 therapy
   c. Expectorants

   d. Continuous aerosol mask
   e. Antibiotics

POST-CHAPTER STUDY QUESTIONS

1. What five conditions are assessed in the Apgar score?
2. Describe the appropriate intervention for the following Apgar scores: 0 to 3; 4 to 6; and 7 to 10.
3. What is often the first sign of respiratory distress in the infant?
4. List the normal ABG levels for an infant.
5. List six indications for nasal CPAP.
6. List five complications of CPAP.
7. List two hazards of O_2 therapy in the neonate.
8. Describe where the tip of the UAC should rest when properly positioned.
9. List four advantages of a UAC.
10. List four complications of a UAC.
11. List six clinical manifestations of infant RDS.
12. List the causes of BPD.
13. List eight clinical manifestations of BPD.
14. Describe the chest x-ray findings in infants with BPD.
15. List the treatment modalities for BPD.
16. List the causes of meconium aspiration.
17. List eight clinical manifestations of meconium aspiration.
18. List eight conditions that accompany PFC.
19. List five clinical manifestations of PFC.
20. List the treatment modalities for PFC.
21. List the causes of epiglottitis.
22. List twelve clinical manifestations of epiglottitis.
23. Describe the classic x-ray finding for diagnosis of epiglottitis.
24. List the treatment modalities for epiglottitis.
25. List twelve clinical manifestations of cystic fibrosis.
26. List the treatment modalities for cystic fibrosis.
27. What drug is most commonly used to treat RSV?

Answers are at the end of the chapter.

REFERENCES

Aloan C: Respiratory care of the newborn, Philadelphia, 1987, JB Lippincott Co.

Barnhart S and Czervinske M: Perinatal and pediatric respiratory care, Philadelphia, 1995, WB Saunders Co.

Carlo W and Chatburn R: Neonatal respiratory care, ed 2, Chicago, 1988, Year-Book Medical Publishers.

Koff P, Eitzman D, and Neu J: Neonatal and pediatric respiratory care, ed 2, St. Louis, 1993, The CV Mosby Co.

Whitaker K: Comprehensive perinatal and pediatric respiratory care, ed 2, Albany, NY, 1996, Delmar Publishers.

PRE-TEST ANSWERS

1. A
2. B
3. B
4. D
5. C
6. B

ANSWERS TO POST-CHAPTER STUDY QUESTIONS

1. Heart rate, respiratory effort, color, reflex irritability, muscle tone
2. Apgar score 0–3: immediate resuscitation with ventilatory assistance; 4–6: stimulation and O_2 administration; 7–10: routine observation, suction upper airway with bulb syringe, dry infant, and place under warmer.
3. Nasal flaring
4. pH, 7.35 to 7.45; $PaCO_2$, 35 to 45 mm Hg; PaO_2, 50 to 70 mm Hg; HCO_3^-, 20 to 26 mEq/L; BE, −5 to +5
5. To improve oxygenation, to increase static lung compliance, to increase FRC, to decrease work of breathing, to decrease intrapulmonary shunting, and to decrease pulmonary vascular resistance
6. Barotrauma, decreased venous return, air trapping, pressure necrosis, loss of CPAP from crying or displacement
7. Neonatal retinopathy, BPD
8. In descending aorta at x-ray level: T6 to T10 or L3 to L4
9. Easily obtained ABG levels, prevents frequent arterial punctures, continuous monitoring of blood pressure, infusion of drugs and fluids
10. Infection, thromboembolism, air embolism, hemorrhage
11. Nasal flaring, grunting, retractions, tachypnea, cyanosis, mixed respiratory and metabolic acidosis with hypoxemia
12. High O_2 concentrations, high ventilatory pressures
13. Increased airway resistance, normal or increased static lung compliance, V/Q mismatching, hypoxemia on room air, tachypnea, barrel chest, retractions, hypercapnia
14. Ground glass appearance, opacification, atelectasis, hyperlucency, bullae
15. O_2 therapy, positive pressure ventilation, adequate humidification of inspired gases, CPT, adequate nutrition, maintenance of fluid balance, bronchodilator therapy, airway suctioning
16. Stress or hypoxia in utero of postmature infants leads to expulsion of meconium into the amniotic fluid, where it may be aspirated with the infant's first breath
17. Long fingernails, peeling skin, hypoxemia, hypercarbia, tachypnea, retractions, nasal flaring, grunting, barrel chest, cyanosis, crackles and rhonchi on auscultation
18. Perinatal asphyxia, meconium aspiration, pneumonia, sepsis, congenital heart defects, diaphragmatic hernia, hypoplastic lungs, hypoglycemia
19. Tachypnea, hypoxemia, cyanosis, more than a 15-mm Hg difference in pre-ductal and post-ductal PaO_2 on 100% O_2, increase in PaO_2 over 100 mm Hg when $PaCO_2$ is maintained between 20 and 25 mm Hg
20. Mechanical hyperventilation, PaO_2 of more than 100 mm Hg, tolazoline, nitroprusside sodium, $NaHCO_3$, dopamine
21. Bacterial infection (*H. influenzae,* streptococci, staphylococci, pneumococci)
22. High fever, drooling, sore throat, dyspnea, tachycardia, inspiratory stridor, retractions, accessory muscle use, hoarseness, swollen epiglottis, hypoxemia, and respiratory alkalosis, followed by respiratory acidosis if not reversed
23. "thumb sign"
24. Intubation, if possible; tracheotomy, if intubation is not possible; O_2 therapy; antibiotics; mechanical ventilation, if necessary
25. Tachypnea, tachycardia, productive cough with thick secretions, increased AP chest diameter, digital clubbing, increased chloride level in sweat, accessory muscle use, hypoxemia with respiratory alkalosis in early stages, chronic ventilatory failure in late stages, cyanosis, cor pulmonale in late stages, decreased result on flow studies, and increased FRC on pulmonary function tests
26. Aerosolized acetylcysteine, CPT, O_2 therapy, expectorants, antibiotics, continuous aerosol therapy
27. Ribavirin via SPAG nebulizer for 12 to 18 hr/day for 3 to 7 days

Chapter 14

Respiratory Medications

PRE-TEST QUESTIONS

Answer the pre-test questions before studying the chapter. This will help you determine your strong and weak areas regarding the material covered.

1. With which of the following lung disorders would acetylcysteine (Mucomyst) be indicated?

    I. Emphysema
    II. Bronchiectasis
    III. Cystic fibrosis
    IV. Pulmonary edema

    A. I and II only
    B. II and III only
    C. III and IV only
    D. I, II, and III only

2. A patient with glottic edema after extubation is in mild respiratory distress. Which of the following medications would be of benefit in this situation?

    A. Cromolyn sodium
    B. Succinylcholine (Anectine)
    C. Racemic epinephrine
    D. Pentamidine

3. You are having difficulty intubating a combative patient in the emergency department. The respiratory therapist should recommend the delivery of which drug to facilitate intubation?

    A. Succinylcholine (Anectine)
    B. Cromolyn sodium
    C. Atropine sulfate
    D. Epinephrine

4. Which of the following aerosolized medications is used in the treatment of RSV.

    A. Succinylcholine (Anectine)
    B. Amoxicillin
    C. Pentamidine
    D. Ribavirin

5. Which of the following airway disorders may be successfully treated with dexamethasone (Decadron)?

    I. Asthma
    II. Glottic edema
    III. Pulmonary edema

    A. I only
    B. II only
    C. I and II only
    D. II and III only

Answers are at the end of the chapter.

REVIEW

> ★ *Exam Note*
>
> Recommending the use of and administering pharmacologic agents appears on the CRT examination only.

I. **CLASSIFICATION OF RESPIRATORY MEDICATIONS**
  A. **Diluents**
    1. **Normal saline solution (0.9% NaCl)**
      a. Used to dilute bronchodilating agents
      b. Used to dilute secretions for improved expectoration. Often instilled through ET tubes and tracheostomy tubes, 3 to 5 mL at a time.
    2. **Hypotonic saline solution (0.4% NaCl)**
      a. Used in ultrasonic nebulizers because smaller particles are produced as result of lower concentration.
      b. More stable than sterile water
    3. **Hypertonic saline solution (1.8% NaCl)**
      a. Larger aerosol particles are produced because of the higher concentration of the solution.
      b. Used to stimulate coughing and induce sputum because it is irritating to the airway.
    4. **Sterile distilled water**
      a. Used to dilute other medications
      b. Used to hydrate secretions, thereby decreasing the viscosity for easier expectoration

c. Used to humidify dry gases
B. **Mucolytics:** Drugs that break the sputum down chemically for more effective expectoration.
   1. **Acetylcysteine (Mucomyst)**
      a. Available in 10% or 20% solutions
      b. It breaks the **disulfide bonds** in the sputum; this decreases the sputum's viscosity.
      c. Often used with bronchodilating agents, since a common side effect of Mucomyst is **bronchospasm.**
      d. Should be used in treating patients with **thick secretions that are difficult to mobilize**
      e. Often used in treating patients with cystic fibrosis or bronchiectasis
      f. May be nebulized (1 to 3 mL, three to four times daily) or instilled directly into the trachea
      ★ g. Should bronchospasm occur, stop the treatment immediately and administer a bronchodilating agent
      h. Is irritating to mucosal tissues; patient should rinse mouth after treatment.
   2. **Sodium bicarbonate (2% NaHCO$_3$)**
      a. Increases the pH of the sputum, thereby decreasing its viscosity.
      b. May be used to improve the mucolytic actions of acetylcysteine
      c. Dosage: 2 to 5 mL via aerosol or 2 to 10 mL instilled directly into the trachea every 4 to 8 hr
C. **Sympathomimetic Bronchodilators**

> **Note**
> These medications stimulate one or more of the following adrenergic receptors.

Receptor	Location	Response
Alpha	Mucosal blood vessels, bronchial smooth muscle	Vasoconstriction, bronchoconstriction
Beta$_1$	Heart muscle	Increased heart rate and cardiac output, arrhythmias
Beta$_2$	Bronchial smooth muscle, peripheral mucosal blood vessels, CNS, and peripheral limb muscles	Bronchodilation, vasodilation, nervousness (CNS), tingling in fingers

> **Note**
> The ideal bronchodilator is one which is a pure adrenergic beta$_2$ receptor stimulator.

1. **Epinephrine hydrochloride (Adrenalin Chloride, Susphrine)**
   a. Stimulates all three adrenergic receptors, but beta$_1$ the strongest
   b. Duration of action is 30 min to 2 hours
   c. Used to stimulate the heart; not commonly used as a bronchodilator
   d. Adverse effects
      (1) Increased heart rate
      (2) Hypertension
      (3) Anxiety
      (4) Mild bronchoconstriction
   e. Dosage: Aerosol, 0.1 to 0.5 mL (1:100 solution) in 3 to 5 mL of diluent
2. **Racemic epinephrine (microNefrin, Vaponefrin)**
   a. Stimulates all three receptors, but beta$_1$ the strongest
   b. Duration of action is 30 min to 2 hours
   ★ c. Used to decrease mucosal edema and inflammation after extubation or in pediatric patients with croup
   d. Has milder effects than epinephrine (½ strength)
   e. Dosage: aerosol, 0.2 to 0.5 mL in 3 to 5 mL of diluent, every 3 to 4 hours
3. **Isoproterenol hydrochloride (Isuprel)**
   a. A strong beta$_1$ and beta$_2$ stimulator
   b. Duration of action is 1 to 2 hours
   c. Used to decrease Raw
   d. Adverse effects:
      ★ (1) Increased heart rate
      (2) Increased blood pressure
      (3) Anxiety
      (4) Tingling in fingers
      (5) Nervousness
   e. Dosage: 0.25 to 0.5 mL in 3 to 5 mL of diluent three to four times daily
4. **Metaproterenol (Alupent, Metaprel)**
   a. Very minor beta$_1$ and mild beta$_2$ stimulator
   b. Duration of action is 4 to 6 hours
   c. Used to decrease Raw
   d. Adverse effects
      (1) Mild cardiac effects
      (2) Mild CNS effects
   e. Dosage: 0.1 to 0.3 mL in 3 to 5 mL of diluent, every 4 hours
5. **Terbutaline sulfate (Brethine, Bricanyl)**
   a. **Very minor beta$_1$ and moderate beta$_2$ stimulator**
   b. Duration of action is 3 to 7 hours
   c. Used to decrease Raw
   d. Adverse effects
      (1) Mild cardiac effects
      (2) Mild CNS effects

e. Dosage: 0.25 to 0.5 mg in 3 to 5 mL of diluent, every 4 to 8 hours
6. **Albuterol (Proventil, Ventolin)**
   a. **Mild beta$_1$ and strong beta$_2$ stimulator**
   b. Duration of action is 4 to 6 hours
   c. Used to decrease Raw
   d. Adverse effects
      (1) Mild cardiac effects
      (2) Mild CNS effects
   e. Dosage: 0.5 mL in 3 to 5 mL of diluent, three to four times daily
D. **Parasympatholytic Bronchodilators**
   1. **Atropine Sulfate**
      a. An anticholinergic drug; it blocks the cholinergic constricting influences on the airway and potentiates the adrenergic influences (beta$_2$ stimulation), resulting in bronchodilation.
      b. Also inhibits secretion production and increases secretion viscosity.

Note

There is more potential for mucus plugging in patients with thick secretions who are administered atropine intravenously. Given as an aerosol, atropine has little effect on lung secretions but may dry out the oral mucosa.

   c. Used to decrease Raw, congestion, and cardiac arrhythmias
   d. Adverse effects
      (1) Increased secretion viscosity
      (2) Dry mouth
      (3) CNS stimulation
   e. Dosage: 1 mg in 3 to 5 ml of diluent, every 4 to 6 hours
   2. **Ipratropium bromide (Atrovent)**
      a. An anticholinergic bronchodilator that acts topically in the lung instead of systemically.
      b. Peak effect of the drug is 1 to 2 hours (compared with 15 minutes to 1 hour with beta-agonists with a duration of action of 3 to 4 hours.
      c. Used to decrease Raw, especially in patients with asthma, bronchitis, and emphysema. Some studies have shown ipratropium to be a more potent bronchodilator than beta-adrenergic agents for the treatment of emphysema and bronchitis.

Note

Ipratropium bromide is faster-acting, longer-lasting, and exhibits fewer side effects than atropine.

d. Adverse effects
   1. Palpitations
   2. Nervousness
   3. Dizziness
   4. Nausea
   5. Tremors
e. Dosage: 0.5 mg in nebulized solution or two inhalations (36 μg) from metered-dose inhaler four times daily.

Note

Current literature shows that up to 10 puffs four times a day is a safe dosage.

E. **Phosphodiesterase Inhibitors:** These drugs are called xanthines, and they inhibit the cellular production of phosphodiesterase, an enzyme that readily breaks down cyclic AMP, another cellular enzyme, which, when produced, results in bronchodilation. It is by the increased production of cyclic AMP that sympathomimetic bronchodilators work.
   1. **Theophylline (Aminophylline)**
      a. Stimulates respiratory rate and depth of breathing, as well as producing pulmonary vasodilation and bronchodilation.
    ★ b. Used to decrease Raw, especially in asthmatics
      c. Duration of action is 4 to 6 hours
      d. Adverse effects
         (1) Cardiac effects
         (2) CNS effects
         (3) Nausea and vomiting
         (4) Diuresis
      e. Dosage: IV loading dose, 6 mg/kg of body weight; maintenance dose, 0.5 mg/kg/hr (average dose is 250 mg every 6 hours)
      d. Theophylline produces effects that provide great benefits for COPD patients.
         (1) Increased right ventricular output (improves cor pulmonale)
         (2) Improves diaphragmatic function
         (3) Produces pulmonary vasodilation, reducing pulmonary hypertension that results from chronic hypoxemia
         (4) Stimulates breathing by altering the hypoxic response curve when PaO$_2$ is elevated above 60 mm Hg.

Note

Therapeutic serum level is 10 to 20 mg/L.

F. **Miscellaneous Respiratory Drugs**
  1. **Cromolyn Sodium (Intal)**
     a. Stabilizes the mast cell, making it less sensitive to specific antigens and inhibiting the release of histamine
     b. Duration of action is 2 to 6 hours
     c. Used as **preventive therapy** for asthma **(not effective during an asthma attack)**
     d. Adverse effects
        (1) Bronchospasm (when delivered in powder form)
        (2) Cough (powder form)
        (3) Local irritation (powder form)

> *Note*
>
> Cromolyn sodium is now available in aerosolized form, which is tolerated much better than in the powdered form. The powdered form is delivered through a device called a spinhaler. The capsule was punctured and placed in the device and the patient inhaled deeply, which delivered the powder into the airway. Bronchospasm is a common complication when Intal is delivered in this form.

     e. Dosage: 1 20-mg capsule four times daily (powder form); nebulized form, 20 mg four times daily

> *Note*
>
> Another mast cell stabilizer similar to cromolyn, but 4 to 10 times stronger, is nedocromil sodium (Tilade), which is available in MDI aerosol only.

> *Note*
>
> Newer oral asthma preventatives called leukotriene inhibitors are becoming popular. The most common leukotriene inhibitors are zafirlukast (Accolate) and zileuton (Zyflo).

  2. **Ethanol (ethyl alcohol)**
     a. An antifoaming agent used to decrease the surface tension of frothy, bubbly secretions that are observed with **pulmonary edema**
     b. **Used in the treatment of pulmonary edema** to disperse the edematous bubbles, making the airway more patent
     c. Adverse effects
        (1) Mucosal irritation
        (2) Dry mouth
     d. Dosage: 3 to 15 mL of a 40% to 50% solution

G. **Neuromuscular Blocking Agents**
  1. **Succinylcholine (Anectine)**
     a. A depolarizing agent that competes with acetylcholine for cholinergic receptors of the motor end plate of a muscle. If these receptors remain occupied by the depolarizing agent, further stimulation cannot occur and paralysis persists.
     b. Onset of action is 1 min with a duration of action of only 5 min
  ★ c. Used as a short-term paralyzing agent to facilitate ET intubation
     d. Adverse effects
        (1) Decreased heart rate
        (2) Decreased blood pressure

> *Note*
>
> Atropine may be administered to counteract these effects.

     e. Dosage: 20 mg IV (2 to 3 mg/min)
  2. **Tubocurarine chloride**
     a. A nondepolarizing agent (related to curare) that blocks the transmission of acetylcholine at the postjunctional membrane.
     b. Onset of action is 3 to 5 min with a duration of action of 40 to 90 min
     c. Used to paralyze patients who are "fighting" mechanical ventilation
     d. Adverse effects
        (1) Bronchospasm (caused by histamine release)
        (2) Decreased blood pressure
  3. **Pancuronium bromide (Pavulon)**
     a. A nondepolarizing agent that is 5 times stronger than curare and much more commonly used.
     b. Onset of action is 2 to 3 min with a duration of up to 1 hour
     c. Used to paralyze patients who are "fighting" mechanical ventilation
     d. Adverse effects:
        (1) Increased heart rate (mild)
        (2) Increased blood pressure (mild)

> *Note*
>
> Pavulon does not cause the release of histamine as curare does, therefore bronchospasm is not a complication.

     e. Dosage: 4 to 5 mg IV at intervals of 1 to 3 hours

H. Antibiotics (aerosolized)

1. **Gentamicin**
   a. Commonly used in cystic fibrosis patients
   b. Effective against *Pseudomonas aeruginosa*
   c. May be combined with carbenicillin
   d. May be instilled directly down the ET tube
2. **Amoxicillin**
   a. Used on patients with bronchiectasis
   b. Reduces the purulence of the sputum
3. **Amphotericin B**
   a. Used for the treatment of fungal infections
   b. Improvement seen in the treatment of pulmonary aspergillosis and the fungus *Candida albicans*
4. **Pentamidine**
   a. An antiprotozoan agent
   ★ b. Used in the treatment of *Pneumocystis carinii* pneumonia (commonly seen in AIDS patients).
   c. Airway side effects of aerosolized pentamidine
      (1) Bronchospasm
      (2) Wheezing
      (3) Bronchial irritation
      (4) Shortness of breath
      (5) Cough

   ★ d. The nebulizer used to deliver pentamidine should incorporate a one-way valve that directs the patient's exhaled air through a scavenging filter to prevent contaminating the personnel and surrounding air with this agent.
5. **Ribavirin (Virazole)**
   a. An antiviral agent

   ★ b. Used specifically to treat RSV in neonatal and pediatric patients
   c. Delivered through a SPAG nebulizer
   d. The medication is delivered continuously for 12 to 18 hours a day for 3 days to 1 week, generally through an oxygen hood, oxygen tent, or face tent.
   e. Hazards of ribavirin
      (1) Worsening of respiratory status
      (2) Bacterial pneumonia (from contamination)
      (3) Occlusion of ET tube or ventilator tubing by the hygroscopic particles; particle filters may decrease the potential of this hazard.

I. **Corticosteroids (aerosolized):** These anti-inflammatory agents are used in respiratory care to prevent or reduce airway inflammation in asthma and upper airway swelling that accompanies glottic edema. Administering these agents via aerosol (usually MDI) reduces the systemic sides effects, such as the cushingoid symptoms (edema, moon-face) and adrenal suppression.
   1. **Dexamethasone sodium phosphate (Decadron)**
      a. One of the first steroids administered successfully as an aerosol
      b. May be administered in MDI or in aerosol solution
      c. Systemic side effects are common even when delivered via aerosol
   2. **Beclomethasone dipropionate (Vanceril, Beclovent)**
      a. Commonly used in asthma and other chronic lung diseases
      b. Less systemic side effects than dexamethasone
      c. Delivered by MDI
   3. **Flunisolide (Aerobid)**
      a. Effective treatment for asthmatics
      b. Delivered by MDI

II. DRUG CALCULATIONS
A. Percentage Strengths
1. Percentage strength is the number of parts of the solute (ingredient) per 100 parts of solution.
2. To convert from ratio strength to percentage strength, use the following instructions.

a. **What is the percentage strength of a 1:2000 solution?**
 (1) Change 1:2000 to a fraction: 1/2000
 (2) Change this to a percentage by dividing 2000 into 1 and multiply by 100.

$$\frac{1}{2000} \times 100 = \textbf{.05\%}$$

b. **What is the percentage strength of a 1:500 solution?**
 (1) Change 1:500 to a fraction: 1/500
 (2) Change this to a percentage by dividing 500 into 1 and multiplying by 100.

$$\frac{1}{500} \times 100 = \textbf{.2\%}$$

3. To convert from percentage strength to ratio strength, use the following instructions.
 a. What is the ratio strength of a 10% solution?
  (1) Change 10% to 10/100 or 10:100.
  (2) 10:100 is the same as 1:10 (10 goes into 100 10 times).
  (3) Therefore a 10% solution has a 1:10 ratio strength.

B. **Dosage Calculations**
 1. **1 mL of a 1% solution (1:100) = 10 mg of solute**
 2. **How many milligrams of a 1:100 solution of isoproterenol make up a dose of 0.5 mL of the drug?**
  a. A 1:100 solution is a 1% solution (1 divided by 100 × 100).
  b. **1 mL of a 1% solution equals 10 mg. (This is a standard rule.)**
  c. But this question is how many milligrams of solution make up **0.5 mL of the drug.**
  d. 1 mL of a 1% solution = 10 mg
  e. 0.5 mL of a 1% solution = 5 mg (half as much)
 3. **How many milligrams in 0.2 mL of a 5% solution of metaproterenol?**
  a. Always go back to the **standard rule:** 1 mL of 1% solution = 10 mg
  b. 1 mL of a 1% solution = 10 mg
  c. 1 mL of a 5% solution = 50 mg (5 times as much)
  d. 0.2 mL of 50 mg = 0.2 × 50 mg = 10 mg

POST-CHAPTER STUDY QUESTIONS

1. What is the primary indication for acetylcysteine?
2. What is racemic epinephrine most commonly used for?

3. List four examples of sympathomimetic bronchodilators.
4. List two examples of parasympatholytic bronchodilators.
5. Which neuromuscular blocking agent is used primarily for short-term paralysis during a difficult intubation?
6. How does cromolyn sodium help in the treatment of asthma?
7. List five antibiotics that are aerosolized and the conditions for which they are indicated.
8. List three corticosteroids that are commonly aerosolized.
9. List the side effects of corticosteroid therapy.

Answers are at end of the chapter.

REFERENCES

Eubanks D and Bone R: Comprehensive respiratory care, ed 2, St. Louis, 1990, The CV Mosby Co.
Oakes D: Clinical practitioner's pocket guide to respiratory care, ed 5, Rockville, MD, 1996, Health Educator Publications.
Rau J: Respiratory care pharmacology, ed 5, St. Louis, 1998, Mosby, Inc.
Scanlan C, Wilkins R, and Stoller J: Egan's fundamentals of respiratory care, ed 7, St. Louis, 1999, Mosby, Inc.

PRE-TEST ANSWERS

1. B
2. C
3. A
4. D
5. C

ANSWERS TO POST-CHAPTER STUDY QUESTIONS

1. Thick secretions
2. Upper airway edema (swelling)
3. Epinephrine, racemic epinephrine, isoproterenol, metaproterenol, terbutaline, albuterol
4. Atropine, ipratropium (Atrovent)
5. Succinylcholine
6. Prevents attacks by stabilizing mast cells
7. Gentamicin, cystic fibrosis (*Pseudomonas* species); amoxicillin, bronchiectasis; amphotericin B, fungal infections; pentamidine, *Pneumocystis carinii;* ribavirin, RSV and bronchiolitis
8. Dexamethasone, beclomethasone, flunisolide
9. Edema, moon face, adrenal suppression, oral candidiasis (thrush mouth)

Chapter 15

Respiratory Home Care

PRE-TEST QUESTIONS

Answer the pre-test questions before studying the chapter. This will help you determine your strong and weak areas regarding the material covered.

1. Which of the following O_2 systems would be indicated for a very active home care patient?

   A. O_2 concentrator
   B. Liquid O_2
   C. H cylinder
   D. E cylinder

2. Which of the following is the *LEAST* important area for the respiratory therapist to discuss with the home care patient?

   A. Pathology of the disease process
   B. Cleaning of equipment
   C. Side effects of prescribed therapy
   D. Importance of proper therapy techniques

3. Which of the following IPPB machines is most convenient for use in the home?

   A. Bird Mark 7
   B. Bird Mark 8
   C. Bennett PR-2
   D. Bennett AP-5

4. Diaphragmatic breathing exercises should result in which of the following?
   I. Increased V_T
   II. Less dependence on the diaphragm during quiet breathing
   III. Increased FRC
   IV. Decreased respiratory rate

   A. I and II only
   B. I and IV only
   C. II, III, and IV only
   D. I, II, and IV only

Answers are at the end of the chapter.

REVIEW

I. **HOME REHABILITATION**
   A. **Goals of Rehabilitation**
      1. Help the patient become independent.
      2. Help the patient improve the ability to cope with the disease.
      3. Help the patient gain an understanding of the disease and the limitations that result from it.
      4. Help the patient to set realistic goals for life and then help them attain those goals.
   B. **Conditions Requiring Pulmonary Rehabilitation**
      1. Chronic lung diseases
         a. Emphysema
         b. Asthma
         c. Chronic bronchitis
         d. Cystic fibrosis
         e. Bronchiectasis
      2. Neuromuscular diseases
         a. Myasthenia gravis
         b. Guillain-Barré syndrome
         c. Poliomyelitis
         d. Muscular dystrophy
      3. Central respiratory center disorders
         a. CNS injury
         b. Hypoventilation syndrome (nonobese or Pickwickian syndrome, sleep apnea)
         c. Ondine's curse (primary alveolar hypoventilation)

II. **CARE OF THE REHABILITATION PATIENT**
   A. **Patient Care Plan**
      1. Humidity therapy
      2. Aerosol therapy
      3. O_2 therapy: **use of reservoir cannulae and pulse dose O_2 delivery systems aid in conserving O_2.**
      4. Bronchodilator therapy
      5. ABG sampling and analysis or pulse oximeter (Sp_{O_2}) monitoring
      6. Oropharyngeal and tracheal suctioning

7. Determination of breath sounds by chest auscultation
8. Chest physical therapy
9. Breathing exercises
10. Sputum induction
11. IPPB therapy: **Bennett AP-5 unit is commonly used since it operates on electricity rather than compressed gas.**

B. **Periodic Evaluations**
   1. Pulmonary function testing
   2. Sputum collection and analysis
   3. ABG collection and analysis
   4. Exercise tolerance testing
   5. Chest x-ray films

C. **Breathing Exercises**
   1. **Pursed-lip breathing**
      a. Should be taught to patients who experience premature airway closure.
      b. Patient should be instructed to inhale through the nose and exhale through pursed lips.
      c. Aids in the patient gaining control of dyspnea.
      d. Provides improved ventilation before a cough effort.
      e. Teaches the patient how to better control rate and depth of breathing.
      f. Prevents premature airway collapse by generating a back pressure into the airways.
      g. Has psychological benefits.
   2. **Diaphragmatic breathing**
      a. Teaches the COPD patient to use the diaphragm during breathing rather than accessory muscles.
      b. The patient or RCP places a hand over the abdomen as the patient, while lying on the back, concentrates on moving the hand upward on inspiration. (A book or weight may be used rather than a hand.)
      c. Increasing the use of the diaphragm will result in a decreased respiratory rate, increased tidal volume, decreased FRC, and increased alveolar ventilation.
   3. **Segmental breathing**
      a. Similar to diaphragmatic breathing exercise, except a hand is placed over a specific lung area in which there is atelectasis, secretions, or decreased air flow.
      b. The patient should concentrate on moving the hand outward on inspiration.

D. **Cough Instruction**
   1. **A FVC of less than 15 mL/kg of ideal body weight indicates inadequate volume for an effective cough.**
   2. **Proper cough instruction:** tell the patient to

a. Inhale slowly and deeply through the nose and hold breath for 3 to 5 sec (in sitting position).
b. Clasp arms across abdomen and give three sharp coughs without taking a breath while pressing arms into the abdomen.
c. Use a pillow to "splint" incision sites (e.g., thorax, abdomen)

E. **Home O$_2$ Administration**

Exam Note

The maintenance and monitoring of home care equipment appears on the RRT examination only. All other areas relating to home equipment (such as setup of equipment) appear on both examinations.

---

1. **O$_2$ cylinders**
   a. Probably the least expensive O$_2$ setup in the home at the present time depending on usage.
   b. Disadvantages of O$_2$ cylinders in the home
      (1) Heavy and difficult to move
      (2) High pressure hazard
      (3) Difficult for older or debilitated patients to change cylinder or attach a regulator
      (4) Small cylinders are difficult to walk with
2. **Liquid O$_2$ system**
   a. May store more O$_2$ in liquid form than in gaseous form (860 times more)
   b. Liquid is safer than gas stored in high-pressure cylinders.
   c. Portable liquid walkers are much more convenient and easier for the patient to handle.
3. **O$_2$ concentrator**
   a. Uses the O$_2$ in the surrounding room air by drawing it into the concentrator and filtering out most of the gases except O$_2$.
   b. Two types of concentrators
      (1) Membrane: produces only about 40% O$_2$ out of the unit
      (2) Molecular sieve: much more commonly used and produces 90% to 95% O$_2$ out of the unit
   c. The concentrator should be placed in the home where air can freely be drawn into it.
   d. The concentrator should not be placed near heat vents.
   e. The RCP, on the routine visit, should analyze the delivered O$_2$ from the concentrator and check all alarms, the flow rate, filters, and batteries.
   f. A backup O$_2$ system with 1 to 3 days' supply should be available in case of a

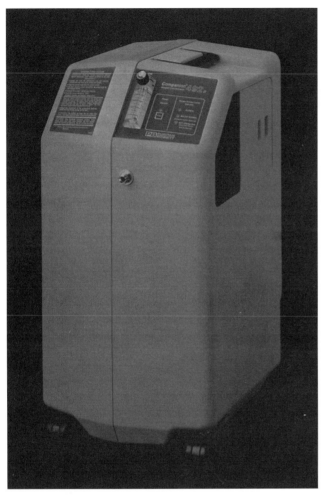

3. Cannulas should be cleaned with mild soap that doesn't leave a soap film and then rinsed before using a disinfectant. They should be replaced every 2 to 4 weeks.
4. Humidifiers and nebulizers should be filled with sterile water and incorporate safety relief devices.
5. If heated moisture is delivered, a thermometer should be placed in the line, close to the patient, to monitor inspired gas temperature.
6. Medication nebulizers should be rinsed with water and dried after each treatment. They should be cleaned every day in a mild soap solution, rinsed, disinfected, rinsed again, dried on a paper towel, and placed in a plastic bag until used again.
7. IPPB circuits (nondisposable) may be cleaned in mild soap, rinsed, disinfected, rinsed again, and dried every 1 to 2 days.
8. IPPB machines may be wiped down with a liquid disinfectant every few days.

G. **RCP Responsibilities in Home Care of Pulmonary Patients**
   1. Help set up and maintain equipment.
   2. Instruct the patient and family on use, care, and safety of all equipment used in the home setting.
   3. Instruct the patient and family in all therapy to be done in the home, including the indications, contraindications, side effects, and hazards of the specific therapy.
   4. Assist in the delivery of therapy to the patient.
   5. Perform simple spirometry tests.
   6. Assess the patient's present cardiopulmonary status and general well-being.
   7. Report to the physician to discuss the present therapy and possible changes needed in current therapy.

III. **HOME APNEA MONITORING**

Exam Note

Home apnea monitoring appears on the RRT examination only.

power outage since concentrators are powered by electricity.
   g. The higher the flow rate used on a concentrator, the less the delivered O_2 percentage.

Note

The patient and family should be instructed in all aspects of the proper care and safety of equipment used in the home.

F. **Cleaning Equipment in the Home**
   1. All equipment designated "single use only" should be considered disposable and discarded after one use.
   2. Nondisposable equipment, such as nebulizers and humidifiers, may be cleaned as follows:
      a. Clean first with mild soap
      b. Rinse
      c. Disinfect with a solution recommended by the manufacturer
      d. Rinse again
      e. Dry the equipment
      f. Repeat the process every 1 to 3 days

A. Apnea monitoring is most commonly used for infants or pediatric patients who have conditions that cause apnea or bradycardia. Also, infants experiencing apnea from unknown causes and siblings of infants who have died from SIDS should be monitored for apnea.
B. Other patients who may require apnea monitoring are those with BPD, neuromuscular diseases, and tracheostomies and those on mechanical ventilation.
C. A soft foam belt with electrodes is fastened around the chest of the infant. The wires of the electrodes send signals of the heartbeat and breathing back to the monitor via a patient cable.
D. Apnea monitors have audible and visual alarms that detect not only apnea and bradycardia but also malfunctions that occur with the patient cable, electrodes, wires, and battery.
E. Caregivers in the home must be trained thoroughly on the use of and troubleshooting for the monitor.

POST-CHAPTER STUDY QUESTIONS

1. List four goals of rehabilitation.
2. List five periodic evaluations that should be conducted by the respiratory therapist on the home care patient.
3. How does pursed-lip breathing benefit patients with emphysema?
4. List two types of O_2 concentrators and the O_2 percentage available with each.
5. What type of evaluations should be made by the RCP on the O_2 concentrators during routine visits?

Answers are at the end of the chapter.

REFERENCES

Eubanks D and Bone R: Comprehensive respiratory care, ed 2, St. Louis, 1990, The CV Mosby Co.

Koff D, Eitzman D, and Neu J: Neonatal and pediatric respiratory care, ed 2, St. Louis, 1993, Mosby-Yearbook, Inc..
McPherson SP: Respiratory home care equipment, St. Louis, 1988, The CV Mosby Co.
Scanlan C, Wilkins R, and Stoller J: Egan's fundamentals of respiratory care, ed 7, St. Louis, 1999, Mosby, Inc.
Shapiro BA: Clinical application of respiratory care, ed 4, St. Louis, 1990, The CV Mosby Co.

PRE-TEST ANSWERS

1. B
2. A
3. D
4. B

ANSWERS TO POST-CHAPTER STUDY QUESTIONS

1. Help the patient to become independent, to cope with the disease, to understand the disease and its limitations, to help set realistic goals and find ways to attain them
2. Pulmonary function tests, sputum collection and analysis, ABG collection and analysis, exercise tolerance testing, chest x-ray films
3. Creates a subtle back pressure into the larger airways, reducing the volume of trapped air and helping to reduce the feeling of dyspnea
4. Membrane concentrator, 40%; molecular sieve concentrator, 90% to 95%
5. FIO_2 analysis, alarm checks, flow measurement, filter and battery checks

Chapter 16

Pulmonary Function Testing

Answer the pre-test questions before studying the chapter. This will help you determine your strong and weak areas regarding the material covered.

1. Reversibility of obstructed airways and improved flow rates after a before-and-after bronchodilator study are considered significant at what minimum percentage of increase?

   A. 5%
   B. 10%
   C. 15%
   D. 25%

2. In which of the following lung conditions would the FRC be increased?

       I. Emphysema
      II. Cystic fibrosis
     III. Pneumonia

   A. I only
   B. I and II only
   C. I and III only
   D. II and III only

3. Which of the following pulmonary function tests would best determine the patient's ability to cough?

   A. V_T
   B. Alveolar minute ventilation
   C. FRC
   D. MIP

4. To evaluate the distribution of ventilation to perfusion with a V/Q scan, the patient is instructed to inhale which of the following substances?

   A. Helium
   B. CO
   C. Xenon
   D. Argon

5. Following are the results of a patient's spirometry test before and after bronchodilator therapy.

	Before	After
FEV_1	32% of predicted	53% of predicted
FVC	38% of predicted	66% of predicted
FEV_1/FVC	50%	64%

Which of the following is the correct interpretation of these results?

A. Mild restrictive disease with significant bronchodilator response
B. Severe obstructive disease with significant bronchodilator response
C. Severe restrictive disease with no significant bronchodilator response
D. Severe obstructive disease with no significant bronchodilator response

Answers are at the end of the chapter.

REVIEW

I. LUNG VOLUMES AND CAPACITIES

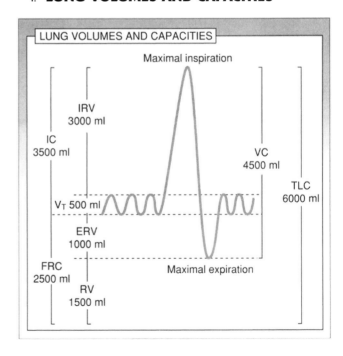

A. Lung Volumes

1. Tidal Volume (V_T)
   a. The volume of air (usually in milliliters) that is inhaled or exhaled during a normal breath.
   b. The exhaled V_T is usually measured with a respirometer at the bedside or by spirometry.

Note

When V_T is measured at the bedside, it is most accurately achieved by the patient being instructed to breathe normally through a mouthpiece connected to a respirometer for 1 full min. The volume reading is then divided by the patient's respiratory rate over that 1 min to obtain the V_T. Noseclips may be used to ensure mouth breathing only.

   ★ c. V_T is decreased or normal in restrictive disease and increased or normal in obstructive disease.
   d. Normal value is 500 mL (or 3 mL/lb of body weight)
2. Residual Volume (RV)
   a. The volume of air left in the lungs after a maximal expiration.
   b. It is derived after FRC is calculated, using either the nitrogen washout test or helium dilution test (see FRC section in this chapter).
   c. Once FRC is calculated, subtract the ERV from FRC; this equals the residual volume (i.e., **RV = FRC − ERV**)
   ★ d. RV is increased in obstructive disease and decreased in restrictive disease.
   e. Normal value is 1500 mL.
3. Inspiratory Reserve Volume (IRV)
   a. The maximum volume of air that can be inspired after a normal inspiration.
   b. Normally not measured during simple spirometry, but if it is, it should be measured from a slow vital capacity.
   c. IRV could be normal in both obstructive and restrictive disease, therefore its measurement is not clinically significant.
   d. Normal value is 3000 mL.
4. Expiratory Reserve Volume (ERV)
   a. The volume of air exhaled after a normal expiration.
   b. ERV measured directly by spirometry from a slow VC (i.e., VC − inspiratory capacity)
   c. ERV may be normal or decreased in obstructive or restrictive disease.
   d. Normal value is 1000 mL and 20% to 25% of the VC.

B. Lung Capacities

1. Functional Residual Capacity (FRC)
   a. The amount of air left in the lungs after a normal expiration (i.e., ERV + RV)
   b. Measured by the helium dilution or nitrogen washout test or body plethysmography.
   c. **Measurement of FRC by helium dilution test**
      (1) Also called the closed-circuit method
      (2) A spirometer is normally filled with about 600 mL of gas with about 10% helium added to the volume. The volume of the gas and the concentration of helium is measured and recorded before the test.
      (3) The patient is instructed to breathe normally and, at the end of a normal exhalation, is connected to the system.
      (4) The patient rebreathes the gas in the spirometer, while carbon dioxide is removed by a CO_2 absorbent.
      (5) Helium is then diluted until equilibrium is reached. This normally takes about 7 min, but in patients with severe lung disease, it may take as long as 30 min for equilibrium to occur. Equilibrium occurs as the helium analyzer falls to a stable level.
      (6) The final concentration of helium is then recorded.
   d. Calculations for FRC

$$\text{System volume} = \frac{\text{helium added (mL)}}{\% \text{ He (first reading)}}$$

$$\textbf{FRC} = \frac{(\% \text{ He}_1 - \% \text{ He}_2)}{\text{He}_2} \times \text{system vol} \times \text{BTPS correction factor}$$

He_1 = helium concentration before patient is connected to the system
He_2 = final helium concentration when equilibrium has occurred
BTPS correction factor = constant to convert volume to body temperature and pressure saturated.

Note

A helium analyzer reads zero when calibrated to room air.

   e. **Measurement of FRC using the nitrogen washout test**
      (1) Also called the open-circuit method

(2) During this test, the patient breathes in 100% oxygen to wash out the nitrogen in the lungs. Nitrogen concentration in the lungs is approximately 79%.

(3) The patient is instructed to breathe normally and, at the end of a normal exhalation, the patient is connected to the 100% oxygen breathing system.

(4) During the procedure, the exhaled volume is monitored and recorded and nitrogen percentages are measured.

(5) Complete nitrogen washout occurs in about 7 min.

f. FRC may now be calculated using this formula:

$$FRC = \frac{\text{expired volume} \times N_2}{N_1}$$

N_1 = nitrogen percentage in lungs at start of test
N_2 = nitrogen percentage in spirometer at end of test

g. **Measurement of FRC using body plethysmography**

(1) The plethysmograph ("body box") is an airtight chamber in which the patient sits during the procedure.

(2) While being tested, the patient is instructed to seal his or her lips tightly around the mouthpiece and to breathe normally. (The patient may also be tested while being instructed to breathe in shallow, panting breaths.)

(3) As the patient breathes, a pressure transducer measures pressure at the airway as well as inside the chamber.

(4) An electrical shutter is used to periodically close the airway, causing the patient to breathe against a closed airway, at which time volume and pressure values are measured.

★ (5) The technique of plethysmography is based on Boyle's law, which states that the volume of gas is inversely proportional to the pressure to which is it subjected.

h. FRC can then be calculated using this formula

$$FRC = \text{atmospheric pressure} \times \frac{\text{volume change}}{\text{pressure change}}$$

i. Body plethysmography also measures thoracic gas volume (VTG), total lung capacity (TLC), and residual volume (RV).

> **Note**
>
> Since body plethysmography actually measures the total amount of gas in the thorax, FRC measurements may be higher than those measured by the helium dilution or nitrogen washout method.

★ j. FRC is increased in obstructive disease and decreased in restrictive disease.

k. Normal value is 2500 mL.

2. Inspiratory Capacity (IC)

a. The maximum amount of air that can be inspired after a normal expiration (i.e., VT + IRV)

b. Measured by simple spirometry from a VC.

c. Usually is decreased or normal in obstructive or restrictive disease.

d. Normal value is 3500 mL (75% to 85% of the VC)

3. Vital Capacity (VC)

★ a. The maximum amount of air that can be exhaled following a maximum inspiration (i.e., VT + IRV + ERV)

b. Measured by simple spirometry or at the bedside using a respirometer.

> **Note**
>
> At the bedside, a mouthpiece connected to a respirometer is used. The patient is instructed to inhale as deeply as possible and then, slowly, completely exhale through the mouthpiece.

★ c. VC is decreased in restrictive disease and normal or decreased in obstructive disease.

d. Normal value is 4800 mL.

> **Note**
>
> A decreased VC may be the result of pneumonia, atelectasis, pulmonary edema, or lung cancer.

4. Forced Vital Capacity (FVC)

a. The maximum amount of air that can be exhaled as **fast and forcefully** as possible after a maximum inspiration.

b. Measured by simple spirometry.

c. Used to measure FEVs and flows.

★ d. FVC is decreased in both obstructive and restrictive disease.

5. Total Lung Capacity (TLC)

a. The amount of air remaining in the lungs at the end of a maximal inspiration.

b. Calculated by a combination of other measured volumes (i.e., FRC + IC, or VC + RV)

★ c. TLC is decreased in restrictive disease and increased in obstructive disease.

d. Normal value is 6000 mL.

Note

TLC decreases as a result of atelectasis, pulmonary edema, and consolidation and increases in emphysema.

---

6. **RV/TLC (ratio)**

a. The percentage of the TLC that remains in the lungs after a maximal expiration.

b. Measured by dividing the RV by TLC and multiplying by 100 to get a percentage.

★ c. RV/TLC is decreased in restrictive disease and increased in obstructive disease.

d. Normal value is 20% to 35%.

II. LUNG STUDIES

A. VEntilation Studies

1. **VT** (discussed previously in chapter)

2. **Respiratory rate**

a. The number of breaths in 1 min

b. Measured by counting chest excursion for 1 min.

c. Increased in hypoxia and hypercarbia and decreased with central respiratory center depression or depressing hypoxic drive on a COPD patient.

d. Normal value is 10/min to 20/min.

3. Minute Volume (MV, $\dot{V}E$)

a. The total volume of air (in liters) inhaled or exhaled in 1 min. Calculated by multiplying the respiratory rate times the VT.

b. Measured by simple spirometry or at bedside with a respirometer.

Note

When measuring $\dot{V}E$ at the bedside, a respirometer with mouthpiece is used. The patient is instructed to breathe normally through the mouthpiece as the practitioner times the breathing for 1 min. The reading on the respirometer after 1 min is the $\dot{V}E$.

---

c. Increased by hypoxia, hypercarbia, acidosis, or decreased lung compliance. Decreases as a result of hyperoxia, hypocarbia, alkalosis, and increased lung compliance.

d. Normal value is 5 to 10 L/min.

B. Flow Studies

1. Forced Expiratory Volume (FEV$_5$, FEV$_1$, FEV$_3$)

★ a. The volume of air that is exhaled over a specific time interval during the FVC maneuver.

b. Measured over 0.5, 1, or 3 sec (shown as subscript to FEV). The FEV$_1$ is the most common measurement.

c. The severity of airway obstruction may be determined, since it is a measurement at specified time intervals. **FEV is usually decreased in both obstructive and restrictive disease.**

Note

FEV may be decreased in restrictive disease because the FVC is below normal and the measurement of FEV is from the FVC. A better indicator of an obstructive or restrictive disorder is determined from the FEV/FVC ratio (discussed next).

---

2. **FEV/FVC (ratio)**

a. A ratio (percentage) of the relationship of FEV to FVC.

b. Normal values are

50% to 60% of the FVC is exhaled in 0.5 sec
75% to 85% of the FVC is exhaled in 1 sec
94% of the FVC is exhaled in 2 sec
97% of the FVC is exhaled in 3 sec

★ c. Obstructive disease is indicated by below normal values of FEV/FVC. Patients with restrictive disease have normal or above normal values.

d. Since the FEV$_1$ is most commonly measured, look for an **FEV$_1$/FVC of less than 75%** to indicate an obstructive disease.

3. **FEF$_{200-1200}$**

a. The average flow rate of the exhaled air after the first 200 mL during an FVC maneuver.

b. Measured on the spirograph tracing between the 200 mL mark and the 1200 mL mark to determine the average flow rate from the FVC.

★ c. Decreased in obstructive disease.

d. Normal value is 6 to 7 L/sec (400 L/min).

4. **FEF$_{25\%-75\%}$**

a. The average flow rate during the middle portion of the FEV.

b. The 25% and 75% points are marked on the spirographic curve from the FVC.

★ c. Values are decreased in obstructive disease.

d. Normal value is 4 to 5 L/sec.

5. **Peak Flow**
   a. The maximum flow rate achieved during an FVC.
   b. Measured from an FVC or by a peak flowmeter.

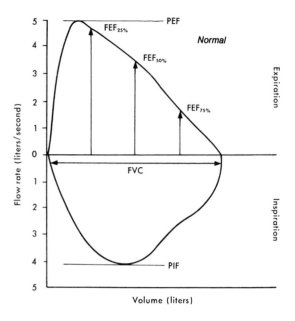

> **Note**
>
> When measured with a peak flowmeter at the bedside, the patient should be instructed to take as deep a breath as possible and exhale quickly as hard and fast as possible through the mouthpiece. This test is often done before a bronchodilating agent is administered and again afterwards to determine the agent's effectiveness.

★ c. Decreased in obstructive diseases
   d. Normal value is 400 to 600 L/min (6.5 to 10 L/sec).

6. Maximum Voluntary Ventilation (MVV)
   a. The maximum volume of air moved into and out of the lungs voluntarily in 10, 12, or 15 sec.
   b. This measurement tests for overall lung function, ventilatory reserve capacity, and air-trapping.
   c. Decreased in obstructive disease and decreased or normal in restrictive disease.
   d. Normal value is 170 L/min.

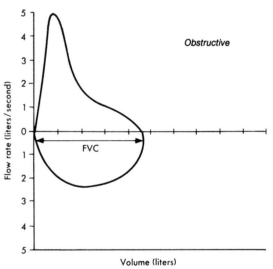

7. **Flow volume loop (curve)**
   a. A flow volume loop is displayed on a graph and represents the flow generated during an FEV maneuver followed by a forced inspiratory volume maneuver, both plotted against volume change.
   b. Using a flow volume loop, the following values may be measured.
      (1) Peak inspiratory flow (PIF)
      (2) Peak expiratory flow (PEF)
      (3) FVC
      (4) $FEV_{0.5}$, FEV_1, FEV_3
      (5) $FEF_{25\%-75\%}$
   c. The three diagrams show comparison of flow volume loops representing normal, obstructive, and restrictive disorders.
      (1) The restriction pattern shows a decreased VC with normal expiratory flow rates.
      (2) The obstructive pattern shows a decreased peak expiratory flow rate with a normal exhaled volume.

8. Diffusion capacity of the lung (DL)
   a. The diffusion capacity is a measurement that represents the gas exchange capabilities of the lungs.

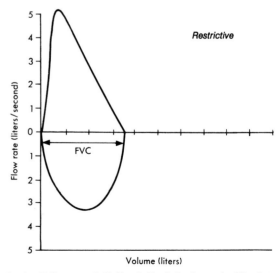

From Scanlan C, Spearman C, Sheldon R: Egan's Fundamentals of Respiratory Care, 5th ed., St. Louis, CV Mosby, 1990.

b. This procedure evaluates how well gas diffuses across the alveolar-capillary membrane into the pulmonary capillaries.

c. The most common method for measuring D_L is the single-breath method.

d. The patient is connected to a system in which the inspired gas contains a mixture of 10% helium and 0.3% CO. CO is used because of its increased affinity for Hb, which keeps the partial pressure of CO in the capillaries low, and also because it diffuses rapidly across the alveolar-capillary membrane.

e. The patient is instructed to exhale completely to the RV level, place the mouthpiece in the mouth, inhale as deeply as possible and hold the breath for 10 sec, and then exhale.

f. The D_{LCO} (carbon monoxide diffusion capacity), or the measurement of the amount of CO diffusing from the alveoli to the pulmonary blood flow, is calculated using this formula

$$D_{LCO} = \frac{mL \text{ of CO diffused per min}}{\text{A-a gradient of CO (mm Hg)}}$$

g. **Normal diffusion capacity is approximately 25 to 30 mL/min/mm Hg.**

h. Diffusion capacity is typically decreased because of either a decreased surface area available for diffusion or thickening of the membrane itself.

i. D_{LCO} is **decreased** as a result of
(1) O_2 toxicity
(2) Emphysema
(3) Sarcoidosis
(4) Edema
(5) Asbestosis

9. **V/Q scanning**

a. This radiograph evaluates the relationship of the distribution of ventilation to pulmonary perfusion in the lungs.

b. To determine gas distribution, the patient inhales the radioactive isotope **xenon** and holds the breath for 10 to 20 sec. Radiographs that are called photoscintigrams are taken to observe how the xenon was distributed in the lung.

c. To determine pulmonary perfusion, the patient is injected with a radioactive iodine preparation and photoscintigrams are taken as the blood perfuses the lungs.

III. **OBSTRUCTIVE VS. RESTRICTIVE LUNG DISEASES**

A. **Obstructive Diseases: These diseases result in decreased flow studies (FEV$_1$, FEV/FVC, FEF$_{25\%-75\%}$, FEF$_{200-1200}$).**
1. Emphysema
2. Asthma
3. Bronchitis
4. Cystic fibrosis
5. Bronchiectasis

B. **Restrictive Diseases or Disorders: These diseases result in decreased volumes (FRC, FVC, IC, IRV).**
1. Fibrotic disease
2. Chest wall disease
3. Pneumonia
4. Neuromuscular disease
5. Pleural disease
6. Postsurgical situations

C. **Severity of disease (by interpretation of pulmonary function tests)**
1. Normal pulmonary function test results: 80% to 100% of predicted value
2. Mild disorder: 60% to 79% of predicted value
3. Moderate disorder: 40% to 59% of predicted value
4. Severe disorder: less than 40% of predicted value

D. **Predicted values are determined from**
1. Age
2. Gender
3. Height
4. Ideal body weight
5. Race

IV. **MISCELLANEOUS PULMONARY FUNCTION STUDIES**

A. **Before-and-After Bronchodilator Studies**
1. Used to determine the reversibility of lung dysfunction and the effectiveness of the bronchodilator.
2. Patients, most commonly asthmatics, are instructed to perform a peak flow test before administration of a bronchodilating agent. The value is recorded. The administration of the agent is followed by another peak flow study.
3. Reversibility of obstructed airways and improved flow rates are considered significant if **increases in flow studies are at least 15%.**

$$\text{Percentage of improvement} = \frac{\text{posttreatment value} - \text{pretreatment value}}{\text{posttreatment value}} \times 100$$

B. **Methacholine Challenge Test**
1. Determines the degree of airway reactivity to methacholine, a drug that stimulates bronchoconstriction.

2. May be performed in a before-and-after bronchodilator study or before exercise-induced asthma studies.

3. The objective of the test is to determine the minimum level of methacholine that illicits **a 20% decrease in FEV$_1$.**

4. A physician should be present during testing and bronchodilators and resuscitation equipment should be readily available.

C. Measurement of maximal inspiratory pressure (MIP)

1. This measurement is also referred to as negative inspiratory force (NIF).

2. This value represents the maximum amount of negative pressure a patient can generate during inspiration.

3. This is measured with the aneroid manometer, which connects to an ET tube via an adaptor. The patient is then instructed to inhale as deeply as possible. The manometer records the negative pressure.

4. An adaptor attached to the manometer, using a one-way valve that allows for exhalation but not for inspiration, is also an effective method for obtaining MIP.

Note

These two methods for determining MIP may cause agitation and anxiety in alert patients. The practitioner should always explain the procedure to the patient before beginning it.

---

5. An MIP may also be obtained in patients who are not intubated by connecting the manometer to a mouthpiece and placing noseclips on the patient.

★ 6. Normal MIP is approximately -50 to -100 cm H$_2$O.

★ 7. A patient who cannot generate at least -20 cm H$_2$O pressure has inadequate respiratory muscle strength. The patient is not capable of generating the necessary negative inspiratory pressures required to cough and maintain a patent airway or to maintain spontaneous ventilation; therefore, mechanical ventilation is most likely indicated.

D. **Positive expiratory pressure (PEP)**

1. Also referred to as maximal expiratory pressure (MEP)

2. An aneroid manometer is attached to the patient's ET tube, and the patient is instructed to inhale as deeply as possible and exhale forcefully and completely.

3. The maximum pressure is observed and recorded.

4. PEP may be obtained in patients who are not intubated by attaching the manometer to a mouthpiece and placing noseclips on the patient.

★ 5. Normal PEP is 90 to 100 cm H$_2$O.

6. Patients unable to generate a PEP of at least **40 cm H$_2$O** pressure are not able to maintain adequate spontaneous ventilation or secretion clearance, making mechanical ventilation necessary.

E. **Exercise stress testing**

1. Exercise stress testing is used to evaluate a patient's cardiopulmonary reserve capacity.

2. The cardiopulmonary stress test is usually conducted with the patient either pedaling a cycle **ergometer** or walking on a treadmill.

3. Before testing a patient, a history and physical examination should be performed. The examination should include
   a. Pulmonary function tests
   b. D$_{LCO}$
   c. ABGs
   d. Blood pressure
   e. Before-and-after bronchodilator study (if airflow obstruction exists)
   f. Resting ECG

4. Some patients are not ideal candidates for cardiopulmonary stress testing. Conditions in which stress testing is contraindicated are
   a. CHF
   b. Recent acute MI
   c. Unstable angina
   d. Acute infection
   e. Uncontrolled cardiac arrhythmias
   f. Dissecting aneurysm
   g. Third-degree heart block
   h. Myocarditis

5. A physician and the following emergency equipment should always be present during a stress test.
   a. Defibrillator
   b. O$_2$ source
   c. Manual resuscitator with mask
   d. Oral airway
   e. Laryngoscope and ET tubes
   f. IV setup with 5% dextrose
   g. Cardiac medications

6. There are two general types of stress tests covered in this chapter.
   a. **The cardiac stress test**
      (1) The patient performs incremental work using either a cycle ergometer or treadmill.

(2) The patient's heart rate, blood pressure, and ECG strip are monitored before the test.

(3) These same parameters are measured at the end of each stage of the test and for at least 15 min after the test or until any cardiopulmonary symptoms subside.

(4) Most healthy individuals are able to complete all four stages of the exercise without difficulty. Patients with coronary artery disease (CAD) may not be able to complete all stages because of dyspnea and angina.

(5) This stress test is very useful in diagnosis and treatment of CAD but has limited efficacy in diagnosis of other cardiopulmonary diseases.

b. **The cardiopulmonary stress test**

(1) This test requires a cycle ergometer or a treadmill, a system for analyzing exhaled gases, a device for recording ventilation parameters, and an oximeter for measuring oxygen saturation or an arterial line for obtaining ABGs.

(2) This test also requires the patient to exercise at certain work load increments.

(3) Values measured during this test include

    (a) Blood pressure

    (b) Heart rate

    (c) ECG

    (d) Respiratory rate

    (e) O_2 saturation by pulse oximetry or arterial blood gases

    (f) V_{O_2}

    (g) V_{CO_2}

    (h) V_{CO_2}/V_{O_2}

    (i) O_2 pulse: volume of O_2 removed from the blood with each heartbeat; calculated by dividing O_2 consumption by the heart rate

    (j) V_D/V_T ratio

    (k) MVV

    (l) Anaerobic threshold: the point at which the O_2 requirements of the exercising muscles cannot be met and anaerobic metabolism begins to provide the O_2 supply.

(4) The test is discontinued when the patient reaches a predetermined heart rate or if the following signs or symptoms occur

    (a) Physical exhaustion

    (b) Excessive chest pain

    (c) Excessive dyspnea

    (d) Excessive fatigue in the legs

    (e) PVCs

    (f) Ventricular tachycardia

    (g) Heart block

    (h) Hypotension

    (i) Patient requests the test to be stopped

F. **Ventilatory Response Test for CO_2** (CO_2 Response Curve)

1. Ventilatory response to CO_2 is the measurement of the increase or decrease in the

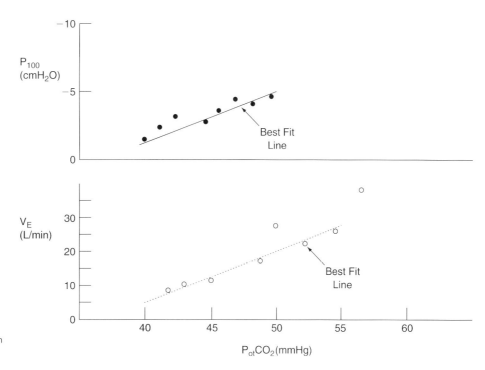

From Ruppell C: Manual of Pulmonary Function Testing, 6th ed., St. Louis, Mosby, 1994.

patient's minute ventilation as the result of breathing various levels of carbon dioxide, usually 1% to 7%, mixed with O_2 to maintain normal PaO2 levels.

★ 2. In a normal individual, there is an increase in $\dot{V}_E$ of about 3 L/min for every 1 mm Hg increase in the P_{CO_2} (there is a range of 1 to 6 L/min/mm Hg). This value is often decreased in COPD patients.

V. INTERPRETATION OF CHART SUMMARY

	Disease	
Function	Obstructive	Restrictive
FVC	Decreased	Decreased
IC	Decreased or normal	Decreased
ERV	Decreased or normal	Decreased
V_T	Increased	Decreased or normal
FRC	Increased	Decreased
RV	Increased	Decreased
RV/TLC	Increased	Decreased
FEV_1	Decreased	Normal or decreased
$FEF_{200-1200}$	Decreased	Normal
$FEF_{25\%-75\%}$	Decreased	Normal
FEV/FVC	Decreased	Normal
MVV	Decreased	Decreased

VI. FLOW-SENSING DEVICES
A. Wright Respirometer

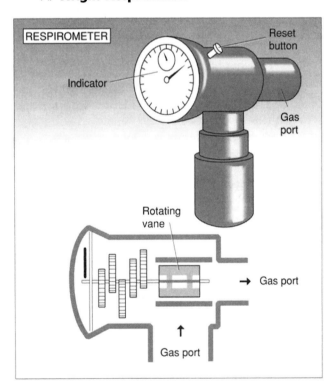

1. This respirometer is a handheld device that is frequently used at the patient's bedside to measure VC, V_T, and $\dot{V}_E$.

2. As the patient's exhaled gas flows through the respirometer, it rotates vanes within the device. Through a gearworks mechanism, the movement of the vane is indicated on a dial calibrated in liters.

3. This device may also be placed in-line to ventilator circuits to measure the patient's exhaled volume. When used for this purpose, it should be placed on the expiratory side of the circuit as close to the patient as possible.

B. Pneumotachometers

1. This type of flow-sensing device integrates flow signals to obtain volume measurements.

2. There are three kinds of pneumotachometers, which use different physical principles to measure flow.

   a. Pressure-drop pneumotachometer: air flows through the tube and meets a resistance, which decreases pressure. The pressure drop is measured by a transducer that converts it into an electronic signal.

   b. Temperature-drop pneumotachometer: uses King's law, which states that the velocity of gas flow over a heated element is proportional to the convective heat loss from the element. It can measure both flow and volume.

   c. Ultrasonic-flow pneumotachometer: this tube has struts inside to cause a turbulence in gas flow. The turbulent flow waves hit the ultrasonic sound waves and change them. The changes in the ultrasonic sound waves are proportional to the flow of gas and are shown as liters per minute or second.

POST-CHAPTER STUDY QUESTIONS

1. Name a condition that results in an increased RV.
2. What type of lung condition may result in a decreased IC?
3. What device may be used at the patient's bedside to measure VC?
4. What pulmonary function test is the best indicator for distinguishing an obstructive lung disorder from a restrictive one?
5. List three tests that aid in determining the severity of obstructive airway disease.
6. An FEV_1/FVC of less than 75% indicates which type of lung disease?
7. What five values may be measured on a flow volume loop?
8. List five conditions in which D_L is decreased.

9. What does a before-and-after bronchodilator test determine?
10. What does MIP, also referred to as NIF, represent?
11. List five parameters that should be obtained from the patient before exercise stress testing.
12. List the emergency equipment that should be present during a stress test.
13. List some of the values that are measured during a stress test.
14. List the signs and symptoms a patient may exhibit that would indicate that the stress test should be discontinued.

Answers are at the end of the chapter.

REFERENCES

Eubanks D and Bone R: Comprehensive respiratory care, ed 2, St. Louis, 1990, The CV Mosby Co.

Levitzky M: Introduction to respiratory care, Philadelphia, 1990, WB Saunders Co.

Ruppell G: Manual of pulmonary function testing, ed 6, St. Louis, 1994, Mosby-Yearbook, Inc.

Scanlan C, Wilkins R, and Stoller J: Egan's fundamentals of respiratory care, ed 7, St. Louis, 1999, Mosby, Inc.

PRE-TEST ANSWERS

1. C
2. B
3. D
4. C
5. B

ANSWERS TO POST-CHAPTER STUDY QUESTIONS

1. Emphysema (or other obstructive lung diseases)
2. Restrictive lung conditions (e.g., pulmonary fibrosis, scoliosis, pneumonia)
3. Respirometer
4. FEV_1/FVC
5. FEV_1, $FEF_{25\%-75\%}$, $FEF_{200-1200}$
6. Obstructive
7. PIF, PEF, FVC, FEV_1, $FEF_{25\%-75\%}$
8. O_2 toxicity, emphysema, pulmonary edema, asbestosis, sarcoidosis, pulmonary fibrosis
9. The response to the bronchodilating agent (increase in flow study results of at least 15% indicates significant response)
10. The maximum amount of negative pressure the patient can generate during inspiration; determines the level of respiratory muscle strength.
11. Pulmonary function tests, including diffusion study, ABGs, blood pressure, before-and-after bronchodilator study, resting ECG
12. Defibrillator, O_2, manual resuscitator with mask, oral airway, laryngoscope, ET tubes, IV with 5% dextrose, cardiac medications
13. Blood pressure, heart rate, ECG, respiratory rate, O_2 saturation by pulse oximetry, ABG levels, O_2 consumption, CO_2 production, respiratory quotient, oxygen pulse, V_D/V_T, MVV, anaerobic threshold
14. Physical exhaustion, excessive chest pain, excessive dyspnea, excessive leg fatigue, PVCs, ventricular tachycardia, heart block, hypotension, request by patient to stop test

Chapter 17

Equipment Decontamination and Infection Control

PRE-TEST QUESTIONS

Answer the pre-test questions before studying the chapter. This will help you determine your strong and weak areas regarding the material covered.

1. Which of the following procedures is most often used to decontaminate a bacterial filter used on a mechanical ventilator?

   A. Ethylene oxide sterilization
   B. Autoclaving
   C. Pasteurization
   D. Glutaraldehyde immersion

2. Diseases that may be transmitted via airborne particles include which of the following?

   I. Tuberculosis
   II. Legionellosis
   III. Histoplasmosis

   A. I only
   B. II only
   C. I and III only
   D. I, II, and III

3. Which of the following procedures are capable of sterilizing equipment?

   I. Pasteurization
   II. Glutaraldehyde immersion
   III. Acetic acid immersion
   IV. Ethylene oxide

   A. I and II only
   B. II and III only
   C. II and IV only
   D. I, II, and IV only

4. Which of the following should be worn as a precautionary measure when changing a patient's ventilator circuit?

   I. Gloves
   II. Eye goggles
   III. Gown

   A. I only
   B. I and II only
   C. I and III only
   D. I, II, and III

5. A HEPA filter should be used in the room of a patient with which type of condition?

   A. Tuberculosis
   B. Adenovirus infection
   C. Epiglottitis
   D. Streptococcal pneumonia

6. Biologic indicators are used in decontamination procedures for which of the following reasons?

   A. They speed up the decontamination process.
   B. They increase the concentration of liquid sterilants.
   C. They indicate what organisms have contaminated the equipment.
   D. They determine if the decontamination process was effective.

Answers are at the end of the chapter.

REVIEW

I. **BASIC TERMINOLOGY**
   A. Vegetative organisms: organisms in active growth. **These organisms pose the greatest hazard for infection via respiratory therapy equipment because the most common equipment contaminants are not spore-forming bacteria.**
   B. Spores: organisms in a resting, resistant stage. They are very difficult to kill but pose little threat for infection via respiratory therapy equipment.
   C. Disinfection: killing of all vegetative forms of organisms but not spores. Agents that disinfect equipment are called disinfectants.
   D. Sterilization: killing of all organisms, both vegetative and spores. An agent that sterilizes equipment is called a sterilant.

E. The suffix "-cidal": meaning to kill, as in **bactericidal,** said of something that kills bacteria.

F. The suffix "-static": meaning to prevent growth of, as in **bacteriostatic,** said of something that prevents the growth of bacteria.

G. Gram's stain method for differential staining of bacteria. Gram-positive bacteria stain a purple-black color and gram-negative bacteria stain a pink color.

H. Nosocomial infection: a hospital-acquired infection. Often caused by *Pseudomonas* species, *Staphylococcus* species, *Candida albicans,* or *Escherichia coli.*

II. CONDITIONS THAT INFLUENCE ANTIMICROBIAL ACTION

A. Chemical concentration: the more concentrated a chemical is, the more rapid the action.

B. Intensity of the physical agent: the more intense a physical agent (e.g., heat), the more rapidly the organisms are killed.

C. Time: the longer the organisms are exposed to the agent, the greater the number killed.

D. Temperature: increasing the temperature of a chemical agent shortens the exposure time required to kill the organisms.

E. Type of organism: vegetative forms of bacteria are more easily killed than spore-forming bacteria. Spores are more resistant to both chemical and physical agents.

F. Number of organisms: the more organisms, the longer the exposure time required to kill them.

G. Nature of material bearing the organism: the presence of blood, sputum, or other medium provides protection for the organisms. It is for this reason that **equipment must be thoroughly washed in soapy water and rinsed off before the decontamination process.**

III. THREE MAIN CLASSES OF BACTERIA

A. Cocci: sphere-shaped bacteria

B. Spirillum: spiral-shaped bacteria

★C. Bacilli: rod-shaped bacteria

1. Bacilli are the bacteria most frequently encountered on respiratory equipment.

2. They **are not** spore-forming bacteria.

3. Examples of bacilli (often causing pneumonia)

a. *Klebsiella pneumoniae:* a gram-negative bacillus

b. *Pseudomonas aeruginosa:* a gram-negative bacillus

c. *Mycobacterium* species: a gram-positive bacillus and causative agent of TB

d. *Legionella* species: gram-negative bacilli

e. *Serratia marcesens:* a gram-negative bacillus and secondary invader in respiratory and burn patients.

f. *Haemophilus influenzae:* a gram-negative bacillus

Note

The gram-negative organisms listed above are often responsible for necrotizing forms of pneumonia.

IV. STERILIZATION AND DISINFECTION TECHNIQUES

A. **Physical Agents**

1. **Moist heat**

a. Boiling water at 100° C for 5 min kills vegetative forms of bacteria, fungi, and most viruses.

b. Kills organisms by coagulation of the cell protein.

c. Since spores are *not* killed, this is a disinfection method.

d. Used mainly at home or in doctor's offices, it is not recommended for use on respiratory therapy equipment.

2. **Autoclave (steam under pressure)**

a. Heat in the form of steam is one of the most dependable and practical methods for decontamination.

b. **Normal operating levels are 15 min at 121° C and 15 psig (2 atm).**

c. **Autoclaving sterilizes equipment.**

d. Kills organisms by coagulation of the cell protein.

e. Bacteria filters are commonly sterilized by this method, but any material made of rubber cannot withstand the intense heat.

f. The tops of nebulizers and humidifiers should be attached loosely to allow exposure to all parts of the device.

g. Equipment to be autoclaved must be thoroughly washed in soapy water, dried, and wrapped in muslin, cloth, or a paper bag.

h. Written on the outside of the wrap should be information including the time and date of processing, what kind of equipment is inside the wrap, and who prepared the equipment for processing.

3. **Pasteurization**

a. Equipment must be washed in soapy water and rinsed off before placement in the pasteurizing machine.

b. Equipment is immersed in hot water at 60° C to 70° C for 20 to 30 min.

c. The hotter the water, the less time needed to clean the equipment.

d. **Pasteurization disinfects equipment,** but spores are not killed.

B. **Chemical Agents**

1. **Ethylene oxide gas sterilization**

a. Equipment must be washed in soapy water, rinsed, **dried completely,** and placed in a sealed plastic bag before being placed in the sterilization chamber.

b. If equipment is not completely dry before the sterilization process, ethylene oxide combines with water to form ethylene glycol, an irritating substance found in antifreeze.

c. Ethylene oxide kills all organisms including spores, therefore it **sterilizes equipment.**

d. It is a highly flammable gas, but by mixing it with approximately 90% carbon dioxide or freon, the explosive danger is minimized.

e. Equipment may be processed in one of two ways.

(1) Warm gas: 50° C to 56° C for 4 hours

(2) Cold gas: 22° C (room temperature) for 6 to 12 hours

f. After exposure to the gas, the equipment must be aerated for about 12 hours at 50° C to 60° C.

g. Most respiratory therapy equipment can be decontaminated by this method.

h. The recommended gas concentration is 800 to 1000 mg/L.

i. Since moisture enhances the action of ethylene oxide, it is recommended that the relative humidity within the sterilizing chamber be maintained at 50% or more.

j. Items placed in sealed plastic bags are suitable for use for up to 1 year after gas sterilization, provided the bag is intact.

2. **Alcohols**

a. Ethyl alcohol (95% concentration) and isopropyl alcohol (70% concentration) are the most commonly used in the clinical setting.

b. Alcohols are bactericidal and fungicidal but not sporicidal, therefore they disinfect (but do not sterilize) equipment.

c. Alcohols kill organisms by destroying the cell protein.

d. Action is intensified if mixed with water.

e. Used as a disinfectant to wipe down respiratory therapy equipment.

3. **Glutaraldehydes**

a. Related to formaldehyde.

b. The most common glutaraldehyde product is Cidex, which is an alkaline glutaraldehyde solution.

c. These agents are **bactericidal in 10 to 15 min and sporicidal in 3 to 10 hours,** depending on the temperature of the solution.

d. Normally used to disinfect equipment but may be used to sterilize. Kills organisms by coagulation of the cell protein.

e. Equipment must be washed in soapy water and rinsed off before placement in the solution bath.

f. On removal from the solution bath (with gloves to prevent skin irritation), the equipment should be rinsed off and thoroughly dried before packaging.

g. Cidex solution remains active for 28 days.

4. **Acetic acid (vinegar)**

a. Kills vegetative bacteria but not spores, therefore it **disinfects equipment.**

b. It is very effective against *Pseudomonas* species.

c. Used as a disinfectant for home care equipment and is often run through room humidifiers for cleaning purposes.

d. Not recommended for use on respiratory therapy equipment in the clinical setting, unless in combination with more effective methods.

V. **IMPORTANT POINTS CONCERNING DECONTAMINATION OF EQUIPMENT**

A. Use only sterile solutions in reservoirs.

B. Solutions left in the reservoir should be discarded before adding fresh solution.

C. Always date the container that holds the solution after it is opened; solutions should be discarded after 24 hours. This reduces the possibility of filling a reservoir with contaminated solution.

D. Condensation in the delivery tubing **should never be drained back into the reservoir.**

E. Provide a method of routine surveillance to determine the effectiveness of the decontamination process. This is referred to as **quality control of equipment.**

1. Processing indicators determine whether the disinfection or sterilization process was effective. There are two types of indicators:

a. Biologic indicators: Strips of paper impregnated with bacterial spores are placed in a glass ampule that contains a growth medium. The ampule is then placed inside the sterilizer. After the sterilization process is complete, the ampule is broken and the spore strip is exposed to the growth medium. After an incubation period, if the spore strip changes color, bacteria are present and the sterilization process was ineffective.

b. Chemical indicators are impregnated on packing tape and change color when exposed to certain conditions. Autoclave and ethylene oxide sterilization both use this type of indicator. These indicators show that the package went through the sterilization process but do not necessarily indicate the equipment is sterile. Ensuring that the equipment is sterile is best accomplished with biologic indicators.

2. Culture sampling: Equipment disinfected by chemical solutions, such as glutaraldehyde, or by pasteurization should be evaluated to determine if the disinfection process is effective.

3. Swab sampling: A sterile swab is used to wipe an area of the equipment and placed in a tube of sterile liquid broth to determine the presence of microorganisms.

F. Use of disposable equipment decreases the potential for cross-contamination. Since warm, moist humidifiers and nebulizers are ideal breeding grounds for bacteria, disposables are for single patient use only.

G. The most cost-effective method of preventing cross-contamination of equipment among patients is by proper **HAND-WASHING techniques.**

H. Disposable equipment should not be refilled or reused.

I. Equipment must be completely dry when packaged and stored to prevent new growth.

VI. INFECTION CONTROL AND STANDARD (UNIVERSAL) PRECAUTIONS

> ### Exam Note
>
> Questions relating to infection control and universal precautions appear on the CRT examination only.

A. **Standard (Universal) Precautions:** All health care providers should practice these precautions, regardless of the patient's diagnosis or presumed diagnosis. They apply to blood, body fluids, secretions, excretions, mucous membranes, and nonintact skin.

1. Hand washing: after every patient, even if wearing gloves

2. Gloves: when treating all patients

3. Gown: should be worn when performing a task that may involve the splashing of fluids or spraying of blood

4. Mask, eye goggles, face shield: should be worn when performing a task that may involve the splashing of fluids or spraying of blood

5. The possibility of bloodborne pathogens requires the proper handling of needles and other sharp instruments.
Use extreme caution when handling needles and other sharp instruments
   a. Never recap used needles.
   b. Used needles and syringes should be placed in puncture-resistant containers.
   c. Never remove used needles by hand.

B. **Transmission-Based Precautions:** These precautions are used when working with patients who have contagious diseases for which standard precautions are inadequate. These precautions are implemented in addition to standard precautions. There are three types of transmission-based precautions.

1. **Precautions against contact**
   a. Decreases the risk of transmission of microorganisms by direct or indirect contact.
   b. Examples of diseases requiring these precautions include hepatitis, AIDS, venereal diseases, and staphylococcal infections.
   c. In addition to standard precautions, the patient should be placed in a private room, and gloves and gowns should be discarded before exiting the room.

2. **Precautions against airborne infections**
   a. Decreases the risk of spread of infectious microorganisms through the air.
   b. Diseases that may be transmitted by this route include tuberculosis, legionellosis, histoplasmosis, and measles.
   c. In addition to standard precautions, the patient should be placed in a private room with the door closed at all times, and anyone entering the room should wear a HEPA mask.
   d. To further aid in the reduction of airborne organisms, the room should have a special (negative pressure) ventilation system from which air is safely discharged or recirculated in the room through a HEPA filter.

3. **Precautions against droplet spread**
   a. Decreases the risk of the transmission of infectious organisms via droplet spread.
   b. Examples of diseases transmitted by this route include *Haemophilus influenzae* infection, streptococcal pneumonia, epiglottitis, pertussis, meningitis, and adenovirus infections.
   c. In addition to standard precautions, the patient should be placed in a private room and a mask should be worn by anyone entering the room.

> **Note**
>
> If private rooms are not available for patients under these three types of special precautions, patients infected with the same organism may share a room. This is referred to as cohorting.

POST-CHAPTER STUDY QUESTIONS

1. List four diseases that are spread by airborne pathogens.
2. What device should be used in the ventilation system through which air is discharged safely from the room of a patient with a disease caused by an airborne pathogen?
3. List three methods that may be used to sterilize respiratory therapy equipment.
4. List three diseases transmitted by droplet spread.
5. What is a nosocomial infection?
6. List four gram-negative organisms that may result in necrotizing pneumonia.
7. What methods are used to determine the effectiveness of the decontamination process?

Answers are at the end of the chapter.

REFERENCES

Barnes TA: Respiratory care practice, Chicago, 1988, Year-Book Medical Publishers.

Eubanks D and Bone R: Comprehensive respiratory care, ed 2, St Louis, 1990, The CV Mosby Co.

The Merck manual, ed 14, St. Louis, 1982, Merck and Company.

Scanlan C, Wilkins R, Stoller J: Egan's fundamentals of respiratory care, ed 7, St Louis, 1999, Mosby, Inc.

PRE-TEST ANSWERS

1. B
2. D
3. C
4. D
5. A
6. D

ANSWERS TO POST-CHAPTER STUDY QUESTIONS

1. Tuberculosis, histoplasmosis, legionellosis, measles
2. HEPA filter
3. Autoclave, ethylene oxide gas, glutaraldehyde solution
4. Streptococcal pneumonia, epiglotittis, adenovirus, meningitis, pertussis, *H. influenzae*
5. Hospital-acquired infection
6. *Pseudomonas, Klebsiella, Serratia,* and *Legionella* species
7. Chemical and biologic indicators, culture and swab sampling

Entry Level Certification Exam: Practice Test

TIME LIMIT: 3 HOURS

> **Note**
>
> 1 torr = 1 mm Hg

Directions: Each of the questions or incomplete statements in this test are followed by four suggested answers or completions. Choose the best answer and circle it on the test.

1. The physician orders a 35% aerosol mask to be set up on a patient who requires an inspiratory flow of 42 L/min. What is minimum flow rate that the flowmeter must be set on to meet this patient's inspiratory flow demands?

   A. 6 L/min
   B. 8 L/min
   C. 10 L/min
   D. 12 L/min

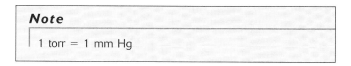

2. A premature infant is receiving O_2 via a 50% O_2 hood and has a PaO_2 of 43 torr and a $PaCO_2$ of 40 torr. The RCP should recommend which of the following?

   A. Increase the O_2 to 70%.
   B. Intubate and institute mechanical ventilation.
   C. Place on CPAP of 4 cm H_2O and 50% O_2.
   D. Increase the O_2 to 100%.

3. A patient arrives in the emergency department after being pulled from a burning house. The RCP should recommend obtaining which of the following measurements to best determine the severity of the patient's smoke inhalation?

   A. SpO_2
   B. HbCO
   C. PaO_2
   D. Hb

4. The physician has ordered 40% O_2 to be administered to an active 3-year-old. Which of the following delivery devices would you recommend for this patient?

   A. O_2 tent
   B. Air entrainment mask
   C. Simple O_2 mask
   D. O_2 hood

5. The ability of the patient to follow instructions would be indicated by which of the following?

   A. Orientation to person
   B. Performance of tasks when asked
   C. Ability to feed himself
   D. Awareness of time

6. The RCP suspects a patient may have a pulmonary embolism. Which of the following would be the most appropriate recommendation for diagnosis of this condition?

   A. Bronchoscopy
   B. V/Q lung scan
   C. Coagulation studies
   D. Shunt study

7. To most effectively increase a patient's alveolar minute ventilation while on a ventilator in the control mode, you would recommend increasing which of the following?

   A. Sigh rate
   B. Inspiratory flow
   C. V_T
   D. Ventilator rate

8. If the RCP fails to hyperoxygenate a patient on a ventilator before ET suctioning, it may result in

   I. Hypocarbia
   II. Hypoxemia
   III. Hypertension
   IV. Bradycardia

   A. I only
   B. I and II only

C. II and III only
D. II and IV only

9. The most reliable method of determining if a mechanically ventilated patient's lungs are getting stiffer and harder to ventilate is by measuring the

A. Static lung compliance
B. Dynamic lung compliance
C. Spontaneous VT
D. PaO₂

λ 10. An RCP is called to the recovery room to transport a patient to the ICU. After attaching the regulator to the E cylinder, gas is heard leaking from the cylinder. The practitioner should do which of the following?

I. Tighten all connections.
II. Lubricate the regulator connection.
III. Replace the washer between the cylinder and regulator connections.

A. I only
B. I and II only
C. I and III only
D. II and III only

11. If not cleaned properly, which one of the following devices is most likely to contaminate a patient's airways with bacteria?

A. Bubble humidifier
B. Heated cascade humidifier
C. Hydrosphere
D. Heated jet nebulizer

12. A baffle is used on a nebulizer to

A. Break the aerosol into smaller particles
B. Entrain room air
C. Alter O₂ concentration
D. Increase the total flow to the patient

13. Which one of the following sets of ABG measurements would be indicative of a renal compensated respiratory acidosis?

A. pH 7.26, PCO₂ 60 torr, PO₂ 68 torr, HCO₃⁻ 24 mEq/L, BE 0
B. pH 7.42, PCO₂ 39 torr, PO₂ 87 torr, HCO₃⁻ 22 mEq/L, BE −1
C. pH 7.25, PCO₂ 61 torr, PO₂ 75 torr, HCO₃⁻ 26 mEq/L, BE +1
D. pH 7.37, PCO₂ 58 torr, PO₂ 60 torr, HCO₃⁻ 31 mEq/L, BE +8

λ 14. The following data has been collected on a patient being ventilated on a volume ventilator.

VT	750 mL	pH	7.29
Mode	SIMV	PaCO₂	50 torr
Ventilator rate	4/min	PaO₂	72 torr
Spontaneous rate	12/min	HCO₃⁻	26 mEq/L
FIO₂	0.35	BE	+1

Based on these data, which of the following should the RCP recommend?

A. Increase the VT to 850 mL.
B. Increase the FIO₂ to 0.40.
C. Increase the ventilator rate to 8/min.
D. Place on assist/control mode at a rate of 15/min.

λ 15. Advantages of low-pressure, high-volume ET tube cuffs include

I. Easier insertion into the airway
II. Less occlusion to tracheal blood flow
III. Improved distribution of alveolar air

A. I only
B. II only
C. I and II only
D. II and III only

16. Tracheal secretions tend to dry out in an intubated patient when inspired air has which of the following characteristics?

I. An absolute humidity of 24 mg/L of gas
II. A water vapor pressure of 47 mm Hg
III. 50 mg of particulate water per liter of gas
IV. A relative humidity of 100% at 25°C

A. II only
B. I and III only
C. I and IV only
D. II and III only

17. It is important to monitor airway pressure on a mechanically ventilated patient because it best reflects

A. Lung compliance
B. PaO₂
C. PaCO₂
D. ICP

18. When a patient is being ventilated in the control mode, how may the PaCO₂ be raised?

A. Increase the VT.
B. Increase the FIO₂.
C. Decrease the mechanical dead space.
D. Decrease the respiratory rate.

19. A patient is being ventilated on a volume-cycled ventilator and the low-pressure alarm suddenly sounds. The corrective action would be to

A. Suction the patient.
B. Begin manual resuscitation.
C. Increase the flow.
D. Determine if the patient is disconnected from the ventilator.

20. After a patient has received bronchodilator therapy, the RCP attempts to perform nasotracheal suction on the patient. As the catheter enters the oropharynx, the following ECG waveform is seen on the oscilloscope monitor.

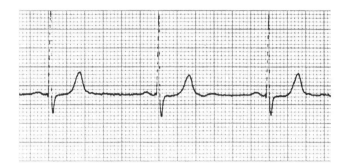

This ECG pattern is most likely the result of which of the following?

A. Excessive suction pressure
B. Hypoxemia
C. Vagal nerve stimulation
D. Hypercarbia

21. If vocal cord trauma is suspected after extubation, the patient would exhibit which one of the following symptoms?

A. Wheezing
B. Rhonchi
C. Stridor
D. Crackles

22. To prevent the obstruction of venous blood flow from the trachea, ET tube cuff pressure should not exceed

A. 5 mm Hg
B. 10 mm Hg
C. 20 mm Hg
D. 25 mm Hg

23. A postoperative 46-year-old, 80-kg (176-lb) patient is breathing spontaneously at a rate of 30/min on an FIO_2 of 0.50. The following ABG results are obtained.

pH	7.29
$PaCO_2$	62 torr
PaO_2	64 torr
HCO_3^-	29 mEq/L
BE	+4

Mechanical ventilation is instituted with a V_T of 800 mL and an FIO_2 of 0.5. The SIMV rate should be set on

A. 4/min
B. 6/min
C. 12/min
D. 16/min

24. The RCP is asked to deliver a medication to a cystic fibrosis patient via an HHN that will improve the mobilization of sputum. Which of the following should be recommended?

A. Acetylcysteine (Mucomyst)
B. Propylene glycol
C. Racemic epinephrine
D. Dexamethasone (Decadron)

25. The therapeutic use of O_2 may aid in accomplishing which of the following?

   I. Decrease the work of breathing
   II. Decrease myocardial work
   III. Prevent ARDS
   IV. Increase the patient's respiratory rate

A. I only
B. I and II only
C. II and III only
D. I, II, and IV only

26. Inspiratory stridor is the major clinical sign of

A. Tracheal malacia
B. Tracheal stenosis
C. Glottic edema
D. Laryngotracheal web

27. A patient on a volume ventilator is ordered to be placed on PEEP. Observation of which of the following values will *best* determine the optimal level of PEEP?

A. Cardiac output
B. PaO_2
C. $PaCO_2$
D. VD/VT

28. Ventilator-induced hyperventilation would be determined in ABG results by

A. Increased pH, decreased $PaCO_2$
B. Increased pH, increased $PaCO_2$
C. Decreased pH, increased $PaCO_2$
D. Decreased pH, decreased $PaCO_2$

29. As inspired air reaches the carina, it should be 100% saturated with water at body temperature,

which represents how many milligrams of water per liter of air?

A. 32
B. 44
C. 47
D. 54

30. Administration of high O_2 concentrations to a neonate for a prolonged period of time may result in which of the following?

   I. Atelectasis
   II. Retinopathy of prematurity
   III. Pneumothorax

A. II only
B. I and II only
C. I and III only
D. I, II, and III

31. The data below pertains to an adult being mechanically ventilated.

Peak inspiratory pressure	50 cm H_2O
Plateau pressure	40 cm H_2O
V_T	800 mL (.8 L)
PEEP	10 cm H_2O

On the basis of this information, this patient's static lung compliance is approximately which of the following?

A. 16 mL/cm H_2O
B. 20 mL/cm H_2O
C. 27 mL/cm H_2O
D. 37 mL/cm H_2O

32. A patient recovering postoperatively is being ventilated in the SIMV mode. The patient has normal ABG levels on 35% O_2 but is still drowsy. The RCP should recommend decreasing the

A. SIMV rate
B. Inspiratory time
C. V_T
D. Sigh volume

33. The RCP is transporting a patient on a nasal cannula running at 6 L/min. To ensure that an E cylinder will last at least 1 hour, what is the minimum amount of pressure it must contain?

A. 1000 psig
B. 1200 psig
C. 1400 psig
D. 1600 psig

34. Which statement(s) relating to uncompensated Thorpe tube flowmeters is (are) *true*?

   I. The Thorpe tube is pressurized to 50 psig when plugged into the gas outlet.
   II. The needle valve is located proximal to the Thorpe tube.
   III. The float will jump up and come back down while the flowmeter is plugged into a wall outlet with the needle valve closed.
   IV. Back pressure into the Thorpe tube does not affect the flow reading.

A. I only
B. II only
C. II and III only
D. III and IV only

35. Which one of these drugs would be best to use to temporarily paralyze a patient to facilitate tracheal intubation?

A. Atropine sulfate
B. Succinylcholine (Anectine)
C. Curare
D. Pancuronium bromide

36. To begin the weaning process from the ventilator, a patient should be able to obtain a MIP of at least

A. 10 cm H_2O
B. 20 cm H_2O
C. 30 cm H_2O
D. 40 cm H_2O

37. While making O_2 rounds you discover that the 6-inch reservoir tubing on a T-piece (Briggs adaptor) setup has fallen off. What may result from this?

   I. Delivered F_{IO_2} would decrease.
   II. Delivered F_{IO_2} would increase.
   III. The patient would entrain room air during inspiration.

A. I only
B. II only
C. I and III only
D. II and III only

38. A patient has been paralyzed with pancuronium (Pavulon) and is being mechanically ventilated. Which of the following ventilator monitoring alarms would be the most important?

A. Low pressure
B. High pressure
C. Inspired gas temperature
D. I:E ratio

39. Use of the inspiratory plateau setting on a ventilator results in

I. Decreasing mean intrathoracic pressure
II. Increasing diffusion of gases
III. Decreasing atelectasis

A. I only
B. II only
C. I and II only
D. II and III only

40. A patient with COPD is in the emergency department and is complaining of shortness of breath. Arterial blood gas results on room air are below.

pH	7.31
$PaCO_2$	62 torr
PaO_2	44 torr
HCO_3^-	34 mEq/L
BE	+10

The most appropriate recommendation for O_2 therapy is which of the following?

A. Simple mask at 10 L/min.
B. Nasal cannula at 6 L/min.
C. Air entrainment mask at 28%
D. Aerosol mask at 40%

41. During CPR, the physician is preparing to administer lidocaine intravenously and discovers the IV is infiltrated. The most appropriate action to take at this time is to

A. Instill the lidocaine down the ET tube.
B. Administer the lidocaine via an HHN.
C. Place a new IV line and administer the lidocaine.
D. Administer the lidocaine sublingually.

42. Which of these devices would be most indicated in the treatment of a patient with large amounts of thick secretions?

A. Bubble humidifier
B. Impeller nebulizer
C. Pass-over humidifier
D. Ultrasonic nebulizer

43. Which of these devices is not a low-flow device?

A. Nasal cannula
B. Venturi mask
C. Partial rebreathing mask
D. Simple O_2 mask

44. You are instructing a patient about the proper procedure for using an MDI. You would instruct the patient to activate the medication in the inhaler

A. Just before inspiration.
B. Just after inspiration has begun.
C. At the end of exhalation.
D. After inhaling as deeply as possible.

45. After the intubation of a patient, the RCP is assessing the chest x-ray films for proper tube placement. The tip of the tube is at the level of the fourth rib. This indicates which of the following?

A. The tube position is too low.
B. The tube is too high.
C. The tube is in the esophagus.
D. The tube is in proper position in the midtrachea.

46. While suctioning through a patient's ET tube, the RCP begins having difficulty removing the thick secretions. Which of the following is the appropriate measure to take?

A. Increase the suction pressure to -160 torr.
B. Use a larger suction catheter.
C. Apply continuous suction while withdrawing the catheter.
D. Instill saline down the ET tube before suctioning.

47. The following ABGs are collected from a patient on a 50% Venturi mask.

pH	7.37
$PaCO_2$	40 torr
PaO_2	70 torr

If the barometric pressure is 747 torr, which of the following represents this patient's $P(A-a) O_2$?

A. 170 torr
B. 230 torr
C. 300 torr
D. 350 torr

48. A patient has just been intubated and the CO_2 detector on the proximal end of the ET tube reads near zero. Which statement is true regarding this situation?

A. The tube is in the trachea.
B. The tube is in the esophagus.
C. The tube should be withdrawn 2 cm.
D. The tube is in the right mainstem bronchus.

49. The following data are collected on a neonate on a pressure ventilator.

Mode	IMV	pH	7.41
Ventilator rate	40/min	$PaCO_2$	43 torr
Inspiratory pressure	28 cm H_2O	PaO_2	41 torr
FiO_2	0.70	HCO_3^-	23 mEq/L
PEEP	4 cm H_2O	BE	0

Based on these data, the RCP should recommend which of the following?

A. Increase ventilator rate to 45/min.
B. Increase PEEP to 6 cm H_2O.
C. Increase inspiratory pressure to 32 cm H_2O.
D. Increase FIO_2 to 0.80.

50. Heavy smokers commonly have HbCO levels as high as

   A. 10%
   B. 20%
   C. 30%
   D. 40%

51. The following data has been collected from a 70-kg (154-lb) patient on a volume ventilator.

Mode	Assist/control	ABGs: pH	7.37
Ventilator rate	12/min	$PaCO_2$	42 torr
V_T	750 mL	PaO_2	161 torr
FIO_2	0.80	HCO_3^-	25 mEq/L
PEEP	10 cm H_2O	BE	0

Based on these data, which of the following ventilator setting changes should the RCP recommend?

   A. Decrease V_T to 700 mL.
   B. Decrease PEEP to 8 cm H_2O.
   C. Increase ventilator rate to 15/min.
   D. Decrease FIO_2 to 0.70.

52. The RCP is assisting the physician with cardioversion on a patient exhibiting atrial fibrillation. The practitioner should recommend which of the following levels of energy to conduct this procedure?

   A. 50 J
   B. 150 J
   C. 200 J
   D. 350 J

53. A 75-kg (165-lb) male patient is being mechanically ventilated in the IMV mode and has the following ABG results.

pH	7.29
$PaCO_2$	59 torr
PaO_2	75 torr
HCO_3^-	27 mEq/L
BE	+2

The ventilator settings are as follows:

FIO_2	0.35
IMV rate	8/min
Spontaneous rate	24/min
V_T	600 mL

The RCP should recommend increasing which two of the following?

   I. Inspiratory flow
   II. IMV rate

III. V_T
IV. FIO_2

   A. I and II
   B. II and III
   C. I and III
   D. II and IV

54. The term purulence in reference to sputum means it is

   A. Yellow or green
   B. Thick
   C. Blood-streaked
   D. Brown

55. An oral ET tube is inserted into an adult patient. A leak is still heard after a large amount of air is placed in the cuff. This problem could be caused by which of the following?

   A. The ET tube is too short.
   B. The ET tube is too long.
   C. The ET tube's internal diameter is too large.
   D. The ET tube's outside diameter is too small.

56. What is the most negative pressure that should supply the suction catheter when suctioning an adult?

   A. −60 mm Hg
   B. −80 mm Hg
   C. −120 mm Hg
   D. −160 mm Hg

57. The following ventilatory parameters are collected from a 68-kg (150-lb) patient on a 2-L/min nasal cannula.

V_T	500 mL
Respiratory rate	10/min

This patient's alveolar minute ventilation is which of the following?

   A. 2.8 L
   B. 3.5 L
   C. 4.3 L
   D. 5.0 L

$VE = 5600$
$5600 mL = 150 + VA$
$5L = 150 + VA$

58. While performing postural drainage and percussion, the RCP palpates subcutaneous emphysema on the patient. The practitioner should postpone the therapy and recommend which of the following?

   A. Measure ABGs
   B. Initiate IPPB therapy
   C. Take chest x-ray films
   D. Do bedside spirometry

59. A patient's PaO_2 increases after being placed on a ventilator at 21% O_2. What accounts for the improved oxygenation status?

    I. Increased distribution of ventilation
    II. Increased V_D/V_T ratio
    III. Decreased venous return to the heart
    IV. Increased $P(A-a)$ O_2 gradient

    A. I only
    B. I and IV only
    C. I, II, and III only
    D. I, III, and IV only

60. You enter a patient's room to administer a treatment and the patient is unresponsive. After opening the airway, what is the next appropriate measure to take?

    A. Give two breaths.
    B. Check for a pulse.
    C. Deliver six abdominal thrusts.
    D. Determine if the patient is breathing.

61. The following data are collected from a patient on a volume ventilator.

PEEP level	PaO_2	PvO_2	V_T
6 cm H_2O	64 torr	35 torr	800 mL
8 cm H_2O	70 torr	38 torr	800 mL
10 cm H_2O	75 torr	43 torr	800 mL
12 cm H_2O	80 torr	37 torr	800 mL

    Which of the following represents optimal PEEP?

    A. 6 cm H_2O
    B. 8 cm H_2O
    C. 10 cm H_2O
    D. 12 cm H_2O

62. During the administration of IPPB with the Bird Mark 7, the RCP notices that the machine repeatedly cycles on shortly after the patient has begun expiration. To correct this problem, the practitioner should check which one of the following controls?

    A. Flow control
    B. Peak pressure control
    C. Sensitivity control
    D. Air mix control

63. Which of the following are advantages of a nasopharyngeal airway?

    I. It will assure lower airway patency during mechanical ventilation.
    II. It provides an adequate route for nasotracheal suctioning.

    III. It is well tolerated by the semicomatose patient.

    A. I only
    B. II only
    C. I and II only
    D. II and III only

64. If the RCP chooses an E cylinder to transport a patient within the hospital and it contains 650 psig of O_2, how long will the cylinder last if the flow is run at 10 L/min?

    A. 18 minutes
    B. 35 minutes
    C. 56 minutes
    D. 1 hour, 45 minutes

65. Which of these airway changes will affect the delivered V_T on a pressure-limited ventilator?

    I. Decreased lung compliance
    II. Increased lung compliance
    III. Increased airway resistance

    A. I only
    B. I and II only
    C. II and III only
    D. I, II, and III

66. The RCP should recommend which of the following first for a patient with a tension pneumothorax?

    A. Obtain a stat chest x-ray film.
    B. Obtain stat ABG levels.
    C. Administer an IPPB treatment.
    D. Release air from the pleural space.

67. A COPD patient on a 50% air entrainment mask becomes drowsy and unresponsive. The patient's reaction most likely is the result of

    A. Insufficient oxygenation
    B. Decreased venous return
    C. Increased $PaCO_2$
    D. Excessive ventilation

68. While performing chest physical therapy on a ventilator patient, the RCP percusses an area of hyperresonance. This assessment is consistent with which of the following conditions?

    A. Pleural effusion
    B. Pneumothorax
    C. Atelectasis
    D. Consolidation

69. A patient's pulse drops from 92 to 54 beats/min when a suction catheter is inserted into the oropharynx. The most likely cause is

A. Hypoxia
B. Vagal stimulation
C. Hypocarbia
D. Coughing

70. After setting up a simple O_2 mask, the RCP kinks the O_2 tubing and the humidifier produces a high-pitched whistling sound. This indicates which of the following?

    A. There are no leaks in the setup.
    B. The O_2 flow to the mask is too low.
    C. There may be a crack in the O_2 tubing.
    D. The capillary tube in the humidifier may be loose.

71. A nebulizer (aerosol generator) is used to

    A. Warm inspired gas
    B. Decrease gas density
    C. Increase the partial pressure of the gas
    D. Facilitate secretion removal

72. The RCP has been asked to deliver a low percentage of O_2 to a patient whose respiratory rate is 30/min with an irregular breathing pattern. Which device would be the best choice?

    A. Nasal cannula at 2 L/min
    B. Venturi mask at 28%
    C. Simple O_2 mask at 5 L/min
    D. Partial rebreathing mask at 8 L/min

73. Which of the following ABG results would be considered normal in a patient with severe COPD?

    A. pH 7.50, P_{CO_2} 40 torr, P_{O_2} 56 torr, HCO_3^- 30 mEq/L, BE +4
    B. pH 7.29, P_{CO_2} 54 torr. P_{O_2} 70 torr, HCO_3^- 23 mEq/L, BE 0
    C. pH 7.36, P_{CO_2} 40 torr, P_{O_2} 85 torr, HCO_3^- 24 mEq/L, BE +1
    D. pH 7.38, P_{CO_2} 60 torr, P_{O_2} 57 torr, HCO_3^- 33 mEq/L, BE +10

74. The following data are collected on a patient on a volume ventilator.

Mode	Control
V_T	800 mL
Ventilator rate	10/min
F_{IO_2}	0.40
Inspiratory flow	40 L/min

    The I:E ratio using these ventilator settings is which of the following?

    A. 1:1
    B. 1:2

C. 1:3
D. 1:4

75. Which of the following is not a hazard of IPPB?

    A. Decreased cardiac output
    B. Increased venous blood return
    C. Excessive ventilation
    D. Gastric insufflation

76. The oropharyngeal airway

    I. Can be inserted orally or nasally
    II. Can cause activation of the gag reflex
    III. Is more suitable for conscious patients

    A. I only
    B. II only
    C. I and II only
    D. II and III only

77. What is the most appropriate ventilator V_T setting on a 75-kg (165-lb) patient?

    A. 450 mL
    B. 650 mL
    C. 750 mL
    D. 950 mL

78. Which of the following parameters, when changed, will alter the inspiratory time on a volume-limited ventilator?

    I. Rate control
    II. Flow control
    III. V_T control
    IV. Expiratory resistance control

    A. I and II only
    B. II and III only
    C. II and IV only
    D. I, II, and III

79. Which of the following situations would result in the high-pressure alarm being activated on a volume-limited ventilator?

    I. Leak in the circuit
    II. Patient disconnected from the ventilator
    III. Patient coughing
    IV. Water in the tubing

    A. I and III only
    B. II and IV only
    C. III and IV only
    D. I, III, and IV only

80. Which statement concerning the inspiratory hold control on a volume ventilator is FALSE?

A. It may be used to improve oxygenation.
B. It will increase intrathoracic pressure.
C. It should result in a decreased P(A-a)O_2 gradient.
D. It is used to calculate tubing compliance.

81. While making O_2 rounds, the RCP notices the mist coming out of the exhalation ports of a patient's aerosol mask completely disappears as the patient inhales. The RCP should recommend which of the following?

    A. Add a heater to the nebulizer.
    B. Decrease the flow.
    C. Analyze the FIO_2.
    D. Increase the flow.

82. A patient who has diabetes enters the emergency department breathing deeply at a respiratory rate of 26/min. This type of breathing pattern is referred to as

    A. Kussmaul's respiration
    B. Biot's respiration
    C. Cheyne-Stokes respiration
    D. Hypopnea

83. The bacterial filter on a ventilator needs to cleaned. Which of the following cleaning methods would be most appropriate to recommend?

    A. Soak in glutaraldehyde solution for 20 min
    B. Ethylene oxide gas sterilization
    C. Autoclave
    D. Pasteurization

84. The following data are obtained from a 32-year-old pneumonia patient in the ICU on a 60% aerosol mask.

Respiratory rate	28/min	ABGs: pH	7.47
Pulse	108/min	PaCO$_2$	32 torr
		PaO$_2$	55 torr

    Which of the following would you recommend at this time?

    A. Intubate and institute mechanical ventilation.
    B. Place on CPAP.
    C. Increase to 70% aerosol mask.
    D. Place on non-rebreathing mask at 15 L/min.

85. The polarographic O_2 analyzer you are using to analyze a patient's aerosol mask is reading inaccurately. Which of the following *would not* result in this inaccurate reading?

    A. No electrolyte gel
    B. Torn membrane
    C. Water on the membrane
    D. Dead fuel cell

86. Which of the following processes or agents can sterilize equipment?

    I. Autoclave
    II. Ethylene oxide
    III. Glutaraldehyde
    IV. Alcohol

    A. I and II only
    B. II and III only
    C. I and IV only
    D. I, II, and III

87. Assuming a patient has an ideal breathing pattern, what is the approximate percentage of O_2 delivered with a nasal cannula at 5 L/min?

    A. 28%
    B. 36%
    C. 40%
    D. 45%

88. Which of the following devices delivers the highest percent body humidity?

    A. Pass-over humidifier
    B. Bubble humidifier
    C. Heated wick humidifier
    D. Jet humidifier

89. After turning the O_2 flowmeter completely off, you notice the water in the humidifier is still slightly bubbling. What is the most likely reason for this?

    A. The humidifier lid is not tight.
    B. There is a crack in the humidifier jar.
    C. The wall outlet is loose.
    D. There is a faulty valve seat in the flowmeter.

90. The following data are collected from a patient on a volume ventilator.

Mode	Assist/control	ABGS: pH	7.29
Ventilator rate	12	PaCO$_2$	55 torr
V$_T$	750 mL	PaO$_2$	68 torr
FIO$_2$	0.40	HCO$_3^-$	25 mEq/L
		BE	−1

    Based on this information, the RCP should recommend which of the following?

    A. Increase the FIO_2.
    B. Add PEEP.
    C. Increase the V$_T$.
    D. Decrease the ventilator rate.

91. A patient has been experiencing a moderate asthmatic attack for 30 min. Which of the following

ABG results would you expect to observe if the patient was on room air?

	pH	Paco$_2$ (torr)	Pao$_2$ (torr)
A.	7.42	44	81
B.	7.08	24	50
C.	7.51	27	60
D.	7.27	52	63

92. Aerosol therapy is ordered for a patient who is producing large amounts of thick, purulent secretions. What device should the RCP recommend?

   A. Ultrasonic nebulizer
   B. HHN
   C. Cascade humidifier
   D. Jet humidifier

93. If a patient's Paco$_2$ decreases to 27 torr, all of the following could have increased EXCEPT

   A. Physiologic dead space
   B. Alveolar ventilation
   C. Respiratory rate
   D. V$_T$

94. Which of the following devices should be recommended for a patient brought into the emergency department who has sustained smoke inhalation injury?

   A. Venturi mask
   B. Nasal cannula
   C. Simple O$_2$ mask
   D. Non-rebreathing mask

95. Hazards associated with aerosol therapy include all of the following EXCEPT

   A. Fluid overload in infants
   B. Bronchospasm
   C. Swelling of dried, retained secretions
   D. Bradycardia

96. If a small hole is present in the exhalation valve diaphragm of an IPPB circuit, the machine

   A. Automatically cycles into exhalation
   B. Cycles into exhalation prematurely on each breath
   C. Delivers an increased inspiratory pressure to the patient
   D. Does not cycle into exhalation

97. Which of the following organisms is most frequently cultured from heated nebulizers and humidifiers?

   A. Staphylococcus aureus
   B. Pseudomonas aeruginosa

C. Mycobacterium tuberculosis
D. Serratia marcesans

98. The following data are obtained from a 36-week-old infant who is receiving mechanical ventilation on a pressure ventilator in the neonatal ICU.

Mode	IMV	ABGs: pH	7.45
Inspiratory pressure	26 cm H$_2$O	Paco$_2$	36 torr
FiO$_2$	0.60	Pao$_2$	98 torr
PEEP	8 cm H$_2$O		
Ventilator rate	35/min		

Which of the following should the RCP recommend at this time?

   A. Increase FiO$_2$ to 0.70.
   B. Decrease PEEP to 6 cm H$_2$O.
   C. Increase ventilator rate to 40/min.
   D. Decrease FiO$_2$ to 0.50.

99. Chest physical therapy is indicated in all of the following EXCEPT

   A. Pulmonary edema
   B. Bronchiectasis
   C. Cystic fibrosis
   D. Chronic bronchitis

100. The RCP is administering IPPB therapy to a postoperative patient using a mouthpiece. During the treatment, the patient is unable to cycle the machine off. What could be done to correct this problem?

   I. Check for a leak in the system.
   II. Check the exhalation valve function.
   III. Decrease the cycling pressure to 10 cm H$_2$O.
   IV. Adjust the sensitivity.

   A. I only
   B. III only
   C. I and II only
   D. II and IV only

101. While delivering a bronchodilating agent to a patient using a HHN, you note the pulse increases from 72/min to 88/min over the first 5 min of therapy. Which of the following is the most appropriate action to take?

   A. Stop the treatment immediately and notify the physician.
   B. Continue the treatment as ordered.
   C. Increase the inspiratory pressure for the remainder of the treatment.
   D. Give the remainder of the treatment with saline only.

102. A postoperative patient is to be treated for the prevention of atelectasis. The patient is still heavily sedated. Which type of therapy should be recommended?

    A. Blow bottles
    B. Incentive spirometry
    C. HHN
    D. IPPB

103. Which of the following can be determined from a forced expiratory spirogram?

    I. FEV_1
    II. $FEF_{200-1200}$
    III. FRC

    A. I only
    B. I and II only
    C. II and III only
    D. I, II and III

104. A patient with COPD is admitted because of fever, cough, and mild confusion. O_2 is administered via a nasal cannula at 5 L/min. One-half hour later the patient is less alert. ABG analysis is as follows:

	On admission (room air)	On nasal cannula (5 L/min)
pH	7.30	7.23
$PaCO_2$	65 torr	76 torr
PaO_2	36 torr	46 torr
HCO_3^-	34 mEq/L	34 mEq/L
BE	+9	+9

    The most appropriate change in the patient's treatment would be to

    A. Use a 28% Venturi mask
    B. Decrease the O_2 flow to 2 L/min
    C. Use a non-rebreathing mask at 10 L/min
    D. Institute mechanical ventilation with an FIO_2 of 0.40

105. A nebulizer is set on the 40% dilution mode and connected to an O_2 flowmeter running at 12 L/min. What is the total flow output of this nebulizer?

    A. 24 L/min
    B. 36 L/min
    C. 48 L/min
    D. 54 L/min

106. A patient on mechanical ventilation has the following ABG values:

pH	7.54
$PaCO_2$	26 torr
PaO_2	102 torr
HCO_3^-	24 mEq/L
BE	0

    All of the following ventilator changes would help correct this *EXCEPT*

    A. Increasing the respiratory rate
    B. Decreasing the V_T
    C. Placement on SIMV
    D. Adding mechanical dead space

107. A humidifier will not bubble if

    A. The capillary tube is plugged
    B. The pop-off valve is open
    C. The O_2 tubing is cracked
    D. The reservoir jar is loose

108. A patient has a V_T of 450 mL and a respiratory rate that fluctuates between 15/min and 25/min. Which of the following is the best device for the administration of a controlled O_2 percentage?

    A. Partial rebreathing mask
    B. Simple O_2 mask
    C. Venturi mask
    D. Nasal cannula

109. A patient is placed on a non-rebreathing mask at 15 L/min. An ABG analysis reveals a PaO_2 of 580 torr. The RCP should recommend which of the following?

    A. Decrease the flow rate to 10 L/min.
    B. Change to a partial rebreathing mask at 10 L/min.
    C. Change to simple O_2 mask at 8 L/min.
    D. Discontinue O_2 therapy.

110. An infant has just been delivered at 30 weeks' gestation and appears cyanotic. While administering O_2, the RCP should recommend doing which of the following?

    A. Obtain a chest x-ray film.
    B. Determine the Apgar score of the infant.
    C. Obtain ABG analysis.
    D. Insert a UAC.

111. While preparing to analyze the O_2 concentration on a patient's aerosol mask, you notice water in the aerosol tubing. What effect does this have on the operation of this device?

    A. Decreases the FIO_2
    B. Increases the FIO_2
    C. Increases air entrainment into the nebulizer
    D. Increases gas flow to the patient

112. The following data are obtained from an infant in the neonatal ICU on a pressure ventilator.

Mode	IMV	ABGs: pH	7.29
PIP	20 cm H_2O	Pa_{CO_2}	51 torr
Ventilator rate	40/min	Pa_{O_2}	53 torr
FI_{O_2}	0.40	HCO_3^-	22 mEq/L
PEEP	5 cm H_2O	BE	+1

On the basis of these data, which of the following would you recommend at this time?

A. Increase FI_{O_2} to 0.60.
B. Decrease ventilator rate to 35/min.
C. Increase PEEP to 8 cm H_2O.
D. Increase PIP to 24 cm H_2O.

113. To minimize an increased airway resistance produced by high-density aerosol inhalation, the RCP should

 A. Use a bronchodilator in conjunction with the aerosol
 B. Instruct the patient to breathe through the nose
 C. Use a heated aerosol
 D. Perform chest physical therapy after the aerosol treatment

114. A patient's heated nebulizer is delivering 41 mg H_2O per liter of gas. The percentage of body humidity delivered by this device is

 A. 32%
 B. 41%
 C. 64%
 D. 93%

115. A patient arrives in the emergency department after being pulled from a burning house. The RCP places a pulse oximeter on the patient's ear lobe and obtains an SpO_2 reading of 93%. An ABG is drawn and the Sa_{O_2} analyzed by co-oximetry is 76%. Which of the following is the most likely reason for the discrepancy in the two saturation readings?

 A. The oximeter needs to be calibrated.
 B. The co-oximeter electrode is out of calibration.
 C. There is an elevated HbCO level.
 D. The pulse oximeter probe is loose.

116. Which of the following aerosol generators depends on the effects of lateral negative pressure to pull fluid over a sphere so that it may be exposed to a high-velocity jet?

 A. Pneumatic jet
 B. Spinning disk
 C. Ultrasonic
 D. Babington

117. A patient with a broken nose and cheekbone is ordered to be placed on 40% O_2. The patient's se-

cretions are thick. Based on this information, which O_2 delivery device would be indicated?

 A. Nasal cannula at 5 L/min
 B. Face tent
 C. Simple O_2 mask at 8 L/min
 D. Aerosol mask

118. The following pulmonary function data are obtained from a patient before and after bronchodilator therapy.

	Before	After
FVC	37% of predicted	53% of predicted
FEV_1	42% of predicted	56% of predicted
FEV_1/FVC	40%	55%

Which of the following is the correct interpretation of these results?

 A. Severe obstructive disease, significant bronchodilator response
 B. Severe restrictive disease, no bronchodilator response
 C. Moderate obstructive disease, no bronchodilator response
 D. Severe restrictive disease, significant bronchodilator response

119. Which piece of equipment is most commonly used for the setup of a tracheostomy collar?

 A. Bubble humidifier
 B. Impeller nebulizer
 C. Ultrasonic nebulizer
 D. Jet nebulizer

120. Choose the device that is not connected to a humidifier.

 A. Simple O_2 mask at 8 L/min
 B. T-piece (Briggs adaptor)
 C. Partial rebreathing mask at 12 L/min
 D. Nasal cannula at 6 L/min

121. Which of the following respiratory medications is not considered a bronchodilating agent?

 A. Metaproterenol (Alupent)
 B. Ipratroprium bromide (Atrovent)
 C. Terbutaline sulfate (Brethine)
 D. Acetylcysteine (Mucomyst)

122. A patient is breathing 16 times per minute and has a V_T of 450 mL. What is this patient's minute ventilation?

 A. 4.2 L
 B. 6.1 L

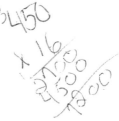

C. 7.2 L

D. 8.6 L

123. A patient is breathing spontaneously on a 50% aerosol mask with the following ABG results:

pH	7.36
Pa_{CO_2}	43 torr
Pa_{O_2}	48 torr
HCO_3^-	24 mEq/L

Based on this information, the RCP should recommend which of the following?

A. Place on CPAP.

B. Increase O_2 percentage to 70%.

C. Place on non-rebreathing mask.

D. Place on simple O_2 mask at 10 L/min.

124. A patient is being mechanically ventilated on the following settings:

V_T	750 mL
Respiratory rate	12/min
Mode	Assist/control
PEEP	10 cm H_2O
F_{IO_2}	0.60

ABG results on these settings are

pH	7.41
Pa_{CO_2}	38 torr
Pa_{O_2}	174 torr

Based on the above information, what would be the appropriate ventilator change?

A. Decrease PEEP to 8 cm H_2O

B. Decrease F_{IO_2} to 0.50

C. Decrease V_T to 650 mL

D. Increase inspiratory flow

125. The reduction in urinary output caused by mechanical ventilation may be the result of

I. Decreased renal blood flow

II. Decreased production of ADH

III. Increased renal blood flow

IV. Increased production of ADH

A. I only

B. I and IV only

C. II and III only

D. III and IV only

126. Which values indicate that a patient is ready to be weaned from mechanical ventilation?

I. V_D/V_T ratio of .45

I. MIP of -31 cm H_2O

III. P(A-a) O_2 of 460 mm Hg on 100% O_2

IV. Vital capacity of 8 mL/kg of body weight

A. I and II only

B. II and III only

C. I, II, and IV only

D. II, III, and IV only

127. Where should a respirometer be placed to most accurately determine the volume being delivered by a ventilator?

A. At the ventilator outlet

B. At the exhalation valve

C. Between the patient's ET tube and the ventilator wye

D. At the humidifier outlet

128. A patient is being mechanically ventilated on a volume ventilator in the control mode. The low-pressure alarm is sounding. Which of the following may be the cause of the alarm activation?

A. Water in the tubing

B. Patient disconnected from the ventilator

C. Secretions in the patient's airway

D. Kink in the ventilator tubing

129. The peak inspiratory pressure has dropped from 34 cm H_2O to 10 cm H_2O on a volume ventilator that is operating in the assist-control mode. You notice the expired volume spirometer is filling during inspiration. Which of the following would be the most likely cause of this problem?

A. There is a leak in the ET-tube cuff.

B. There is a malfunction of the exhalation valve.

C. There is a malfunction of the pressure manometer.

D. This is a normal occurrence.

130. You have just obtained blood from the patient's radial artery to determine ABG results. As you run the blood through the blood gas analyzer you notice you failed to remove an air bubble from the sample. The blood gas results will most likely reflect values with a

A. High pH and low P_{O_2}.

B. Low P_{CO_2} and low P_{O_2}.

C. Low P_{CO_2} and high P_{O_2}.

D. High P_{CO_2} and high P_{O_2}.

131. The RCP is monitoring a patient with Guillain-Barré syndrome for signs of respiratory impairment. Which one of the following parameters would signal the earliest indication?

A. Pa_{O_2}
B. Pa_{CO_2}
C. MIP
D. V_T

Questions 132-134 relate to the following situation.

A 36-year-old, 65-kg (143-lb) unconscious man is admitted to the emergency department. His breathing rate is 8/min and very shallow. A drug overdose is suspected.

132. To maintain a patent airway, what type of device should be employed?

    A. Bite block
    B. Oropharyngeal airway
    C. Tongue depressor
    D. Esophageal obturator airway

133. The patient becomes apneic and mechanical ventilatory support is required. How would the airway best be maintained at this time?

    A. CPAP mask
    B. Cuffed ET tube
    C. Uncuffed ET tube
    D. Fenestrated tracheostomy tube

134. The most appropriate ventilator settings would be which of the following?

    A. V_T 600 mL, rate 8, control mode
    B. V_T 800 mL, rate 6, control mode
    C. V_T 700 mL, rate 12, assist-control mode
    D. V_T 1000 mL, rate 14, assist-control mode

Questions 135-137 relate to the following situation.

A 48-year-old, 75-kg (165-lb) woman is in the ICU after coronary bypass surgery. The patient is to be placed on mechanical ventilation.

135. As you connect the patient to the ventilator you notice the peak inspiratory pressure is registering only 10 cm H_2O on the manometer and the exhaled volume display is showing 300 mL less than the dialed-in volume setting. Which of the following could be causing this problem?

    I. There is a leak around the humidifier.
    II. The medication nebulizer is not connected tightly.
    III. There is no water in the humidifier.

    A. I only
    B. II only
    C. I and II only
    D. II and III only

136. During ventilator checks 6 hours later, you notice the peak inspiratory pressure has been gradually

increasing. What could be the cause of this occurrence?

    I. Bronchospasm
    II. Accumulation of secretions
    III. Increasing pulmonary compliance
    IV. Decreasing airway resistance

    A. I and II only
    B. II and III only
    C. III and IV only
    D. I, II, and III only

137. The following day, the patient is placed on T-tube flow-by for weaning purposes. During this time the patient's respiratory rate increases to 30/min and her blood pressure begins to drop. What is the appropriate measure to take at this time?

    A. Place on SIMV rate of 10/min.
    B. Obtain stat chest film.
    C. Place on CPAP.
    D. Place on control mode at a rate of 10/min.

Questions 138-140 relate to the following situation.

A 17-year-old boy with multiple rib fractures is admitted to the emergency department after a motor vehicle accident. An ABG analysis reveals the following results on room air:

pH	7.50
Pa_{CO_2}	30 torr
Pa_{O_2}	44 torr
HCO_3^-	25 mEq/L
BE	+1

138. These data indicate which of the following?

    I. Decreased $P(A-a)_{O_2}$
    II. Hyperventilation
    III. Respiratory acidosis

    A. I only
    B. II only
    C. I and II only
    D. II and III only

139. The patient's condition has deteriorated and mechanical ventilation is initiated. What parameters should the RCP determine at this time?

    I. V_T required by patient
    II. Patient's FVC
    III. Patient's NIF
    IV. Minute ventilation required by patient

    A. I and II only
    B. II and III only
    C. I and IV only
    D. I, II, and III only

140. Six days later, the physician is considering weaning this patient from the ventilator. The following data are collected:

MIP	-30 cm H_2O
VC	3.0 L
Mode	Assist/control
Ventilator rate	12/min
V_T	650 mL
FIO_2	0.35
pH	7.38
$PaCO_2$	41 torr
PaO_2	86 torr
HCO_3^-	24 mEq/L
BE	0

Based on this information, the practitioner should recommend which of the following?

A. Institute SIMV.
B. Continue mechanical ventilation on assist/control.
C. Increase the V_T.
D. Add PEEP of 4 cm H_2O.

END OF ENTRY LEVEL PRACTICE EXAM

GO TO THE ANSWER KEY/EXPLANATION SECTION AND GRADE YOUR TEST

Entry Level Certification Exam: Practice Test

Passing score: 105 correct answers
After each answer is the explanation for why the choice is correct.
Questions on the NBRC exams fall into three complexity levels.

- Recall questions: These questions require "the ability to recall or recognize specific respiratory care information." The Entry-Level Certification Exam contains 36 recall questions.
- Application questions: These questions require "the ability to comprehend, relate, or apply knowledge to new or changing situations." The Entry-Level Certification Exam contains 72 application questions.
- Analysis questions: These questions require "the ability to analyze information, to put information together to arrive at solutions, or to evaluate the usefulness of the solutions." The Entry-Level Certification Exam contains 32 analysis questions.

1. B, The air/O_2 ratio for a 35% oxygen mixture is 5 : 1. To calculate total flow output from this device, add the ratio parts together and multiply by the liter flow: $6 \times 6 = 36$ L/min, $6 \times 8 = 48$ L/min, $6 \times 10 = 60$ L/min, $6 \times 12 = 72$ L/min. Total flow needed: 42 L/min. The minimum flow necessary is 8, giving a total flow of 48 L/min. (Application)
2. C, As with adults, if the infant is hypoxemic with a normal or low $PaCO_2$, increase the PaO_2 by increasing oxygen to no more than 60%. If 60% doesn't reverse the hypoxemia, place the infant on CPAP. Notice in this question that there is not a choice for 60%. But do not choose 70%, since it exceeds 60%. (Analysis)
3. B, To best determine the severity of smoke inhalation, an HbCO level should be determined with a co-oximeter. (Analysis)
4. A, An active 3-year-old generally tolerates an oxygen tent much more than any kind of mask and is too large for an O_2 hood. (Application)
5. B, If the patient is able to perform simple tasks when asked, this best determines his or her ability to follow instructions. This is important before administering an incentive spirometry or IPPB treatment, which require the patient to be able to follow instructions well or the treatment will not be effective. (Recall)
6. B, The best diagnostic test to determine if a pulmonary embolism is present is the V/Q lung scan. (Application)
7. C, To increase a patient's alveolar minute ventilation, the V_T must be increased. If only the ventilator rate is increased, the same V_T is delivered, even though the minute ventilation also increases. (Recall)
8. D, It is important during ET suctioning that the PaO_2 be maintained within a normal range or hypoxemia will occur, which may lead to cardiac arrhythmias, such as bradycardia. (Application)
9. A, When lungs get stiffer and harder to ventilate, greater pressure is required to move the same volume of air. Since peak inspiratory pressure will increase when Raw increases, for example, when airway secretions are present or there is water in the ventilator tubing, this pressure does not reflect how stiff the lungs actually are. We determine the plateau or static pressure by holding the volume in the patient's lungs for 1 to 2 sec. This pressure closely relates to alveolar pressure. PEEP (if used) is subtracted from the plateau pressure and this number is divided into the V_T. The results will determine how compliant the lungs are. (Application)
10. C, A leak may be heard around the cylinder outlet as a result of a loose connection or if the washer between the cylinder outlet and regulator inlet is cracked or missing. (Recall)
11. D, A warm moist environment is a breeding ground for bacteria to grow. A heated nebulizer and heated humidifier both have an increased potential for growing bacteria. But nebulizers produce particles in approximately the same size range as bacteria and therefore have a greater chance of transporting the bacteria to the patient. Humidified

particles are smaller and are less likely to serve as a transport medium. (Recall)

12. A, A baffle is an object placed in the path of the aerosol particles so that when the particles strike it, the particles break up, forming smaller particles. Even the walls of the nebulizer are considered baffles. (Recall)

13. D, A blood gas is considered compensated when both the $PaCO_2$ and HCO_3^- are abnormal and the pH level is normal. Respiratory acidosis is caused by an elevated $PaCO_2$, which drops the pH to below normal levels. If the patient is not ventilated better to decrease the $PaCO_2$, the HCO_3^- levels in the blood begin to increase (renal compensation), which increases the pH toward normal. When the pH reaches the normal range, it is called fully compensated. The most common example of this type of blood gas is the patient with severe COPD who chronically retains CO_2 and remains in a constant state of renal compensation. (Application)

14. C, This patient's increased $PaCO_2$ level indicates hypoventilation, which can be reversed by increasing the $\dot{V}E$. This can be accomplished by increasing the ventilator rate or VT, both of which are choices. Since this patient is being weaned from the ventilator (SIMV rate of 4), we must assume he has ventilated well on higher rates and the same VT. This patient is not tolerating this low rate at this time. Therefore, the best choice is increasing the rate. (Analysis)

15. B, Since this type of cuff contains residual air when fully deflated, less pressure is required to inflate it, resulting in less pressure exerted on the tracheal wall. The lower the pressure placed on the tracheal wall while still preventing a leak, the less potential of decreasing blood flow to the trachea in the area of the cuff. (Recall)

16. C, When air that is not fully saturated at body temperature is delivered to an intubated patient, a humidity deficit exists and secretions get thicker because of lack of inspired water. The inspired air must contain at least 44 mg H_2O per liter of gas or exert a water vapor pressure of 47 torr. This represents 100% body humidity. Even though choice IV has a relative humidity of 100%, it is at 25°C (room temperature), so it holds less water than 100% at body temperature and also creates a humidity deficit. (Analysis)

17. A, Lung compliance is determined by dividing the VT by the inspiratory pressure. Therefore, monitoring airway pressure is essential in the measurement of compliance. Remember, however, that the most accurate pressure to measure is the static or plateau pressure, not PIP. (Application)

18. D, Decreasing the respiratory rate will decrease $\dot{V}E$, resulting in an increase in $PaCO_2$. (Application)

19. D, The low-pressure alarm will sound if there is a leak in the ventilator tubing or around the ET-tube cuff, the patient is disconnected from the ventilator, or the low-pressure alarm is set too high. (Analysis)

20. C, The ECG strip indicates sinus bradycardia, which results from vagal stimulation from suctioning. The vagus nerve runs through the oropharynx. When the vagus nerve is stimulated, bradycardia and hypotension result. So, a catheter placed in the oropharynx during suctioning may illicit this response. Hypoxemia may also result in bradycardia, but with the catheter in the oropharynx, hopoxemia is unlikely. (Application)

21. C, Stridor is a loud, high-pitched sound heard in the upper airway, generally around the glottic area, where air flow is partially obstructed. (Recall)

22. C, Venous blood pressure in the trachea is approximately 18 to 20 mm Hg. A cuff exerting a pressure of more than 20 mm Hg will obstruct venous blood flow. Cuff pressures should be kept below this pressure. (Recall)

23. C, Even though clinically it may not always be true, an **initial ventilator rate** on the examination should be 8/min to 12/min. Do not select a rate that is below 8 or above 12 for the **initial** rate setting. (Analysis)

24. A, Cystic fibrosis is a lung disease characterized by production of large amounts of thick secretions. Mucomyst is commonly administered to these patients, since the mucolytic effects help thin the secretions, making them easier to mobilize. (Recall)

25. B, Since hypoxemia results in an increase in both the respiratory rate and heart rate, administration of oxygen will increase PaO_2 levels, thereby reducing the work of breathing and tachycardia. Oxygen percentages of over 60% lead to oxygen toxicity, which may result in ARDS. (Recall)

26. C, Refer to explanation for question 21. (Application)

27. A, Optimal PEEP is the level of PEEP that improves lung compliance without decreasing the cardiac output. When a PEEP study is done, the cardiac output is measured at different PEEP levels. When the cardiac output drops after an increase in PEEP, the PEEP should be decreased to the previous level. In other words, use the PEEP level that renders the best cardiac output. Or, if measuring the static lung compliance at various PEEP levels, use the level that produces the best lung compliance. (Application)

28. A, Hyperventilation refers to a pH level above normal (> 7.45) that results from a decreased $PaCO_2$ level (< 35 mm Hg). (Application)

29. B, Inspired air fully saturated at body temperature holds 44 mg H_2O per liter of gas. Should the air hold less than 44 mg H_2O per liter at the carina,

the airway's own humidification system will add water to the air but at the expense of drying out the airway, resulting in thicker pulmonary secretions. (Recall)

30. B, If the high O_2 concentration results in high PaO_2 levels (>100 torr), retinal detachment may occur, leading to blindness in the premature neonate. Remember, it is the high PaO_2 that causes the damage, not the FIO_2. In other words, a neonate on 100% oxygen and a PaO_2 of 60 torr will most likely not develop retinopathy of prematurity because the PaO_2 is below 100 torr. High FIO_2 levels, on the other hand, will lead to atelectasis because of nitrogen washout of the lung and the suppression of surfactant production by the alveolar type 2 cells. (Recall)

31. C

$$\text{Compliance} = \frac{V_T}{\text{Plateau pressure} - \text{PEEP}} = \frac{800}{30}$$
$$= 27 \text{ mL/cm H}_2\text{O}$$

(Application)

32. A, To facilitate weaning this postoperative patient off the ventilator, the SIMV rate should be reduced. This will stimulate the patient to begin breathing more on his own. (Analysis)

33. C, When working a problem like this, don't worry about arranging the equation to solve for pressure. Use the equation you are most familiar with.

$$\frac{\text{cylinder pressure} \times \text{cylinder factor}}{\text{liter flow}}$$

Start with the (B) choice and determine if this is enough pressure to run the tank for at least 1 hour. Since the answer is only 56 minutes, use the next pressure to calculate cylinder running time. By starting with the (B) choice you won't have to do more than two calculations.

$$\frac{1400 \times .28}{6} = 65 \text{ min}$$

(Analysis)

34. B, Location of the needle valve is what makes a flowmeter compensated or uncompensated. The needle valve is located proximal to or before the Thorpe tube on an uncompensated flowmeter. When the flowmeter is plugged into a wall outlet with the needle valve closed, gas goes only as far as the needle valve. This means atmospheric pressure is in the Thorpe tube since the needle valve is before the tube. When a device is attached to the outlet of the flowmeter, back pressure is generated back into the Thorpe tube, pushing the float down

and compressing gas molecules in the tube, so that more of them get by the float. This causes the flowmeter to read a lower flow than what the patient is actually receiving. (Application)

35. B, Succinylcholine is a fast-acting, short-term muscle relaxant used to aid in the intubation of combative patients. The patient will be paralyzed for only about 5 min. (Recall)

36. B, Although normal MIP level is -50 to -100 cm H_2O, an MIP of at least -20 cm H_2O is an indication that the patient can take deep enough breaths to produce an adequate cough and maintain secretion clearance. MIP is also referred to as negative inspiratory force (NIF). (Recall)

37. C, The purpose of the 50-mL reservoir tubing is to prevent the patient from drawing in room air through the distal end of the T-piece. If the reservoir falls off, room air will be entrained during inspiration, which results in a drop in the O_2 percentage delivered to the patient. (Application)

38. A, Since the patient will not be able to breathe on his/her own, it is essential that the therapist is aware when the patient is disconnected. The low-pressure alarm is activated if this occurs. (Application)

39. D, Using an inspiratory plateau permits the V_T to be held in the lungs for 1 to 2 sec. This helps open up areas of atelectasis, while allowing for a longer diffusion time for gases to cross the alveolar-capillary membrane. This will also cause an **increased** intrathoracic pressure, since the pressure is maintained in the lungs for an extra 1 to 2 sec, which may result in barotrauma and cardiovascular side effects. (Application)

40. C, The COPD patient in this problem is a chronic retainer of CO_2, as evidenced by the elevated HCO_3^- level on admission. This indicates compensation has occurred and also suggests this patient is chronically hypoxemic. The PaO_2 should be maintained between 50 and 65 torr to prevent knocking out the patient's hypoxic-drive stimulus to breathe. The oxygen device of choice for these patients is an air entrainment mask at, initially, 25% to 35%. (Analysis)

41. A, Although lidocaine is normally given intravenously to counteract arrhythmias during CPR, it is permissible to instill it directly down the ET tube. (Application)

42. D, An ultrasonic nebulizer is capable of producing 6 mL of H_2O per minute and is therefore indicated for patients with thick secretions to aid in the thinning and mobilization of the secretions. (Application)

43. B, A Venturi (air entrainment) mask is considered a high-flow oxygen delivery device because it is capable of delivering flows that can meet or exceed the patient's inspiratory flow demands. Its ability to

deliver high flows is the result of entrainment of large volumes of air, which mixes with the oxygen flow to deliver fairly precise and consistent oxygen percentages. (Recall)

44. B, Studies show that a better distribution of the aerosol with be delivered if the MDI is activated shortly after the patient has begun the deep breath. (Application)

45. A, On an inspiratory chest film, the carina is located at the level of the fourth rib. The ET-tube tip should rest about 2 to 7 cm above this level. (Application)

46. D, Instilling saline down the ET tube may stimulate coughing and may help loosen secretions for easier mobilization. Although some studies clearly disagree with this, it has appeared as a correct answer on the examination. (Application)

47. B, P(A-a) O_2, or the A-a gradient, is the difference between alveolar PO_2 (PAO_2) and arterial PO_2 (PaO_2).

$$PAO_2 = (BP - 47 \text{ torr}) \times FIO_2 - (PaCO_2 + 10)$$

Note: 47 torr represents water vapor pressure

$$PAO_2 = (747 - 47) \times 0.50 - (40 + 10)$$
$$= 700 \times 0.5 = 350 - 50$$
$$= 300 \text{ torr}$$

$$PAO_2 - PaO_2 = 300 - 70 = 230 \text{ torr}$$

(Application)

48. B, Exhaled air contains around 6% to 7% CO_2. If the tube is in the airway, exhaled gas passing through the airway and on through the CO_2 detector should read approximately 7%. If it reads near zero, it must be in the esophagus, since no air is flowing through this area. The CO_2 detector does not indicate where in the airway the tube is located, only that it is in the airway. There is one exception: In a full cardiac arrest in which blood pressure is very low, gas exchange is extremely compromised, and therefore there may be little CO_2 in the exhaled air; even if the tube is in the airway, the detector would not indicate that it is. (Analysis)

49. B, Normal PaO_2 for a neonate is 50 to 70 torr. To increase the PaO_2 in this question, either the FIO_2 or PEEP may be increased. Since the FIO_2 is above 0.60 and the infant still remains hypoxemic, the likelihood of atelectasis and right-to-left shunting is high. Increasing the PEEP to help open up atelectatic lung areas will increase the PaO_2 more than an increase in the FIO_2. (Analysis)

50. A, Studies have shown this level of HbCO in heavy smokers. (Recall)

51. D, Since the patient is hyperoxygenating, the PaO_2 may be decreased by reducing FIO_2 or PEEP. Since the FIO_2 is over 0.60, it should be reduced first.

Once the FIO_2 is 0.60, the PEEP should then be decreased. (Analysis)

52. A, Normal energy levels used to convert atrial fibrillation back to a normal sinus rhythm are between 25 and 100 J. (Recall)

53. B, The blood gases indicate hypercarbia (increased $PaCO_2$), and this condition can be corrected by increasing the patient's $\dot{V}_E$. This is done by increasing the respiratory rate or volume. Notice also the patient's V_T in relation to his/her weight. Remember to use a minimum of 10 mL/kg of ideal body weight for the V_T setting. (Analysis)

54. A, The yellow or green color of sputum is the result of an increased WBC count, which indicates infection. When yellow or green sputum is observed, a CBC count, chest film, sputum culture, and sensitivity test should be ordered. (Recall)

55. D, The ET-tube cuff should be inflated to a point where only a slight leak is heard during inspiration with a stethoscope placed over the larynx. This is called the minimal leak technique. If a large volume of air is placed in the cuff to obtain minimal leak or if an audible leak is heard, the tube is too small and should be replaced with a larger one. (Application)

56. C, Appropriate suction levels for the adult are −80 to −120 mm Hg. (Recall)

57. B, Alveolar $\dot{V}_E$ is calculated:

$$\dot{V}_E = (V_T - V_D) \times \text{rate}$$

In a nonintubated patient, V_D is equal to 1 mL/lb of body weight (or 1 mL/kg of body weight in an intubated patient).

$$\dot{V}_E = (500 - 150) \times 10 = 3.5 \text{ L}$$

(Application)

58. C, Subcutaneous emphysema is air present in the subcutaneous tissues. If air leaks out of the lung, it often finds its way into the subcutaneous tissues. It is common after a tracheotomy is done to observe subcutaneous emphysema in the neck area. But to observe it at any other time indicates a pulmonary air leak and a pneumothorax should be suspected. A chest film should be ordered for confirmation while the therapist assesses the patient for asymmetrical chest movement, tracheal deviation, diminished breath sounds, tachycardia, tachypnea, and SpO_2 value. (Application)

59. A, Even on room air, positive pressure to the lungs will increase PaO_2 as a result of increased distribution of ventilation. Positive pressure ventilation will increase the diameter of the alveoli, providing a larger surface area for the diffusion of gases at the

alveolar-capillary membrane. This will decrease P(A-a) O_2 and V_D/V_T. (Application)

60. D, Always read all the choices before marking an answer. Many students will see choice A and choose it, since it seems correct. But before initiating ventilation, we first determine if the patient is breathing. The patient may have been apneic as a result of airway obstruction by the tongue and, once the airway is opened, the patient may resume breathing. (Recall)

61. C, Optimal PEEP is that level of PEEP that improves lung compliance without reducing cardiac output. In this question, compliance is not the issue. A decrease in cardiac output is observed when the mixed venous P_{O_2} ($P\bar{v}_{O_2}$) starts decreasing. $P\bar{v}_{O_2}$ is the partial pressure of O_2 in the pulmonary artery obtained via Swan-Ganz catheter. It represents blood at the end of the venous circuit. Even though cardiac output is reduced, the tissues will extract O_2 from the blood at the same rate. By the time the blood reaches the pulmonary artery, less O_2 will be present, as evidenced by a low $P\bar{v}_{O_2}$. In this question, notice how as the PEEP level is increased from 6 to 10 cm H_2O, $P\bar{v}_{O_2}$ likewise increases. But as PEEP is increased from 10 to 12 cm H_2O, $P\bar{v}_{O_2}$ drops. This indicates the cardiac output has decreased. Therefore, the optimal PEEP level is that level just before the $P\bar{v}_{O_2}$ decreased, which is 10 cm H_2O. (Analysis)

62. C, When the IPPB machine cycles on prematurely, the sensitivity control is not set appropriately. In this case, it is set too sensitive and cycles the machine into inspiration before the patient is ready. The sensitivity should be decreased to where the patient has to pull -1 to -2 cm H_2O to initiate inspiration. Notice this question appears to be asking about the Bird Mark 7 specifically. But the answer would be the same no matter what IPPB machine was mentioned in the question. Although this is not a choice, another situation that might cause the machine to cycle prematurely is when the rate control has been left on inadvertently. It should always be off during IPPB. (Application)

63. D, The most common use for a nasopharyngeal airway (nasal trumpet) is to facilitate nasotracheal suctioning. It is tolerated well by all patients, whether unconscious, semiconscious, or conscious. (Analysis)

64. A, Duration of minutes remaining in a cylinder is calculated as follows:

$$\frac{\text{cylinder pressure} \times \text{factor}}{\text{liter flow}} = \frac{650 \times .28}{10} = 18 \text{ min}$$

Note: The cylinder factor for an E tank is .28 and for an H tank is 3.14. (Some therapists remember it more easily as 0.3 for E, 3.0 for H.) (Application)

65. D, Anytime a change in compliance or airway resistance occurs, the inspiratory pressure will also change. For example, say a patient is on a pressure ventilator and an inspiratory pressure of 25 cm H_2O. If an airway resistance problem occurs, such as secretions in the airway or bronchospasm, or the patient's lungs get stiffer (decreased compliance), more pressure will be needed to deliver the same volume. But on a pressure-limited ventilator, pressure is limited, in this case to 25 cm H_2O, and it cannot increase. Therefore, V_T must decrease. (Application)

66. D, When a tension pneumothorax occurs, inspired air becomes trapped in the pleural space. Air enters the space during inspiration but cannot get out because the opening between the lung and pleural space acts like a one-way valve. Pressure begins to increase in the pleural space, which pushes the mediastinal contents to the opposite side. The blood vessels returning blood to the heart become compressed, reducing venous return and decreasing cardiac output. The heart itself may become compressed, drastically reducing its contracting ability. The trachea may be pushed to the opposite side. This is a life-threatening condition. A needle placed in the second or third intercostal space will decompress the pleural space and allow the lung to reexpand. (Application)

67. C, A patient with severe COPD who chronically retains CO_2 and is chronically hypoxemic, breathes on a different drive than other patients. When any person's Pa_{O_2} drops below 60 to 65 torr, peripheral chemoreceptors located in the carotid arteries and aortic arch sense this low Pa_{O_2} and trigger responses that increase heart rate and respiratory rate to improve oxygenation. Once O_2 is administered and Pa_{O_2} levels increase above 65 torr, these receptors stop triggering and we return to our normal central respiratory center breathing stimulus. But in a COPD patient who is constantly hypoxemic, with Pa_{O_2} levels below 65 torr, the primary breathing stimulus is from the peripheral chemoreceptors. This is called the "hypoxic drive" breathing stimulus. If oxygen is given and results in a Pa_{O_2} above 65 torr, the potential of knocking out this drive increases. The patient's respiratory rate or V_T will begin to diminish, resulting in a decreased $\dot{V}_E$, leading to increased Pa_{CO_2} levels. As CO_2 increases, it causes a narcotic effect, known as "CO_2 narcosis," causing the patient to become drowsy. This is best treated by simply decreasing the delivered O_2 concentration. Some studies are questioning the validity of the "hypoxic drive" phenomenon but you should still understand its characteristics for this examination. (Application)

68. B, A hyperresonant percussion note is heard over areas of the lung that contain a higher proportion of air than tissue. When a pneumothorax is present, air enters and collects in the pleural space away from normal blood flow or tissue. Another instance where a hyperresonant note is heard is over a hyperinflated chest, such as with emphysema. (Application)

69. B, Refer to explanation for question 20. (Application)

70. A, After an O_2 delivery device is attached to the humidifier, the tubing should be kinked to check for leaks in the system. When the O_2 tubing is kinked, back pressure enters the humidifier. When the pressure builds to 2 psi, the pressure pop-off valve opens to release the built-up pressure. That is the whistling noise heard. This indicates the setup has no leaks. If, after kinking the tubing, the pop-off valve fails to open, there is a leak somewhere in the setup. The most common leak occurs when the humidifier bottle is not screwed on tight to the top. Other sources are small holes in the tubing or loose-fitting tubing on the humidifier outlet. (Application)

71. D, A nebulizer, or aerosol generator (as they are often called), delivers water in particulate form or in a mist. This increased water delivery to the airway plays a role in aiding in the mobilization of pulmonary secretions by loosening and thinning the secretions. (Recall)

72. B, This question appears to not give adequate information to answer the question. But the idea is that a low-flow O_2 device should not be set up on a patient who has an irregular breathing pattern or a respiratory rate of more than 25/min, because of inconsistent O_2 concentrations. A high-flow device (Venturi mask) is indicated in this situation, since more consistent O_2 concentrations are delivered regardless of the patient's ventilatory pattern. (Application)

73. D, Refer to explanation for question 13. (Application)

74. D

$$I:E \text{ ratio} = \frac{\text{inspiratory flow}}{\text{minute ventilation}} = \frac{40}{8} = 5$$

Subtract 1 from 5 and you get a 1:4 I:E ratio. (Application)

75. B, IPPB can result in a **decreased** cardiac output. This results from positive pressure being transferred from the airways onto the vessels around the heart, restricting venous blood flow back into the heart. (Recall)

76. B, The major hazard of the oropharyngeal airway is the activation of the gag reflex, which could lead to vomiting and aspiration of the stomach contents into the lungs resulting in aspiration pneumonia.

That is why this airway should only be placed in unconscious patients. (Application)

77. C, Ventilator V_T should be set at 10 to 12 mL/kg of ideal body weight. The most appropriate volume would be 750 mL. (Application)

78. B, When flow is increased, inspiratory time decreases, and vice versa. When V_T is increased, inspiratory time increases, and vice versa. Respiratory rate and expiratory resistance alter the expiratory time. (Analysis)

79. C, Decreasing lung compliance and increased Raw results in higher inspiratory pressures. If the pressure increases enough to reach the high-pressure limit, an alarm sounds and inspiration ends at that time. The pressure limit should be set 5 to 15 cm H_2O above the average peak inspiratory pressure. Choices I and II would result in the low-pressure alarm being triggered. (Application)

80. D, This control is used to calculate **static** lung compliance by generating a plateau pressure. (Application)

81. D, The volume of mist exiting the exhalation ports of an aerosol mask should diminish as the patient inspires, but if it totally disappears, the patient is not only taking all the flow from the mask, but also entraining air through the ports. This reduces the oxygen concentration. The flow to the mask must be increased. (Analysis)

82. A, Kussmaul's respirations are a deep and rapid breathing pattern encountered in patients with severe metabolic acidemia (low pH, low HCO_3^-). The lungs are making an effort to increase the pH back toward normal by removing CO_2 from the blood, which results in an increased pH. (Recall)

83. C, In-line bacterial filters are most effectively decontaminated by sterilization in an autoclave. (Application)

84. B, Refer to explanation for question 47. (Analysis)

85. D, A polarographic O_2 analyzer uses a battery, not a fuel cell. (Application)

86. D, Autoclave, ethylene oxide gas, and glutaraldehyde solution (Cidex) can all sterilize equipment. (Recall)

87. C, Generally, to calculate the approximate percentage of O_2 delivered by a nasal cannula, add 4% for each liter of oxygen flow (e.g., 1 L, 24%; 2 L, 28%; and so on) (Recall)

88. C, A heated humidifier will always deliver a higher percent body humidity because warm air can hold more water than cooler air. Body humidity is the relative humidity of the air at body temperature. A device delivering 100% body humidity will deliver all the water the patient's airway requires (44 mg of H_2O per liter of gas). (Recall)

89. D, The needle valve, when completely closed, fits into a valve seat. If the valve seat is damaged and

lets gas past it, the humidifier will bubble, but the flow is so low it will not show a reading on the flowmeter. The flowmeter should be replaced. (Application)

90. C, The blood gases reveal hypercapnia (high P_{CO_2}), which is corrected by increasing the patient's minute ventilation. This is accomplished by increasing the ventilator rate or V_T. By increasing the V_T, more volume is made available to the alveoli for gas exchange to occur, thereby decreasing the Pa_{CO_2}. (Analysis)

91. C, Since the attack has been for only 30 min, the patient will most likely be hyperventilating as a result of hypoxemia. If this condition is not reversed, the patient will begin to tire, resulting in a decreasing minute ventilation accompanied by rising Pa_{CO_2} levels. (Application)

92. A, The ultrasonic nebulizer is capable of delivering approximately 6 mL of H_2O per minute. This is a much higher volume than any other nebulizer, which is why it is indicated for patients with thick retained secretions. (Application)

93. A, Be sure to read these questions carefully. This question is asking for "all of the following EXCEPT." When physiologic dead space increases, it indicates less air is getting to the normally functioning alveoli for gas exchange, while more is occupying the anatomic deadspace. This would result in increased Pa_{CO_2} levels, not decreased. (Application)

94. D, Whenever a patient is suspected of having sustained smoke inhalation, as close to 100% O_2 should be delivered. Our goal should be to achieve the highest Pa_{O_2} possible because, the higher the Pa_{O_2}, the less affinity hemoglobin has for CO; therefore, the sooner it will release the CO making more binding sites available for O_2. Of the choices, the non-rebreather is capable of delivering the highest percentage of O_2 (70% to 80%). (Analysis)

95. D, Bradycardia is not a hazard of aerosol therapy. (Recall)

96. D, The exhalation diaphragm will not be able to close effectively if a hole is present. There will be a leak in the system, preventing it from pressurizing and cycling to the expiratory phase. (Application)

97. B, The most frequently encountered bacteria found in our heated devices are *Pseudomonas* species. (Recall)

98. B, The normal Pa_{O_2} for a neonate is 50 to 70 torr; therefore, this neonate is overoxygenating. To reduce Pa_{O_2}, either the F_{IO_2} or PEEP needs to be reduced. Remember the 60% rule. Since the F_{IO_2} is 0.60, do not reduce it further: reduce the PEEP level. If the F_{IO_2} had been above 0.60, then it should be reduced before decreasing the PEEP level. (Analysis)

99. A, Chest physical therapy is indicated for patients with thick pulmonary secretions that are difficult to remove. The fluid with pulmonary edema is thin and frothy and mobilizes very easily, therefore CPT is not indicated. (Recall)

100. C, If the IPPB machine will not cycle into the expiratory phase, there is usually a problem with the exhalation valve or there is a leak somewhere in the system. The most common areas for leaks are at the tubing connections and around the mouth; other causes are the patient breathing through the nose or, if the patient is intubated or has had a tracheostomy, leaks around the cuff. (Application)

101. B, The pulse rate increased only 16 beats/min. If the pulse increased 20/min or more, the treatment should be stopped and the physician notified. (Application)

102. D, The key to this question is that the patient is "still heavily sedated." The best treatment modality for postoperative atelectasis in a patient who cannot follow commands is IPPB. If a patient is alert and able to follow commands, incentive spirometry should be tried first. (Analysis)

103. B, The FVC maneuver is used to obtain FEV_1, $FEF_{200-1200}$, and $FEF_{25\%-75\%}$.

104. D, If you are like many of my students and attendees of my review workshops, it is not unlikely that you chose either choice A or B. It is all in the way the question is written. After placing this COPD patient on a 5 L/min cannula, the patient becomes less alert and the Pa_{CO_2} begins climbing. Automatically, many people assume the patient's "hypoxic drive" has been knocked out. But to do that, the patient's Pa_{O_2} would have to be above 60 to 65 torr, and it is only 46 torr. This patient is simply deteriorating and needs to be placed on mechanical ventilation. If there was a choice for noninvasive ventilation, this also would be correct. Make sure you read all the data carefully and never anticipate where you think the question is going. That can get you in trouble. If you got this question right, good job, because more people miss this one than get it right. (Analysis)

105. C, Total flow is calculated as follows:

Sum of air/O_2 ratio parts $\times$ liter flow

Two methods of calculating air/O_2 ratios
First method:

$$\frac{100 - x = \text{parts air}}{x - 20^* = 1 \text{ part } O_2}$$

$$\frac{100 - 40 = 60}{40 - 20 = 20} = 3:1$$

*Use 21 if solving for a percentage of less than 40%

Second method:
If math equations make you nervous, try tic-tac-toe. Draw a tic-tac-toe box and place the number 20 (or 21) in the upper left hand box to represent air. In the lower left hand box, place 100 to represent O_2. In the middle box in the middle column, write the number of the percentage you are solving for. Then subtract diagonally.

$$40 - 20 = 20$$

Write 20 in the lower right hand box.

$$100 - 40 = 60$$

Write 60 in the upper right box.
Then divide 60 by 20 and you get 3, or a 3:1 air:O_2 ratio.
To calculate total flow:

$$3 + 1 = 4$$
$$4 \times 12 = 48 \text{ L/min}$$

(Application)

106. A, This blood gas represents alveolar hyperventilation. The only choice that will not start bringing the CO_2 level back to normal is increasing the respiratory rate. This would further decrease the CO_2. (Analysis)

107. A, If the capillary tube is plugged, gas will not be able to exit the diffuser and make contact with the water so that bubbling can take place. (Application)

108. C, Refer to explanation for question 72. (Application)

109. D, A PaO_2 of 580 torr on 100% oxygen is normal, indicating the patient is not in need of supplemental O_2. A good rule of thumb to determine normal PaO_2 at various O_2 percentages is to multiply the percentage of O_2 the patient is on by 5. This gives a ballpark figure for the normal PaO_2. (Analysis)

110. B, An Apgar score should be obtained at 1 and 5 min after delivery to assess the overall status of the neonate. (Analysis)

111. B, When gas flow from a nebulizer meets a resistance, such as H_2O, in the aerosol tubing, a back pressure is generated into the nebulizer. The pressure inside the nebulizer increases, reducing the pressure gradient from the inside of the nebulizer to the entrainment port, thereby decreasing the amount of air entrained from the room. This reduces the total flow put out by the nebulizer, while the delivered O_2 percentage increases. (Application)

112. D, This neonate's primary problem is ventilation, not oxygenation. The blood gas reveals a normal PaO_2 but an elevated $PaCO_2$. To treat the hypercapnia, minute ventilation must be increased and this is accomplished on a pressure ventilator by increasing peak inspiratory pressure or ventilator rate. (Analysis)

113. A, A bronchodilator should be administered with the aerosol to any patient who is susceptible to bronchospasm, such as patients with hyperactive airway disease (asthma). (Application)

114. D, Percentage of body humidity is calculated:

$$\frac{\text{Absolute humidity}}{44 \text{ mg } H_2O/L \text{ of gas}} \times 100 = \frac{41 \text{ mg/L}}{44 \text{ mg/L}} = .93 \times 100 = 93\%$$

Note: Absolute humidity is defined as the amount of water in a given sample of gas. (Application)

115. C, A pulse oximeter does not read accurately when HbCO is present in the blood. The pulse oximeter cannot determine whether O_2 or CO is bound to Hb. The reading may be 100% when the actual saturation level is much lower. A pulse oximeter should never be used to determine the oxygenation status of a patient who has sustained smoke inhalation, since it will give a false high reading. (Application)

116. D, The Babington nebulizer is the only nebulizer that operates in this fashion. It produces about the same amount of H_2O content as a jet nebulizer and is most commonly used with O_2 tents. (Recall)

117. B, Since the face tent is open at the top, it is well tolerated by patients with facial trauma or those who feel confined with a tight-fitting mask. Since this question stated that the patient has thick secretions, a mask with a nebulizer should be used. (Analysis)

118. A, These data show poor results on flow studies along with a reduced FVC. But the determining factor for obstructive versus restrictive disease is the FEV_1/FVC. Any time this value is less than 75%, the disease process is obstructive. A patient with restrictive lung disease will have reduced FVC and FEV_1 values. But the restrictive patient's FEV_1 is reduced only because the FVC is reduced. In other words, the patient did not get as much air in and, therefore, doesn't get as much air out. If you compare the patient's FEV_1 to his/her FVC (not the predicted value), which is what the FEV_1/FVC is, the value will be normal, or above 75%. However, the patient with obstructive disease gets plenty of air in during inspiration, but the FEV_1 is reduced because of airflow obstruction. Since the values after a bronchodilator was administered improved by at least 15%, the condition is said to respond to a bronchodilator. Remember, patients with obstructive disease generally do not have problems getting air in, but getting air out. Patients with restrictive disease have problems getting air in, not getting air out. (Application)

119. D, The most common device used to deliver H_2O to the tracheostomy is a jet nebulizer. Studies vary on whether the H_2O should be heated or unheated. But remember that warmer air can hold more H_2O than cold, and this may make a difference in the thickness of the secretions. If the secretions are thick and difficult to mobilize, a heater should be added to the nebulizer. (Recall)

120. B, The T-piece, or Briggs adaptor, has 22-mm adaptors on each side that allow for the connection of large-bore aerosol tubing, not the small-bore tubing that connects to humidifiers. (Recall)

121. D, Acetylcysteine (Mucomyst) is a mucolytic agent that chemically breaks sputum down, making it less viscous and easier to mobilize. Patients with lung conditions that produce thick secretions, such as bronchiectasis and cystic fibrosis, often are administered Mucomyst. (Recall)

122. C, Minute ventilation is calculated:

$$V_T \times RR$$

Convert V_T from mL to L by dividing by 1000.

$$0.45 \times 16 = 7.2\ L$$

(Application)

123. A, Refer to explanation for question 47. (Analysis)

124. A, Refer to explanation for question 51. (Analysis)

125. B, Positive pressure ventilation has the potential for decreasing venous blood return to the heart. This results from this pressure being transferred to the superior and inferior vena cavae, restricting blood flow back into the heart. Baroreceptors (pressure receptors) sense this lower pressure in the right atrium and send signals to the brain, which causes an increased production of ADH by the pituitary gland. This causes the body to hold on to more fluid as a compensatory mechanism, since the right heart is sensing a low pressure. The decreased cardiac output results in decreased perfusion to the kidneys, which also reduces urine output. (Recall)

126. A, A V_D/V_T of less than 0.60 and an MIP of at least -20 cm H_2O indicate weaning should be attempted. For weaning to be attempted, the P(A-a) O_2 on 100% oxygen should be less than 350 torr and the VC more than 10 to 15 mL/kg of body weight. (Recall)

127. A, The respirometer should be placed on the ventilator outlet, because if placed anywhere else in the circuit and a leak is present, the reading will not be accurate. (Application)

128. B, The pressure alarm on a volume ventilator will be activated if the patient becomes disconnected from the circuit or if leaks are present in the system. Choices A, C, and D could result in the high pressure alarm being activated as a result of increased airway resistance. (Application)

129. B, If the expiratory spirometer is filling during inspiration instead of emptying, the problem indicates the expiratory valve is malfunctioning. Because the exhalation valve is failing to block the expiratory limb of the circuit during a positive pressure breath, the V_T produced by the ventilator is bypassing the patient, flowing directly into the expiratory limb, and causing the spirometer to rise. Therefore, the spirometer fills during the inspiratory phase of the ventilatory cycle, instead of emptying as it should. This results in a drastic decrease in inspiratory pressure and a loss of delivered V_T to the patient. (Application)

130. C, Since air contains little CO_2 and a much higher amount of O_2, these values will be reflected if an air bubble is in the sample. (Application)

131. C, MIP, sometimes referred to as NIF, measures the patient's respiratory muscle strength. It is obtained by having the patient inhale as deeply as possible through a mouthpiece or mask that is attached to a pressure manometer. The MIP is measured periodically on patients with neuromuscular disease to determine weakness in the ventilatory muscles. Normal MIP is -50 to -100 cm H_2O. (Application)

132. B, An oropharyngeal airway is indicated for unconscious patients to prevent the tongue from falling back against the back of the throat and obstructing the airway. (Application)

133. B, Cuffed ET tube should be used to help prevent aspiration and prevent volume leaks around the tube. (Application)

134. C, The initial ventilator rate should be between 8 and 12 breaths/min and the V_T should be 10 to 12 mL/kg of body weight. (Application)

135. C, When less volume is being recorded on the exhaled volume display than the set machine volume, a leak is present. Leaks can occur at tubing connections, the humidifier, the medication nebulizer, the ET-tube cuff, or through chest tubes. A low H_2O volume in the humidifier will not cause the exhaled volume display to read low, although the patient does not receive as much volume as when the humidifier has the appropriate amount of H_2O. The reason less volume gets to the patient is because the lower the H_2O level, the more of the humidifier jar is exposed to the volume flowing through the humidifier. This causes more volume to be compressed against the sides of the humidifier jar. But, just like volume compressed in the ventilator tubing, when exhalation occurs, the volume leaves the humidifier and is measured on the exhaled volume display. (Application)

136. A, Increased inspiratory pressures on a volume ventilator indicate decreasing lung compliance (stiffer lungs) or increasing airway resistance. Increased airway resistance results as the gas meets a resistance to flow caused by H_2O in the tubing circuit, secretions in the airway, bronchospasm, or coughing. It is important to understand that an increasing peak pressure by itself does not indicate a decreasing lung compliance. Static pressure must be determined by a 1-sec inspiratory hold, noting the plateau pressure. If the plateau pressure is likewise increasing, compliance is indeed decreasing. But if plateau pressure is unchanged when peak pressure is increasing, it is an airway resistance problem, not a compliance problem. Remember, plateau or static pressure is registered when no air is flowing through tubing and airways. The pressure drop that occurs from peak to plateau pressure is the pressure exerted against the walls of the ventilator circuit and patient's airways as the gas flows to the patient's lungs. (Analysis)

137. A, The patient was not ready for T-tube weaning and should be placed on SIMV to allow for spontaneous breathing along with ventilator breaths. A postoperative patient such as this one should not be on the ventilator for long unless unforeseen problems arise, therefore SIMV is indicated. (Analysis)

138. B, These data reveal an increased, not decreased, P(A-a) O_2 and a low $PaCO_2$, indicating alveolar hyperventilation and respiratory alkalosis. This patient is hyperventilating in response to hypoxemia. (Application)

139. C, Since mechanical ventilation is to be initiated, it is not important to determine the patient's FVC or NIF. Most important is to determine the required minute ventilation (rate and V_T) necessary for the patient. (Application)

140. A, Based on the ABG levels, MIP, and VC, this patient is a good candidate for beginning the weaning process. Placing the patient on the SIMV mode will best accomplish this. (Analysis)

Maximum Score: 140

Incorrect answers: _____

Correct answers: _____

Minimum passing score: 105

Advanced Practitioner Written Registry Exam: Practice Test

TIME LIMIT: 2 HOURS

Note: torr = 1 mm Hg

Directions: Each of the questions or incomplete statements below are followed by four suggested answers or completions. Select the best answer.

1. While evaluating a patient's cardiopulmonary status, the respiratory therapist determines the patient has a 6-sec capillary refill time. This reflects which of the following conditions?

   A. Increased Q_T
   B. Decreased peripheral perfusion
   C. Hypertension
   D. Sufficient perfusion to the extremities

2. While making O_2 rounds, the respiratory therapist notices that the reservoir bag on the patient's non-rebreathing mask completely deflates as the patient inspires. Which of the following should the therapist recommend at this time?

   A. Change to partial rebreathing mask.
   B. Instruct the patient to take more shallow breaths.
   C. Increase flow to the mask.
   D. Remove the one-way valve between the bag and the mask.

3. Continuous monitoring of a neonate's PaO_2 is best achieved by using which of the following methods?

   A. Transcutaneous monitoring
   B. Pulse oximetry
   C. Capnography
   D. Pulmonary artery catheter

4. The respiratory therapist palpates no pulse on a patient, but the ECG oscilloscope monitor shows QRS complexes on the tracing. The therapist should

   A. Get stat ABG studies
   B. Administer a stat IPPB treatment with atropine
   C. Begin cardiac compressions
   D. Recommend a stat chest radiograph

5. A patient is being administered CPAP via mask at 8 cm H_2O. The low pressure alarm is sounding, and the manometer is reading 2 cm H_2O. Which of the following may be causing this situation?

   I. Excessive flow
   II. Loose-fitting mask
   III. Leak around tubing connection
   IV. Inappropriate low-pressure alarm setting

   A. I and II only
   B. II and III only
   C. II and IV only
   D. II, III, and IV only

6. Which of the following statements regarding a pulse-dose O_2 system is true?

   A. O_2 is delivered to the patient only as the patient inspires.
   B. Higher flows are required for equivalent O_2 concentrations.
   C. A nasal cannula cannot be used as an O_2 delivery device with this system.
   D. The system cannot be incorporated with O_2 cylinders.

7. A SPAG nebulizer is indicated for the delivery of aerosolized medication with which of the following pulmonary conditions?

   A. Bronchiectasis
   B. Acute infectious bronchiolitis
   C. Bacterial pneumonia
   D. Cystic fibrosis

8. While reviewing a patient's chart, the respiratory therapist notices the patient's Hb level is 20 g/dL and SpO_2 is 80%. Which of the following is true regarding this situation?

   A. The patient is most likely cyanotic.
   B. The patient is hypoxic.
   C. The patient is hyperventilating.
   D. The patient has a normal HbO_2 level.

9. A patient enters the emergency department after a motor vehicle accident in mild respiratory distress and complaining of soreness on the left side of the chest. Auscultation of breath sounds reveals diminished breath sounds in the left lung. After placing the patient on O_2, the respiratory therapist should recommend which of the following first?

   A. IPPB with a bronchodilator
   B. Stat chest radiograph
   C. CBC count
   D. CPAP at 4 cm H_2O

10. A patient is on a 30% air-entrainment mask with an O_2 flow of 4 L/min. The total flow being delivered by this O_2 setup is which of the following?

    A. 16 L/min
    B. 24 L/min
    C. 36 L/min
    D. 44 L/min

11. A patient is having difficulty cycling the IPPB machine into the inspiratory phase. The respiratory therapist should adjust which of the following controls?

    A. Sensitivity
    B. Flow rate
    C. Inspiratory pressure
    D. Air dilution

12. The following ABG results are obtained from an adult patient on a 50% aerosol mask.

pH	7.45
$PaCO_2$	34 torr
PaO_2	57 torr
HCO_3^-	25 mEq/L
BE	+2

    Based on these data, the respiratory therapist should recommend which of the following?

    A. Administer a stat IPPB treatment.
    B. Increase to O_2 to 70%.
    C. Institute CPAP mask.
    D. Place on 100% non-rebreathing mask.

13. A 58-year-old emphysema patient enters the emergency department on a 2 L/min nasal cannula. ABGs are drawn and after the results are evaluated, the O_2 flow is increased to 5 L/min. Below are ABG results for both flow rates.

	(2 L/min)	(5 L/min)
pH	7.34	7.28
$PaCO_2$	62 torr	77 torr
PaO_2	44 torr	52 torr
HCO_3^-	35 mEq/L	35 mEq/L
BE	+10	+10

Based on these data, which of the following should the respiratory therapist recommend?

A. Decrease the liter flow to 3 L/min.
B. Place on CPAP of 4 cm H_2O and 60% O_2.
C. Increase the liter flow to 6 L/min.
D. Institute noninvasive ventilation.

14. A 34-year-old female patient enters the emergency department complaining of severe chest pain. The patient is placed on a 50% air-entrainment mask. Thirty minutes later, ABGs are drawn and the results are

pH	7.50
$PaCO_2$	31 torr
PaO_2	253 torr
HCO_3^-	24 mEq/L
BE	−1

    Which of the following is a true statement regarding these ABG results?

    A. The results appear to be accurate and consistent with the FIO_2.
    B. The PaO_2 is too high for the FIO_2.
    C. The $PaCO_2$ is not consistent with the pH.
    D. The results represent a metabolic alkalosis.

15. A patient in the cardiac ICU is intubated and receiving mechanical ventilation on 40% O_2. The following data have been collected:

pH	7.41	HCO_3^-	23 mEq/L
$PaCO_2$	37 torr	$C(a-v)O_2$	8.1 vol%
PaO_2	81 torr	PCWP	2 mm Hg
		BE	−2

    Based on these data, the respiratory therapist should recommend which of the following?

    A. Administer a diuretic.
    B. Institute PEEP at 5 cm H_2O.
    C. Administer fluids.
    D. Increase the FIO_2.

16. The physician wants to wean a patient from a ventilator. Which of the following parameters obtained by the respiratory therapist indicate weaning will most likely be successful?

    I. MIP of −28 cm H_2O
    II. $P(A-a)O_2$ of less than 200 torr on 100% O_2
    III. Vital capacity of 19 mL/kg body weight

    A. I only
    B. I and III only
    C. II and III only
    D. I, II, and III

17. The respiratory therapist is calibrating a helium analyzer. When calibrated to room air, the analyzer should read

    A. 0%
    B. 21%
    C. 79%
    D. 100%

18. A 43-year-old patient in ICU is receiving 40% O_2 by air-entrainment mask. His Pao_2 is 58 torr and his shunt has been calculated to be 6%. Which of the following is most likely causing his hypoxemia?

    A. Pulmonary edema
    B. Lobar pneumonia
    C. Pneumothorax
    D. Hypoventilation

19. A V/Q scan is conducted on a patient in whom pulmonary embolism is suspected. The scan shows normal ventilation with the absence of perfusion in the left upper lobe. The respiratory therapist should estimate the V/Q ratio in this area to be which of the following?

    A. less than 0.5
    B. 0.8
    C. 1.0
    D. more than 2.0

20. While making ventilator checks, the respiratory therapist measures the ET-tube cuff pressure to be 40 mm Hg. At peak inspiratory pressure, air is passing around the cuff. Which of the following actions should the therapist take at this time?

    A. Decrease cuff pressure to 20 mm Hg.
    B. Add more air to the cuff to stop the leak.
    C. Recommend changing to a larger tube.
    D. Maintain the cuff pressure at 40 mm Hg.

21. The respiratory therapist is monitoring a patient on IMV that employs an H-valve circuit to provide air for the patient's spontaneous breaths. During spontaneous inspiration, the reservoir bag on the H-valve completely collapses. The therapist should do which of the following?

    A. Increase the ventilator flow.
    B. Increase the ventilator sensitivity.
    C. Increase flow to the H-valve.
    D. Decrease the IMV rate.

22. The following data are collected from an infant on a pressure ventilator.

Mode	IMV
Ventilator rate	35/min
Inspiratory pressure	26 cm H_2O
PEEP	6 cm H_2O
FIO_2	0.40
pH	7.27
$Paco_2$	52 torr
Pao_2	47 torr
HCO_3^-	22 mEq/L

Based on these data, the respiratory therapist should recommend which of the following?

    A. Decrease PEEP to 4 cm H_2O.
    B. Increase ventilator rate to 40/min.
    C. Decrease inspiratory pressure to 22 cm H_2O.
    D. Decrease inspiratory flow.

23. After assisting the physician with a bronchoscopy, the respiratory therapist should disinfect the bronchoscope with which of the following techniques?

    A. Wipe down with alcohol.
    B. Wipe down with Betadine solution.
    C. Soak in glutaraldehyde for 15 to 20 min.
    D. Steam autoclave for 15 min.

24. A patient with a peak inspiratory flow of 40 L/min is to be set up on a 30% air-entrainment mask. What is the minimum O_2 flow required to meet the patient's inspiratory flow demands?

    A. 3 L/min
    B. 5 L/min
    C. 8 L/min
    D. 10 L/min

25. The RCP is performing postural drainage and percussion on a patient with right lower lobe atelectasis and observes the tracing below on the cardiac monitor.

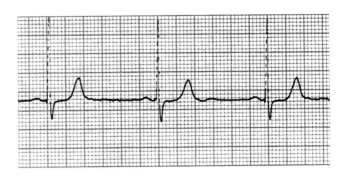

This heart rhythm is most likely the result of which of the following?

    A. Vagal stimulation
    B. Hypoxemia
    C. Loose ECG lead
    D. Artifact from patient movement

26. The respiratory therapist has just completed assisting the physician with a bronchoscopy on a venti-

lator patient and notices the high-pressure alarm is activated. This increased pressure could be the result of all of the following *EXCEPT*

A. Pneumothorax
B. Bronchospasm
C. Hypotension
D. Pulmonary hemorrhage

27. The following data have been collected from a patient in the cardiac ICU.

pH	7.42
Pa_{CO_2}	42 torr
Pa_{O_2}	70 torr
HCO_3^-	25 mEq/L
Sa_{O_2}	93%
Pv_{O_2}	34 torr
Sv_{O_2}	72%
$P(A-a)O_2$	100 torr
Hb	14 g/dL

Based on these data, which of the following represents this patient's intrapulmonary shunt?

A. 4%
B. 7%
C. 9%
D. 12%

28. Following a cardiac arrest, a 48-year-old female is placed on a mechanical ventilator. A Swan-Ganz catheter is in place. The following data are obtained.

BP	94/52 mm Hg
Pulse	116/min
PCWP	6 mm Hg
PAP	40/22 mm Hg
Q_T	3.5 L/min

Based on these data, which of the following has increased?

A. Pulmonary vascular resistance
B. Left atrial pressure
C. Stroke volume
D. Systemic vascular resistance

29. An otherwise healthy 24-year-old, tall, thin man enters the emergency department complaining of chest pain with mild respiratory distress. A chest radiograph reveals a spontaneous pneumothorax of approximately 10%. Which of the following should the respiratory therapist recommend?

    I. O_2 therapy
    II. Needle aspiration
    III. Chest tube insertion
    IV. Continuous pulse oximetry

A. II and III only
B. I and IV only

C. I, II, and III only
D. I, III, and IV only

30. The respiratory therapist is having difficulty intubating a patient who is in respiratory failure. In place of an ET tube, which of the following should be inserted to facilitate the most effective manual ventilation?

A. Esophageal tracheal combitube
B. Nasopharyngeal airway
C. Oropharyngeal airway
D. Nasogastric airway

31. A patient with bronchiectasis has been receiving postural drainage and percussion for 2 days. The patient's chest radiograph has not shown improvement, and he still is having difficulty expectorating sputum. Which of the following therapies may be of benefit in the treatment of this patient?

    I. Intrapulmonary percussive ventilation (IPV)
    II. Flutter valve device
    III. PEP therapy

A. I only
B. I and II only
C. II and III only
D. I, II, and III

32. A patient with chest trauma is on a volume ventilator and a V_T of 800 mL. The returned exhaled volume is 500 mL. Which of the following could be causing this problem?

A. Inadequate inspiratory flow
B. Leak around chest tube
C. Excessive ET-tube cuff pressure
D. Low humidifier H_2O level

33. The respiratory therapist is having difficulty calibrating a transcutaneous O_2 monitor to room air. This is most likely because of which of the following?

A. The membrane is torn.
B. The sensor won't stick to the infant's skin properly.
C. There is poor perfusion to the sensor site.
D. The infant is hemodynamically unstable.

34. After administering 200 J with a defibrillator, ventricular fibrillation continues. Which of the following is the appropriate measure to recommend at this time?

A. Administer $NaHCO_3^-$.
B. Repeat defibrillation with 300 J.
C. Administer intracardiac epinephrine.
D. Repeat defibrillation at 400 J.

35. The following data have been recorded from a patient on a volume ventilator.

Mode	Assist/control	pH	7.51
Ventilator rate	10/min	$PaCO_2$	30 torr
V_T	750 mL	PaO_2	57 torr
FIO_2	0.60	HCO_3^-	25 mEq/L
PEEP	6 cm H_2O		

Based on this information, the respiratory therapist should recommend which of the following?

A. Increase PEEP to 8 cm H_2O.
B. Decrease V_T to 700 mL.
C. Decrease rate to 8/min.
D. Increase FIO_2 to 0.70.

36. The following data have been obtained from a patient on a volume ventilator.

PEEP	Peak pressure	Plateau pressure	V_T
4 cm H_2O	32 cm H_2O	24 cm H_2O	600 mL
6 cm H_2O	37 cm H_2O	24 cm H_2O	600 mL
8 cm H_2O	43 cm H_2O	28 cm H_2O	600 mL
10 cm H_2O	47 cm H_2O	31 cm H_2O	600 mL

Optimal PEEP is which of the following?

A. 4 cm H_2O
B. 6 cm H_2O
C. 8 cm H_2O
D. 10 cm H_2O

37. The respiratory therapist is assisting the physician in the insertion of a Swan-Ganz catheter. The patient is hemodynamically stable at the time. The therapist would know the catheter tip has entered the pulmonary artery when which of the following pressures is observed?

A. 12/4 mm Hg
B. 24/10 mm Hg
C. 40/0 mm Hg
D. 110/75 mm Hg

38. A postoperative patient is to be weaned from mechanical ventilation. He is on the following ventilator settings.

Mode	SIMV
Ventilator rate	6/min
V_T	700 mL
FIO_2	0.40
Pressure support	25 cm H_2O
ABG values: pH	7.44
$PaCO_2$	37 torr
PaO_2	97 torr

Which of the following should the respiratory therapist recommend to begin weaning this patient?

A. Decrease the FIO_2.
B. Decrease pressure support.
C. Decrease V_T.
D. Increase inspiratory flow.

39. A patient has the following pulmonary function results.

FVC	56% of predicted
FEV_1	53% of predicted
FEV_1/FVC	86%
TLC	75% of predicted
Peak flow	108% of predicted

The most appropriate interpretation of these results is which of the following?

A. Obstructive disease only
B. Restrictive disease only
C. Mixed obstructive and restrictive disease
D. Normal pulmonary function results

40. A patient with severe COPD is on a 2 L/min nasal cannula. ABGs are drawn and, after interpreting the results, the liter flow is increased to 5 L/min, and another ABG sample is drawn 1 hour later. The ABG results are

	(2 L/min)	(5 L/min)
pH	7.34	7.28
$PaCO_2$	62 torr	81 torr
PaO_2	46 torr	84 torr
HCO_3^-	35 mEq/L	35 mEq/L
BE	+12	+12

While on the 5 L/min cannula, the patient seems lethargic and drowsy. Based on this information, the respiratory therapist should recommend which of the following?

A. Institute noninvasive ventilation.
B. Place on non-rebreathing mask at 12 L/min.
C. Decrease liter flow to 3 L/min.
D. Place on CPAP of 4 cm H_2O and FIO_2 of 0.40.

41. A COPD patient is extubated after being on mechanical ventilation for 2 weeks. For several hours after extubation, the patient complains of progressively worsening shortness of breath while on a 2 L/min nasal cannula. His respiratory rate has increased from 16/min to 26/min. The most appropriate recommendation is which of the following?

A. Initiate noninvasive positive pressure ventilation.
B. Reintubate and place on mechanical ventilation.
C. Place on non-rebreathing mask.
D. Begin postural drainage and percussion every 4 hours.

42. Independent lung ventilation is indicated with which of the following conditions?

I. Unilateral bronchopulmonary fistula
II. Single lung transplantation
III. ARDS with pulmonary edema

A. I only
B. I and II only
C. II and III only
D. I, II, and III

43. After increasing a ventilator patient's PEEP level from 8 cm H_2O to 12 cm H_2O, the PvO_2 drops from 37 torr to 33 torr. This indicates which of the following?

A. Venous return has increased.
B. Tissue oxygenation has increased.
C. Static CL has increased.
D. Q_T has decreased.

44. A patient's pulmonary function study shows an FRC of 127% of predicted. The patient most likely has which of the following conditions?

A. Pulmonary fibrosis
B. Atelectasis
C. Emphysema
D. Pneumonia

45. The high-pressure alarm is activated on a patient's volume ventilator. Which of the following should the respiratory therapist do to help correct this problem?

I. Add air to the ET-tube cuff.
II. Suction the patient's ET tube.
III. Make sure the expiratory drive line is connected.

A. I only
B. II only
C. II and III only
D. I, II, and III

46. The following data are collected from a patient on mechanical ventilation.

	08:00 PM	**11:00 PM**
PAP	24/12 mm Hg	42/20 mm Hg
PVR	2.1 mm Hg/L/min	4.2 mm Hg/L/min
PCWP	6 mm Hg	7 mm Hg

Based on this information, these changes are most likely the result of which of the following?

A. Pulmonary embolus
B. Left ventricular failure
C. Aortic stenosis
D. Overhydration

47. Hyperbaric O_2 therapy is indicated in which of the following clinical conditions?

A. Pulmonary embolism
B. CO poisoning
C. Bronchopleural fistula
D. Tension pneumothorax

48. The following data are collected from a 43-year-old patient breathing room air at a PB of 747 torr.

pH	7.24
$PaCO_2$	68 torr
PaO_2	60 torr
HCO_3^-	26 mEq/L
BE	+1

All of the following statements are true about this situation *EXCEPT*

I. The patient is hypoventilating.
II. The $P(A-a)O_2$ is increased.
III. The patient has chronic hypoxemia.

A. II only
B. III only
C. I and II only
D. II and III only

49. A 5-ft 5-inch, 120-kg (264-lb) woman is brought to the emergency department and is being ventilated with a manual resuscitator and mask on 100% O_2. A drug overdose is suspected. After intubating the patient, the respiratory therapist is asked to recommend initial ventilator settings. What are the most appropriate settings for this patient's ventilator?

A. SIMV, rate 10/min, V_T 1.0 L, FIO_2 1.0
B. Assist/control, rate 16/min, V_T 800 mL, FIO_2 1.0
C. Assist/control, rate 12/min, V_T 1.2 L, FIO_2 1.0
D. SIMV, rate 12/min, V_T 650 mL, FIO_2 1.0

50. Below is a volume waveform from a patient on a volume ventilator.

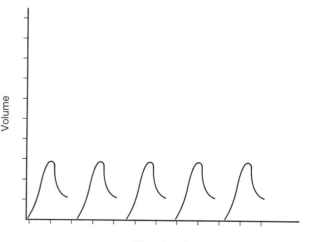

Time (secs)

This waveform indicates which of the following?

A. *It represents a normal volume waveform.*
B. *The patient has obstructive lung disease.*
C. *There may be a leak around the ET-tube cuff.*
D. *The patient is coughing or agitated.*

51. A patient with ARDS is on a volume ventilator with a PEEP of 15 cm H_2O and an FiO_2 of 1.0 and remains hypoxemic. Which of the following ventilator modifications is the most appropriate recommendation at this time?

    A. *Increase the PEEP to 20 cm H_2O.*
    B. *Place on pressure control ventilation.*
    C. *Sedate the patient and place ventilator in the control mode.*
    D. *Begin in-line bronchodilator therapy using a MDI.*

52. A malnourished COPD patient is having difficulty being weaned from mechanical ventilation. The respiratory therapist recommends conducting an indirect calorimetry study. This procedure will determine which of the following?

    I. Patient's nutritional status
    II. CO_2 production
    III. O_2 cost of breathing

    A. *I only*
    B. *I and II only*
    C. *II and III only*
    D. *I, II, and III*

53. The following data are collected from patient on a volume ventilator.

PEEP	Pao$_2$	Pvo$_2$
4 cm H_2O	68 torr	36 torr
6 cm H_2O	73 torr	38 torr
8 cm H_2O	77 torr	34 torr
10 cm H_2O	80 torr	32 torr

    Optimal PEEP is which of the following?

    A. *4 cm H_2O*
    B. *6 cm H_2O*
    C. *8 cm H_2O*
    D. *10 cm H_2O*

54. The respiratory therapist has just completed assisting the physician with a thoracentesis when the patient becomes anxious and complains of shortness of breath. The therapist finds the patient is also tachycardic. Which of the following should the therapist recommend at this time?

    A. *Chest radiograph*
    B. *V/Q scan*

C. *Bronchoscopy*
D. *Echocardiogram*

55. The following ABG results are recorded for a patient on a volume ventilator.

pH	7.26
Paco$_2$	25 torr
Pao$_2$	89 torr
HCO$_3^-$	27 mEq/L
BE	+2

    The respiratory therapist should recommend which of following?

    A. *Decrease ventilator VT.*
    B. *Administer $NaHCO_3^-$.*
    C. *Get repeat ABG samples, since this indicates laboratory error.*
    D. *Increase ventilator rate.*

56. A patient is receiving helium/O_2 therapy through a simple O_2 mask. The patient is experiencing shortness of breath. The respiratory therapist should

    A. *Increase flow to the mask*
    B. *Discontinue the treatment*
    C. *Instruct the patient to take deeper breaths*
    D. *Change to a non-rebreathing mask*

57. The following data are collected from a patient on a 60% aerosol mask.

pH	7.42
Paco$_2$	45 torr
Pao$_2$	90 torr
HCO$_3^-$	25 mEq/L

    If the PB is 747 torr, this patient's P(A-a)o$_2$ is approximately which of the following?

    A. *150 torr*
    B. *275 torr*
    C. *305 torr*
    D. *365 torr*

58. Which of the following indicate that the patient should not be extubated?

    A. *VC 18 mL/kg, MIP −37 cm H_2O, VD/VT 28%*
    B. *VC 15 mL/kg, MIP −25 cm H_2O, VD/VT 40%*
    C. *VC 16 mL/kg, MIP −15 cm H_2O, VD/VT 50%*
    D. *VC 20 mL/kg, MIP −24 cm H_2O, VD/VT 35%*

59. The following pulmonary function data was obtained from a 51-year-old man who is 5 ft 10 inches tall and weighs 77 kg (169 lb).

FVC	2.7 L
FEV$_1$	2.3 L
FEV$_1$/FVC	85%
DLCO	44% of predicted

This patient most likely has which of the following conditions?

A. Bronchiectasis
B. Pulmonary fibrosis
C. Emphysema
D. Chronic bronchitis

60. A 2-week-old infant is being ventilated with a pressure-limited, time-cycled ventilator. The peak inspiratory pressure is 24 cm H_2O, inspiratory time is 0.5 sec, and the mean airway pressure (MAP) is 14 cm H_2O. If the inspiratory time is increased to 0.8 sec, which of the following responses will most likely occur?

A. MAP will increase.
B. Peak inspiratory pressure will increase.
C. V_T will decrease.
D. F_{IO_2} will increase.

61. The patient is having difficulty cycling the IPPB machine into the inspiratory phase. Which of the following modifications should the respiratory therapist make to correct this problem?

I. Increase the sensitivity.
II. Make sure the patient's lips are sealed tight around the mouthpiece.
III. Make sure all tubing connections are tight.

A. I only
B. I and II only
C. II and III only
D. I, II, and III

62. The respiratory therapist notes that the patient's $C(a-v)O_2$ increases from 4.0 vol% to 8.5 vol% after increasing the PEEP level from 5 to 10 cm H_2O. This suggests that which of the following has occurred?

A. Static C_L increased.
B. Raw decreased.
C. Q_T decreased.
D. MAP decreased.

63. The respiratory therapist has just intubated the patient and the CO_2 detector on the proximal end of the ET tube reads 6%. This indicates which of the following?

A. The tube is in the airway.
B. The patient is hyperventilating.
C. The tube is in the esophagus.
D. The patient's V_T is not adequate.

64. The following data are obtained from a patient on a volume ventilator.

Mode	SIMV	pH	7.44
Ventilator rate	6/min	$PaCO_2$	34 torr
V_T	700 mL	PaO_2	89 torr
F_{IO_2}	0.35	HCO_3^-	23 mEq/L
		BE	−1

Based on this information, the respiratory therapist should recommend which of the following?

A. Administer $NaHCO_3^-$.
B. Add mechanical V_D.
C. Extubate and place the patient on a 35% Venturi mask.
D. Decrease ventilator rate to 4/min.

65. While making O_2 rounds, the respiratory therapist notices that the reservoir tubing on a patient's T-piece setup has fallen off. How could this affect the operation of this device?

A. The total flow will increase.
B. The F_{IO_2} will decrease.
C. Less room air will be entrained.
D. The temperature of the inspired air will increase.

66. A 2-month-old infant is being mechanically ventilated by a pressure-limited, time-cycled ventilator. The ventilator rate is 30/min and the I:E ratio is 1:3. Based on this information, the inspiratory time is which of the following?

A. 0.3 sec
B. 0.5 sec
C. 0.8 sec
D. 1.0 sec

67. The following ECG strip appears on the cardiac monitor.

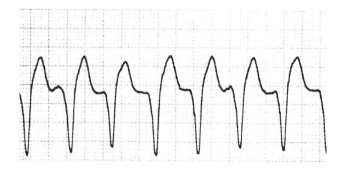

Which of the following should be done *first*?

A. Defibrillate the patient.
B. Order a stat chest radiograph
C. Order serum electrolyte studies.
D. Obtain an ABG sample.

68. A patient has an arterial catheter in place and a "damped" pressure tracing appears on the monitor.

Which of the following should the respiratory therapist recommend at this time?

    I. Reposition the catheter.
    II. Flush the line with heparinized saline solution.
    III. Disconnect the transducer and flush out any air bubbles.

A. I only
B. I and II only
C. II and III only
D. I, II, and III

69. A 75-kg (165-lb) patient on a 2 L/min nasal cannula has a respiratory rate of 15/min and a V_T of 550 mL. This patient's $\dot{V}_E$ is which of the following?

A. 5.8 L
B. 7.1 L
C. 8.3 L
D. 9.6 L

70. Obstructive sleep apnea is suspected in a patient. The respiratory therapist should recommend which of the following to help diagnose this condition?

A. ABG studies
B. Polysomnogram
C. V/Q scan
D. CT scan

71. Two hours after the insertion of a UAC in a 1-day old infant, cyanosis of the lower extremities is noted. The respiratory therapist should recommend which of the following?

A. Withdraw the catheter to the level of T8 on radiograph.
B. Advance the catheter until the extremities turn pink.
C. Withdrawn the catheter to the level of T2 on radiograph.
D. Discontinue the UAC.

72. The respiratory therapist is ventilating an intubated patient with a self-inflating manual resuscitator. When the bag is squeezed, there is little resistance met and the patient's chest does not rise. Which of the following should the therapist do at this time?

A. Check the bag intake valve for proper function.
B. Make sure the reservoir is attached to the bag properly.
C. Make sure the O_2 tubing has not fallen off the flowmeter.
D. Increase the liter flow to the bag.

73. While transporting a patient on a 4 L/min nasal cannula with an E cylinder, the cannula tubing becomes kinked between the mattress and the bedrail. The Bourdon gauge flow-metering device would

A. Show a decreased liter flow.
B. Continue to display an accurate flow reading.
C. Show a higher flow reading than the patient is actually receiving.
D. Show a lower flow than what the patient is actually receiving.

74. After setting up a 6 L/min cannula, the respiratory therapist kinks the cannula tubing and a high-pitched whistle is heard coming from the humidifier. The therapist should

A. Replace the humidifier
B. Make sure the jar is connected tightly to the humidifier top
C. Decrease the liter flow
D. Place the cannula on the patient as ordered

75. A patient's chest radiograph shows hyperinflation, right ventricular hypertrophy, and diffuse infiltrates. Which of the following would most likely be observed during a pulmonary assessment of this patient?

    I. Pedal edema
    II. Paradoxical respirations
    III. Barrel chest
    IV. Distended neck veins

A. I and III only
B. II and III only
C. I, III, and IV only
D. I, II, III, and IV

76. An 34-year-old unconscious patient, admitted because of a drug overdose, is intubated and placed on a volume ventilator. Average peak inspiratory pressure is 30 cm H_2O. The high-pressure limit is set at 40 cm H_2O. One hour later, the patient becomes agitated and combative, and the high-pressure alarm sounds with each breath. The respiratory therapist should recommend

A. Increasing the pressure limit to 50 cm H_2O
B. Decreasing the inspiratory flow
C. Increasing the V_T
D. The administration of Pavulon

77. A patient enters the emergency department on a 5 L/min nasal cannula. Although the patient is not cyanotic, ABG results reveal a PaO_2 of 45 torr and an SpO_2 of 98%. The respiratory therapist should

recommend which of the following to better assess this patient's oxygenation status?

A. Hb level
B. V_D/V_T
C. P_{VO_2}
D. $P(A-a)_{O_2}$

78. While making O_2 rounds, the respiratory therapist observes H_2O bubbling in the aerosol tubing connected to a jet nebulizer set on 40%. Which of the following statements is true regarding this situation.

A. Total flow will increase.
B. F_{IO_2} will decrease.
C. Air entrained into the nebulizer will increase.
D. This is a heated nebulizer.

79. A 2-week-old infant is being ventilated on a time-cycled, pressure-limited ventilator. The physician wants to increase the MAP. Which of the following could be increased to accomplish this?

    I. PEEP
    II. PIP
    III. Inspiratory time

A. I only
B. II only
C. II and III only
D. I, II, and III

80. A 34-year-old, 80-kg (176-lb) man with a history of cardiac disease has been intubated, and the physician wants your recommendation for initial ventilator settings. Which of the following would be most beneficial in preventing cardiac side effects?

A. SIMV mode, rate 14/min, V_T 850 mL, F_{IO_2} 0.50
B. Control mode, rate 12/min, V_T 900 mL, F_{IO_2} 0.60
C. Assist/control mode, rate 14/min, V_T 800 mL, F_{IO_2} 0.50
D. SIMV mode, rate 10/min, V_T 800 mL, F_{IO_2} 0.50

81. The following data are obtained from a patient on a volume ventilator with a V_T of 750 mL.

	Peak pressure	Plateau pressure
200 PM	34 cm H_2O	16 cm H_2O
300 PM	38 cm H_2O	19 cm H_2O
400 PM	44 cm H_2O	23 cm H_2O

Based on this information, the respiratory therapist should conclude which of the following?

A. The patient is experiencing bronchospasms.
B. Raw is increasing.
C. Static C_L is decreasing.
D. H_2O has accumulated in the ventilator tubing.

82. The most accurate method of determining how well an emphysema patient is ventilating is by

A. Measuring peak flow.
B. Measuring FRC.
C. Obtaining ABG samples.
D. Measuring SpO_2.

83. After repeated attempts to wean a patient from mechanical ventilation without success, the respiratory therapist should recommend obtaining which of the following values?

A. Serum electrolytes
B. Peak flow studies
C. Cardiac enzymes
D. BUN level

84. A ventilator patient is on a PEEP of 8 cm H_2O and an F_{IO_2} of 0.50. After increasing the PEEP to 10 cm H_2O, his Q_T drops from 4.8 L/min to 3.3 L/min. The respiratory therapist should recommend which of the following?

A. Increase the PEEP to 12 cm H_2O.
B. Decrease the PEEP to 8 cm H_2O and increase the F_{IO_2} to 0.60.
C. Discontinue PEEP.
D. Maintain the PEEP at 10 cm H_2O and increase the F_{IO_2} to 0.60.

85. Which of the following could cause an increase in peak inspiratory pressure on a volume ventilator?

    I. Decreased C_L
    II. Decreased Raw
    III. Partially occluded ET tube
    IV. High inspiratory flow setting

A. I and II only
B. II and III only
C. I, III, and IV only
D. I, II, III, and IV

86. Before administering IPPB, the respiratory therapist notes subcutaneous emphysema around the neck tissues of the patient. Which of the following should the therapist do at this time?

A. Administer the IPPB and recommend a chest radiograph.
B. Measure the patient's SpO_2.
C. Administer the IPPB using a lower inspiratory pressure.
D. Withhold the IPPB and recommend a chest radiograph.

87. The following ventilator settings are recorded on a patient.

Mode	Control
Ventilator rate	10/min
V_T	800 mL
FIO_2	0.40
PEEP	6 cm H_2O
Inspiratory flow rate	40 L/min

Based on this information, the I:E is which of the following?

A. 1:1
B. 1:2
C. 1:3
D. 1:4

88. The I:E ratio alarm is sounding on a volume ventilator. Which of the following is the most appropriate ventilator setting change to correct this problem?

A. Increase the flow rate.
B. Decrease the V_T.
C. Add a 1-sec inspiratory hold.
D. Increase the ventilator rate.

89. The following data have been recorded for a patient on a volume ventilator.

CVP	10 mm Hg
PAP	48/26 mm Hg
PCWP	10 mm Hg
Q_T	5.8 L/min

Based on these data, the patient most likely has

A. Pulmonary hypertension.
B. Mitral valve regurgitation.
C. Aortic stenosis.
D. Right ventricular failure.

90. Which of the following indicates a ventilator patient is most likely ready to be weaned?

    I. V_D/V_T of 0.65
    II. MIP of −28 cm H_2O
    III. VC of 17 mL/kg of body weight

A. II only
B. I and II only
C. II and III only
D. I, II, and III

91. A ventilator patient suddenly becomes tachycardic and agitated, and the high-pressure alarm begins sounding. The respiratory therapist auscultates diminished breath sounds in the right lung and palpates the trachea left of midline. Which of the following should the therapist recommend at this time?

A. Get a stat chest radiograph.
B. Increase the ventilator rate.
C. Insert a needle into the second intercostal space.
D. Suction the patient's ET tube.

92. The H_2O in the H_2O-seal bottle of a chest-tube drainage system fluctuates 5 to 10 cm H_2O as the patient is breathing. This is most likely the result of which of the following?

A. A leak in the system.
B. A clot in the tubing.
C. The chest tube has slipped out of the pleural space.
D. This is a normal occurrence with chest-tube drainage systems.

93. A patient enters the emergency department complaining of shortness of breath with a respiratory rate of 32/min and a V_T that fluctuates between 350 mL and 500 mL. Which of the following is the most appropriate device to deliver approximately 40% O_2 to this patient?

A. Nasal cannula at 5 L/min
B. Simple O_2 mask at 6 L/min
C. Partial rebreathing mask at 8 L/min
D. Air-entrainment mask

94. A patient is on a volume ventilator with an HME. Over the past 4 hours, the respiratory therapist notes that the patient's sputum has become thicker and more difficult to suction through the catheter. Which of the following should the therapist recommend at this time?

A. Replace the HME with a heated humidifier.
B. Suction the patient more frequently.
C. Increase the suction pressure to −140 mm Hg.
D. Use a larger suction catheter.

95. While making O_2 rounds, the respiratory therapist notices very little mist being produced by a jet nebulizer attached to an aerosol mask. Which of the following may be causing this?

    I. The capillary tube filter is clogged.
    II. The jet is obstructed.
    III. The liter flow is too low.

A. I only
B. I and II only
C. II and III only
D. I, II, and III

96. The respiratory therapist is using a size 12 French suction catheter to suction a female patient who is intubated with a 6.5-mm ET tube. The therapist is

having difficulty aspirating the thick secretions. Which of the following is the most appropriate action to take?

A. *Change to a coudé suction catheter.*
B. *Increase the suction pressure to −150 mm Hg.*
C. *Instill 5 mL of normal saline down the ET tube.*
D. *Change to a size 14 French suction catheter.*

97. The respiratory therapist has instilled air into a ventilator patient's ET-tube cuff so that a slight leak is heard with a stethoscope at peak inspiration. The peak inspiratory pressure is 30 cm H_2O at the time. Four hours later, after suctioning the patient and draining H_2O out of the ventilator tubing, the therapist notes the peak inspiratory pressure is 40 cm H_2O. Which of the following is true regarding this patient's ET-tube cuff care?

   I. The leak around the cuff is larger.
   II. Air should be removed from the cuff.
   III. Minimal leak technique should be used at 40 cm H_2O.

A. *I only*
B. *II only*
C. *I and III only*
D. *II and III only*

98. While ventilating a patient with a manual resuscitator, ABG results indicate a PaO_2 of 50 torr. Which of the following would increase the O_2 being delivered by the bag?

   I. Add a reservoir to the bag.
   II. Increase the O_2 flow to the bag.
   III. Increase the ventilation rate.

A. *I only*
B. *I and II only*
C. *II and III only*
D. *I, II, and III*

99. The peak inspiratory pressure has dropped from 34 cm H_2O to 5 cm H_2O on a volume ventilator operating in the assist/control mode. The respiratory therapist notices the exhaled volume spirometer is filling during inspiration. Which of the following is the most likely cause of this?

A. *The exhalation valve is malfunctioning.*
B. *There is a leak around the ET-tube cuff.*
C. *The pressure manometer is malfunctioning.*
D. *No problem exists because this is a normal occurrence.*

100. A patient is on a volume ventilator set on a V_T of 700 mL, but the exhaled volume display reads 400 mL. After finding no leaks in the tubing and connections, the respiratory therapist wants to determine the volume the ventilator is actually delivering. To most accurately measure this volume, the therapist should place a respirometer

A. *At the exhalation valve.*
B. *At the ventilator outlet.*
C. *At the humidifier outlet.*
D. *At the patient wye connector.*

END OF ADVANCED PRACTITIONER (RRT) WRITTEN PRACTICE EXAM

GO TO THE ANSWER KEY/EXPLANATION SECTION AND GRADE YOUR TEST

Advanced Practitioner Written Registry Exam: Practice Test

Passing Score: 70 correct answers
After each answer is the explanation for why the choice is correct and the complexity level of the question. For an explanation of each complexity level, see page 208.

1. B, Capillary refill is determined by compressing the nailbed of the patient and, after releasing it, observing the time required for the nail to return to its original color. Normal refill time is less than 3 sec. The result in the problem indicates decreased perfusion to the extremities, which could be caused by decreased Q$_T$. Both extremities should be checked, since reduced perfusion to one extremity could be the result of vasospasm or a clot. (Analysis)

2. C, The reservoir bag of a partial or non-rebreathing mask should remain $\frac{1}{2}$ to $\frac{1}{3}$ full at all times during the breathing cycle. If it collapses at any time, it is an indication of inadequate flow to the mask. (Recall)

3. A, Transcutaneous monitoring reflects Pao$_2$, while the other choices monitor other parameters. (Pulse oximetry, Spo$_2$; capnography, PETco_2; pulmonary artery catheter, Pvo$_2$) (Application)

4. C, Regardless of what the ECG monitor is recording, if the patient has no pulse, compressions must be started immediately. An example of this rare situation is electromechanical dissociation (EMD), also referred to as pulseless electrical activity (PEA), in which the ECG monitor does not reflect the actual mechanical activity of the heart. (Analysis)

5. B, If the low pressure alarm is sounding, either leaks are present somewhere in the system or the alarm is not set appropriately. It should be set about 2 to 4 cm H$_2$O below the CPAP level. (Analysis)

6. A, This type of O$_2$ system conserves O$_2$ by sensing the patient's inspiratory effort and delivering O$_2$ during inspiration only. (Recall)

7. B, The SPAG nebulizer is used to deliver the antiviral drug ribavirin for the treatment of RSV infec-

tion, often referred to as acute infectious bronchiolitis. (Recall)

8. D, The patient has an abnormally high Hb level of 20 gm/dL of which 80% is saturated with O$_2$. That is 16 gm/dL of saturated Hb, which is a normal value. The tissues should be receiving adequate O$_2$ supply. For cyanosis to be present, there must 5 g/dL of unsaturated Hb. In this example, there are only 4 g/dL of unsaturated Hb, therefore the patient would not be cyanotic. (Application)

9. B, The symptoms this patient exhibits suggest a pneumothorax. A stat chest radiograph should be ordered to confirm the diagnosis so that proper treatment may be instituted. (Analysis)

10. C, The air/O$_2$ ratio for 30% is 8:1. Add the ratio parts together and multiply by the flow rate to determine the total flow rate.

$$8 + 1 = 9$$
$$9 \times 4 = 36 \text{ L/min}$$

(Application)

11. A, The sensitivity control determines the inspiratory effort required to cycle the machine into the inspiratory phase. If more than -2 cm H$_2$O is required by the patient to cycle the machine on, the sensitivity should be increased. (Application)

12. C, If the patient's hypoxemia requires more than 60% O$_2$, CPAP should be initiated to open up more alveoli for improved oxygenation. (Analysis)

13. D, This COPD patient is clearly chronically hypoxemic and hypercapnic, as evidenced by the initial ABG results on 2 L/min. When the ABG results reveal elevated HCO$_3^-$ levels on admission, compensation of the respiratory acidosis is occurring. This patient's primary problem is his Pao$_2$, which should be maintained in the 50-to-65-torr range. As the liter flow was increased, the patient's ABG results worsened, as reflected by an increasing Paco$_2$ and a decreasing pH. Automatically, the thought of knocking out the patient's "hypoxic drive" comes to mind. But for this to occur, the Pao$_2$ must be higher than 65 torr. The Pao$_2$ is

only 52 torr, which is normal for this patient. The cause of the patient's deteriorating ventilatory status is not the result of the removal of the hypoxic drive stimulus but of a worsening pulmonary condition. The patient needs to be ventilated more effectively and this may be done initially with noninvasive ventilation, such as BiPAP with a nasal mask. The patient avoids being intubated, yet still receives positive pressure ventilation. It buys some time for the patient, so the pulmonary problem may be treated to prevent the patient from being intubated and placed on mechanical ventilation. Since COPD patients are typically difficult to wean from the ventilator, it is to their advantage to attempt noninvasive mask ventilation first. (Analysis)

14. A, To approximate the normal PaO_2 on a given O_2 percentage, multiply the percentage times 5. This patient is on 50% O_2. So: $50 \times 5 = 250$, therefore the PaO_2 of 253 is consistent with the FiO_2 the patient is on. (Analysis)

15. C, The $C(a-v)O_2$ is the difference between the O_2 content in arterial and venous blood. The normal value is 4 to 6 vol%. An elevated $C(a-v)O_2$ indicates a greater difference between the two, suggesting less O_2 in the venous blood. This results from a decreased QT. Even though blood is flowing through the circulatory system at a slower rate (decreased QT) the tissues will extract the O_2 at the same rate. This causes less O_2 content in the venous blood, resulting in an increased $C(a-v)O_2$. Another value measured in this question that is not normal is the PCWP, sometimes referred to as PAWP. The normal value is 4 to 12 mm Hg. A decreased value, as in this problem, means a lower pressure in the left side of the heart as a result of the decreased venous return caused by the decreased QT or hypovolemia. This is best treated by increasing fluids. (Analysis)

16. D, All three of these parameters meet the criteria for the initiation of ventilator weaning.
    A. MIP of more than 20 cm H_2O
    B. $P(A-a)O_2$ of less than 350 torr on 100% O_2
    C. VC of more than 15 mL/kg of body weight
    (Recall)

17. A, Helium is a trace element in atmospheric air, therefore a helium analyzer would read zero when calibrated to room air. (Recall)

18. D, This patient has a slightly higher measured shunt than normal (2% to 5%). Pulmonary edema, lobar pneumonia, and pneumothorax would all cause shunts of more than 6%. Hypoventilation is an example of a V/Q mismatch, which will not result in increased shunt levels. (Analysis)

19. D, To determine V/Q ratio, ventilation (represented by the numerator) is divided by perfusion (represented by the denominator). Normal alveolar ventilation is approximately 4 L/min, with an average pulmonary blood flow of about 5 L/min. Divide ventilation by perfusion (4/5); the result is a 0.8 V/Q ratio. In the normal individual in the upright position, the upper portion of the lung receives greater ventilation than perfusion and therefore has an increased V/Q ratio (more than 0.8). Perfusion is greater than ventilation in the lower portions of the lung as a result of gravity, therefore the V/Q ratio is decreased (less than 0.8) in those areas. In this question, perfusion is decreased while ventilation remains normal, therefore the V/Q ratio is increased (more than 0.8). This is a classic example of a pulmonary embolism, in which pulmonary blood flow is obstructed while ventilation remains normal. (Application)

20. C, Pressure in the cuff should be maintained at no more than 20 mm Hg. If there is twice that amount of pressure and a leak is still present, the tube is too small and should be replaced with a larger one. (Analysis)

21. C, The reservoir bag should never completely collapse as the patient inspires. If it does, it indicates inadequate flow to the H-valve setup. (Analysis)

22. B, This infant's ABG results reveal respiratory acidemia as the result of an increased $PaCO_2$. This indicates ventilatory failure that may be reversed by increasing minute ventilation. On a pressure ventilator, this is accomplished by either increasing the inspiratory pressure or ventilator rate. (Analysis)

23. C, Total immersion in a liquid disinfectant and sterilant, such as Cidex, is necessary to expose both the inside and outside of the bronchoscope to the cleaning agent. Submerging the bronchoscope for 10 to 15 minutes in Cidex will produce disinfection; soaking for 3–10 hours produces sterility and is also common practice. This should be done after each use. (Application)

24. B, The air/O_2 ratio for 30% is 8:1. Add the two ratio parts together and multiply by the lowest choice of the flow rates given that results in a total flow of at least 40 L/min. (Analysis)

25. B, The ECG shows sinus bradycardia, which is most likely the result of hypoxemia caused by placing the patient in a head-down (Trendelenburg) position to drain the right lower lobe. (Analysis)

26. C, This question is asking what complications of bronchoscopy would result in high peak inspiratory pressures. All of the choices are complications of bronchoscopy, but only hypotension **would not** result in high peak ventilatory pressures. (Analysis)

27. B, Using the clinical shunt equation:

$$QS/QT = \frac{(PAO_2 - PaO_2) \times 0.003}{(CaO_2 - CvO_2) + (PAO_2 - PaO_2) \times 0.003}$$

The P(A-a)O_2 is given as 100 torr. The arterial to venous O_2 content difference must be determined.

$$CaO_2 = 1.34 \times 14 \text{ (Hb)} \times 0.93 \text{ (}O_2 \text{ sat)} = 17.45 \text{ vol\%}$$

(This represents O_2 bound to Hb.)

$$0.003 \times 70 \text{ (Pa}O_2\text{)} = 0.21 \text{ vol\%}$$

(Represents O_2 dissolved in plasma.)

$CaO_2 = 17.45 + 0.21 = 17.66$ vol%
$CvO_2 = 1.34 \times 14 \times 0.72$ (SvO_2) $= 13.51$ vol%
0.003×34 (PvO_2) $= 0.10$
$CvO_2 = 13.51 + 0.10 = 13.61$ vol%
$CaO_2 - CvO_2 = 17.66 - 13.61 = 4$ vol%

Now, plug into the shunt equation:

$$\frac{100 \times 0.003}{4 + (100 \times 0.003)} = \frac{0.3}{4.3} = 7\%$$

(Analysis)

28. A. The patient is hypotensive, which indicates a decreased SVR. PCWP, a measure of left atrial pressure, is normal; therefore, left atrial pressure cannot be increased. Since QT is decreased, SV would also be decreased. The PAP is elevated, which indicates an **increased** resistance to blood flow in the pulmonary vasculature. (Analysis)

29. B, A 10% pneumothorax is relatively small. A chest tube is not indicated; a needle aspiration is indicated only when a tension pneumothorax is present, which is not the case here, based on the patient's respiratory status. O_2 therapy is indicated because the patient is in mild respiratory distress, and O_2 will help absorb the air in the pleural space. Pulse oximetry should be employed to continuously monitor the SpO_2 level to help determine the patient's oxygenation status. (Analysis)

30. A, The ETC is easy to insert and may be used temporarily in place of an ET tube if intubation is difficult. Intubation should be reattempted but, until then, the ETC serves as an adequate tube through which to manually ventilate. See chapter on management of the airway for further discussion. (Analysis)

31. D, All three of these therapies aid in secretion mobilization and should be considered when secretion removal is difficult. (Analysis)

32. B, Leaks of any kind result in reduced exhaled volume readings. A low H_2O level in the humidifier will result in more volume being compressed into the walls of the device, resulting in less volume being delivered to the patient. But the volume leaves the humidifier during expiration and is measured as part of the exhaled V_T. (Analysis)

33. A, The transcutaneous O_2 monitor is calibrated to room air while off the infant. Therefore, the cause could not be related to the infant's hemodynamic status. The problem must be with the monitor itself. (Application)

34. B, The initial amount of energy is 200 J and, if defibrillation is not reversed, a maximum of 360 J may be used. (Analysis)

35. A, Since the patient remains hypoxemic on 60% O_2, the PEEP level should be increased, not the FiO_2. The patient is hyperventilating, but in response to hypoxemia. Therefore, the respiratory rate or V_T should not be decreased. As oxygenation improves, hyperventilation should subside resulting in the PaCO_2 returning to normal. (Analysis)

36. B, The PEEP level that produces the best static C_L indicates the optimal PEEP level. There is no need to calculate static compliance at each PEEP level in this question. Simply subtract the PEEP level from its corresponding plateau pressure, and the lowest number of the four choices will produce the highest number when divided into the 600-mL V_T. The difference in the PEEP and plateau pressure for each choice is: A, 20; B, 18; C, 20; D, 21. Therefore, choice B represents optimal PEEP, because 18 divided into 600 results in the highest compliance of the four choices. (Analysis)

37. B, 24/10 mm Hg is a normal value for PAP; therefore, when this value is observed during the insertion of a Swan-Ganz catheter, you would know it was in the pulmonary artery. (Recall)

38. B, A pressure support of 25 cm H_2O is too high to begin the weaning process. The pressure support needed to overcome resistance to breathing through the ventilator tubing and ET tube is only about 5 to 10 cm H_2O, which is ideally the level we should target in the weaning process. (Analysis)

39. B, An FEV_1/FVC above 75% indicates obstructive disease is not present. Even though the FEV_1 is decreased, when coupled with a normal FEV_1/FVC, a restrictive process is the cause. Patients with restrictive disease have no trouble exhaling air normally but have difficulty getting air in on inspiration. The reason the FEV_1 is decreased is not because of airway obstruction during exhalation, but because the patient did not get the predicted normal volume of air in to begin with; therefore, a normal volume of air is not exhaled out in 1 sec. But when the FEV_1 is compared to the **patient's** FVC (not the predicted value), which is what the FEV_1/FVC is, a normal value is observed. Also ruling out obstructive disease is a normal TLC (which would normally be increased in obstructive

disease) and a peak flow higher than the predicted value (which would normally be below normal in obstructive disease). (Analysis)

40. C, This question is much like question 13, with the same type of scenario but with one distinct difference. When the O_2 flow was increased from 2 L/min to 5 L/min, the patient's $PaCO_2$ not only increased, but the PaO_2 increased dramatically to 84 torr. This high PaO_2 (more than 65 torr) is sufficient to reduce the drive for this COPD patient to breathe, therefore the $PaCO_2$ level began increasing resulting in the patient becaming drowsy and lethargic. This is called CO_2 narcosis, which refers to higher levels of $PaCO_2$ having a narcotic-like effect on the patient. By decreasing the liter flow to 3 L/min, PaO_2 should decrease and, as long as the PaO_2 is maintained in the 50-to-65-torr range, CO_2 narcosis will subside and the patient's ventilatory status will improve. Again, as mentioned earlier, there is some debate about the validity of the "hypoxic drive" breathing mechanism, but you should understand it for the examination. (Analysis)

41. A, It is appropriate in COPD patients to attempt noninvasive ventilation initially, because if it is successful, intubation can be avoided. (Analysis)

42. B, With unilateral lung disease or other conditions where only one lung is affected (e.g., single lung transplantation), damage is often done to the good lung by positive pressure ventilation. By using special ET tubes and separate ventilators for each lung, this damage to the unaffected lung can be avoided. (Recall)

43. D, A drop in mixed venous PO_2 is indicative of a decreased Q_T. This drop in PvO_2 occurs because the tissues extract O_2 from the blood at the same rate, even though the blood is flowing slower past the tissues (decreased Q_T). Therefore, more O_2 is extracted and by the time the blood reaches the pulmonary artery, which is where PvO_2 is measured, there is less O_2 in the blood. (Application)

44. C, FRC is the amount of air remaining in the lungs following a normal exhalation. Since emphysema patients trap air during exhalation, more air stays in the lungs after exhalation and FRC increases. (Analysis)

45. B, The high-pressure alarm indicates resistance to gas flow through the tubing or airways. Secretions can cause an increased Raw and, by suctioning the patient, Raw can be decreased, with a corresponding decrease in peak inspiratory pressure. (Analysis)

46. A, This patient's pulmonary wedge pressure (PCWP) is normal (e.g., 4 to 12 mm Hg), which indicates normal left heart function. Both the PAP and PVR are increased, which indicates restriction to blood flow through the pulmonary arterial system, most likely the result of a pulmonary em-

bolism. Overhydration should not be suspected because the PCWP is normal, not elevated as seen in overhydration. (Analysis)

47. B, The affinity of Hb for CO is 200 to 250 times greater than for O_2. High PaO_2 levels will decrease this affinity, so that Hb will release CO more readily. This is the reason a patient exposed to CO should be placed on a non-rebreathing mask initially. The higher the PaO_2, the more CO is released from the Hb. By placing the patient in an HBO chamber, 100% O_2 can be delivered at 2 to 3 atm. This means PaO_2 levels of 2 to 3 times normal on 100% O_2 can be achieved. Normal PaO_2 on 100% O_2 is 500 to 600 torr. This means PaO_2 levels on 2 to 3 times atmospheric pressure may reach 1000 to 1800 torr. This enhances CO release from Hb. (Recall)

48. D, You are looking for the false statements in this question. It is easy to start looking for untrue choices, then select a true choice. Choice A is true since the $PaCO_2$ is 68 torr, which indicates hypoventilation. By calculating the $P(A-a)O_2$, you will find it to be normal:

$$PAO_2 = (747 - 47) \times 0.21 - (PaCO_2 + 10)$$
$$= 700 \times 0.21 - 78$$
$$= 69 \text{ torr}$$
$$PAO_2 - PaO_2 = 69 - 60 = 9 \text{ torr}$$

Normal $P(A-a)O_2$ on room air is less than 15 torr. This patient does not have ABG values that reflect chronic hypoxemia, or the HCO_3^- would be elevated to compensate for the chronic hypercapnia that accompanies chronic hypoxemia. Therefore, choices II and III are the false statements. (Analysis)

49. D, Remember, on the **initial** ventilator setup, to select a ventilator rate between 8/min and 12/min. Based on the recorded height and weight, this female patient is obese and we need to calculate ideal body weight to determine the correct V_T setting.

$$105 + 5 \text{ (height in inches} - 60)$$
$$105 + 5 \text{ } (65 - 60)$$
$$105 + 25 = 130 \text{ lb}$$

To convert 130 lb to kg:

$$\frac{130 \text{ lb}}{2.2 \text{ lb/kg}} = 59 \text{ kg}$$

The initial V_T setting should be 10 to 12 mL/kg. (Analysis)

50. C, This volume tracing shows the volume not returning to baseline, indicating a low exhaled V_T.

Respiratory Care Exam Review

This results from a leak somewhere in the tubing circuit, around the ET-tube cuff or out the chest tube drainage system. (Analysis)

51. B, Pressure control ventilation is a useful mode for patients with noncompliant (stiff) lungs, such as those seen in patients with ARDS. Volume ventilation on ARDS patients leads to high peak pressures and an increased potential of barotrauma by overdistention of the alveoli. This leads to pneumothorax. Using inspiratory pressures that deliver lower V_T (6–8 mL/kg) and maintaining plateau pressures at 35 cm H_2O or less will reduce the risk of overdistention of alveoli. (Analysis)

52. D, All three of these can be obtained by using indirect calorimetry and are all important in predicting how successful weaning might be. (Recall)

53. B, Optimal PEEP is determined in this PEEP study as the level that produces the highest $P\overline{v}O_2$. As the PEEP level is increased, $P\overline{v}O_2$ will increase. But the PEEP level at which $P\overline{v}O_2$ decreases is the point at which QT has decreased. Go back to the PEEP level **before** the drop in $P\overline{v}O_2$. (Analysis)

54. A, One complication of thoracentesis is pneumothorax. A patient exhibiting these signs and symptoms, especially after a thoracentesis, should make you suspect a pneumothorax, which needs to be confirmed by chest radiograph. (Application)

55. C, An acidic pH (7.26) is caused by either an increased $PaCO_2$ level or a decreased HCO_3^- level, neither of which are observed in the ABG values. Therefore, we must assume laboratory error and repeat the ABG sample. (Analysis)

56. D, Because He/O_2 mixtures are lighter than oxygen mixtures, leaks around the mask and exhalation ports are more prevalent. A tight-fitting nonrebreathing mask reduces the potential for leaks. (Analysis)

57. B,

$$PAO_2 = [(PB - 47) \times FiO_2] - PaCO_2 + 10$$
$$= [(747 - 47) \times 0.60] - 45 + 10$$
$$= 420 - 55 = 365 \text{ torr}$$

$$PAO_2 - PaO_2 = 365 - 90 = 275 \text{ torr}$$

Be careful working a problem like this. If you look at the choices after calculating PAO_2, you notice choice D is 365 torr. But the question is asking what the A-a gradient is, not the alveolar PO_2. On almost all of the mathematical calculations on the test, there will be choices for the most commonly made errors. So check your work carefully before moving to the next question. (Application)

58. C, Even though the patient's VC is acceptable (16 mL/kg), the MIP should be at least -20 cm H_2O and the V_D/V_T is still too high (normal value is 25% to 35%). (Analysis)

59. B, The only abnormal PFT value in this question is the diffusion capacity (D_{LCO}). The D_{LCO} is a measurement of the diffusion of CO across the alveolar capillary membrane into the pulmonary capillaries. Although it is typically decreased in patients with emphysema as well as patients with pulmonary fibrosis, a patient with emphysema will not have a normal FEV_1 or FEV_1/FVC ratio, as seen in this question. The formation of fibrous tissue in the lung results in decreased C_L as well as decreased capacity of gas to cross the alveolar capillary membrane. (Analysis)

60. A, The longer the time that positive pressure is in the airways, the higher the MAP. (Analysis)

61. D, The patient should never have to initiate more than -2 cm H_2O to cycle the machine into inspiration. The sensitivity control adjusts the amount of negative pressure the patient must generate to cycle the IPPB machine on. Any leaks in the system or around the mouth can make it difficult for the patient to cycle the machine into inspiration as well. (Analysis)

62. C, Refer to explanation for question 15. (Analysis)

63. A, The normal $P_{E}CO_2$ is 6% to 7%. If the CO_2 reads in this range, it indicates the ET tube is in the airway. If the tube is in the esophagus, the reading would be near zero. (Analysis)

64. D, The patient's $PaCO_2$ is slightly decreased, indicating mild hyperventilation. This may be corrected by decreasing the patient's V_T or ventilator rate. Since this patient is obviously being weaned, reducing the rate will continue the weaning process. (Analysis)

65. B, The 50-cc tubing attached to the opposite end of the T-piece (Briggs adaptor) serves as a reservoir for the O_2 that is continuously flowing through the T-piece past the patient. When the patient inspires, gas flowing through the T-piece as well as from the reservoir will enter the ET tube or tracheostomy tube for the patient's inspired gas supply. If the reservoir falls off, room air will likely be drawn in, diluting the supplemental O_2, resulting in a decrease in the delivered O_2 percentage. (Analysis)

66. B, Inspiratory time is calculated as follows:
Total cycle time divided by total I:E ratio parts.

$$\text{Total cycle time} = \frac{60}{\text{rate}}$$
$$= \frac{60}{30} = 2 \text{ sec}$$

If the I:E ratio is 1:3:

$$1 + 3 = 4$$
$$\text{Inspiratory time} = \frac{2 \text{ sec}}{4} = \textbf{0.5 sec}$$

To check your work, go back and determine the expiratory time. If total breath time is 2 sec and inspiratory time is 0.5 sec, the expiratory time is 2 sec minus 0.5 sec, or 1.5 sec. Three times 0.5 is 1.5, therefore the I : E ratio is 1 : 3, which is stated in the question, and therefore you know you have made a correct calculation. (Application)

67. A, This ECG strip shows ventricular tachycardia, which is a life-threatening arrhythmia and must be reversed immediately. This is accomplished by defibrillation. (Analysis)

68. D, A "damped" wave form renders inaccurate pressure readings making proper troubleshooting measures important. This type of wave may be caused by air bubbles or clots in the transducer or tubing or by the catheter resting against the wall of the artery. (Analysis)

69. C

$$\dot{V}_E = RR \times V_T$$
$$= 15 \times 0.55 \text{ L}$$
$$= 8.25, \text{ or } 8.3 \text{ L}$$

Remember, if the question asks to determine **alveolar** minute ventilation, subtract about 1 mL/lb of body weight from the V_T to estimate anatomic V_D, then multiply by the respiratory rate (RR). (Application)

70. B, A polysomnogram is a sleep study that continuously measures the patient's O_2 saturation, EEG, ECG, apnea periods, eye movement, and chest and abdominal movement and traces them on a graph. (Analysis)

71. A, The distal tip of the UAC should rest at the level of T6 to T10. If the catheter is placed too low, interference with blood flow to the lower extremities may occur and would be detected by cyanosis of the legs or feet. (Analysis)

72. A, If there is a leak around the bag intake valve, the bag will not pressurize as O_2 leaks out of the valve. Since all the bags we use to manually ventilate are self-inflating bags, even if there is no O_2 flowing into the bag, and if there are no leaks in the system, the bag will pressurize when compressed. The only problem is that the patient is receiving only room air from the bag, not supplemental O_2. (Analysis)

73. C, The Bourdon gauge measures pressure, not flow. The gauge is recalibrated in liters per minute when used as a flow-metering device. If the tubing becomes kinked, back pressure builds in the gauge and the reading goes up. (Analysis)

74. D, After setting up a cannula and kinking the tubing, a whistle should be heard coming from the humidifier. This is the pressure pop-off valve indicating that there are no leaks in the setup. If the

pop-off valve is not heard, there is a leak present, and the therapist should check for leaks around the jar top or in the tubing itself. (Analysis)

75. C, This chest radiograph is typical for a patient with severe emphysema. The hyperinflation seen on the radiograph will result in an increased AP chest diameter (barrel chest). Right ventricular hypertrophy (enlarged right heart) is caused from chronic pulmonary hypertension, which results from chronic hypoxemia, which, in turn, results in right-sided heart failure (cor pulmonale). Because of this, blood from the right heart backs up into the venous system, leading to distended neck veins and pooling of blood in the ankles (pedal edema). (Analysis)

76. D, Muscular paralysis should be initiated when the patient fights the ventilator. Each time the high-pressure alarm is activated, inspiration ends without delivering the set V_T. If this continues, the patient's $PaCO_2$ will begin to increase and the patient will go into ventilatory failure. By paralyzing the patient with pancuronium bromide (Pavulon), ventilation can continue uninterrupted. (Analysis)

77. A, A patient who is anemic (low Hb level) may have a normal SpO_2 value. But if the patient's Hb level is only 8 g/dL (normal value is 12 to 16 g/dL), the tissues are not receiving an adequate amount of O_2. Notice this patient is not cyanotic. For cyanosis to be present, there must be 5 g/dL of unsaturated Hb. This patient may have a Hb level of 8 g/dL and be 98% saturated, meaning the patient is not be cyanotic, but the patient is most likely hypoxic. Do not be deceived by a normal SpO_2 reading. Always check the Hb level. Remember, 99% of O_2 delivery to the tissues is accomplished bound to Hb. (Analysis)

78. D, It must be heated because condensation forms in the tubing when heated aerosol travels through the tubing, which is exposed to room temperature. Since the tubing is cooler and can't hold as much water, condensation forms in the tubing. H_2O in the aerosol tubing causes a resistance to gas flow, resulting in back pressure into the nebulizer. As pressure increases in the nebulizer, less air is able to be entrained into the nebulizer through the entrainment ports. This results in an increased O_2 percentage delivered from the nebulizer. (Analysis)

79. D, Higher pressures and a longer time with positive pressure in the airway will increase the MAP. (Analysis)

80. D, The lower the peak pressure and number of positive pressure breaths, the fewer cardiac side effects. In the assist/control mode, every breath is a positive pressure breath, even if the patient breathes above the set rate. SIMV and the control mode will deliver the same number of positive

pressure breaths if set on the same rate, but in this problem, the control mode rate was 12/min (choice B), while the SIMV mode rate was 10/min (choice D). Also, the SIMV rate of 10/min had a V_T of 800 mL, rather than 900 mL in the control mode. The lower the V_T, the lower the PIP. (Analysis)

81. C, Plateau pressures are getting progressively higher, which indicates more pressure is required to ventilate the alveoli on the same volume. This means that the lungs are getting stiffer and harder to ventilate, indicating a decreasing static C_L. (Analysis)

82. C, The effectiveness of any patient's ventilation is measured by the Pa_{CO_2}. This is best accomplished by ABG analysis. (Analysis)

83. A, Determination of the level of specific electrolytes that affect muscle strength, such as potassium, magnesium, phosphorus, sodium, and chloride, is essential. If the levels of these electrolytes are low, the muscles of ventilation may be too weak for the patient to be weaned from the ventilator. Supplemental IV administration of these electrolytes should be included in patient care to increase muscle strength. (Analysis)

84. B, The increased PEEP level decreased Q_T; therefore, the PEEP should be reduced back to its original level. The hypoxemia should be treated by increasing the Fi_{O_2}. (Analysis)

85. C, A decreased C_L indicates the lungs are stiffer and harder to ventilate; therefore, more pressure is required to ventilate the lungs. Any resistance to flow, such as a partially plugged ET tube, increases inspiratory pressure, and the higher the inspiratory flow, the more resistance to flow as it rubs against the sides of the ventilator tubing, causing an increased inspiratory pressure. (Analysis)

86. D, Subcutaneous emphysema, or air in the subcutaneous tissues, indicates an air leak from the lung. Positive pressure should not be introduced into the airway because this may further complicate the potential pneumothorax. A chest radiograph should be ordered to confirm the diagnosis and determine the severity of the leak. (Analysis)

87. D
I:E ratio is calculated as follows:

$$I:E = \frac{\text{inspiratory flow}}{\dot{V}_E}$$
$$= \frac{40}{0.8\ L \times 10} = \frac{40}{8} = 5$$

Subtract 1 from 5 to get the ratio.
I:E ratio = 1:4
(Application)

88. A, An inverse I:E ratio alarm indicates that inspiration is longer than expiration. To shorten the inspi-

ratory time on a volume ventilator, the V_T may be decreased or the flow rate may be increased. We do not want to alter alveolar ventilation by decreasing V_T to shorten inspiratory time, so getting the volume to the patient faster by increasing the flow will end inspiration sooner, decreasing the inspiratory time. This will return the I:E ratio back to a more normal ratio of 1:2 or 1:3. (Application)

89. A, Both the CVP and PAP are abnormal values in this question. Since the PCWP is normal, indicating adequate left heart function, mitral valve regurgitation and aortic stenosis can be ruled out. (These conditions would cause an elevated PCWP.) The CVP is elevated (normal value is less than 6 mm Hg). Since PAP is also elevated, we must suspect pulmonary hypertension. Pulmonary vasoconstriction causes an increase in CVP as the right side of the heart must work harder to pump blood through constricted pulmonary vessels. The CVP would be much higher than 10 mm Hg if right ventricular failure was present. (Analysis)

90. C, V_D/V_T should be less than 0.60; MIP should be at least -20 cm H_2O; and VC should be more than 15 mL/kg. (Recall)

91. C, The patient is exhibiting symptoms of a tension pneumothorax. Taking the time to get a chest radiograph is detrimental. This is a life-threatening situation, which requires immediate treatment. Inserting a needle into the second intercostal space will relieve pressure in the pleural space and mediastinum and allow the lung to reexpand. (Analysis)

92. D, During normal breathing, pleural pressure increases and decreases: this is indicated by the H_2O fluctuating in the H_2O-seal bottle. If the H_2O level is not fluctuating, a clot in the tube should be suspected. (Analysis)

93. D, Low-flow devices (choices A, B, and C) should never be set up on a patient with a respiratory rate of more than 25/min or an inconsistent V_T. We cannot determine what O_2 percentage we are delivering with these devices, either. A high-flow device, such as the air-entrainment mask, should be used. It can deliver more consistent O_2 percentages at higher flows than a low-flow device can. (Analysis)

94. A, An HME, or "artificial nose," provides less H_2O to the patient's airway than a conventional heated humidifier. HMEs are fine for some patients, but if secretions begin getting thicker, more H_2O must be delivered and a heated humidifier is indicated. (Analysis)

95. D, If the capillary tube is clogged, H_2O cannot be drawn up into it, so H_2O output diminishes. If the jet is obstructed, gas cannot pass through it as readily to create the pressure drop necessary to draw the H_2O up the capillary tube; therefore,

H_2O output decreases. An excessively low liter flow delivers less H_2O per minute, which is indicated by a decreased mist output. (Application)

96. C, Instilling saline down the ET tube will help loosen the secretions, making them easier to aspirate. The suction pressure should not exceed -120 mm Hg. A size 14 French suction catheter is too large for a 6.5-mm ET tube. To determine the proper size of catheter, multiply the ET tube size by two, then select the next smaller size (lower numbered) catheter. For example: 6.5 mm $\times$ 2 = 13. The next lowest numbered catheter size is a 12 French. Therefore, a No. 14 French catheter is too large. Suction catheter sizes: (Fr) 6 1/2, 8, 10, 12, 14, 16. (Analysis)

97. C, Minimal leak technique was initially performed when PIP was 30 cm H_2O. If the PIP increases to 40 cm H_2O, less pressure is exerted on the tracheal wall around the cuff at peak inspiration; this results in a larger leak around the cuff. Minimal leak technique should be done at the higher peak pressure so that not as much volume is lost around the cuff. (Analysis)

98. B, As a manual resuscitator is compressed, the O_2 inlet valve closes, preventing O_2 from entering the bag. As the bag is released, a negative pressure is created inside the bag, which draws air into it. If a reservoir filled with O_2 is attached at the O_2 inlet valve, O_2 enters the bag instead of room air. This increases the delivered O_2 percentage. A higher flow rate provides O_2 to the bag at a faster rate, making more O_2 available with each breath. Increasing the ventilation rate decreases the delivered O_2 percentage because less time is allowed for the bag to refill. Also, if the ventilation rate is too high, excessive amounts of CO_2 will be blown off, leading to respiratory alkalosis. Alkalosis results in a leftward shift of the HbO_2 dissociation curve. This causes Hb to have a greater affinity for O_2, meaning it will pick up O_2 more easily but will not release it as readily to the tissues. Alkalosis may also result in electrolyte imbalances. This is obviously detrimental during manual resuscitation. (Analysis)

99. A, The expiratory volume spirometer should receive gas during expiration only. The expiratory side of the circuit should be blocked by the exhalation valve during inspiration so that all the volume from the ventilator is delivered through the inspiratory side and on to the patient. If the spirometer is rising during inspiration, gas is flowing past a malfunctioning exhalation valve. Because of this leak around the valve, the peak pressure drops dramatically and the patient does not receive adequate ventilation. (Analysis)

100. B, To most accurately measure the volume delivered from the ventilator, the respirometer should be placed on the ventilator outlet (before the bacterial filter). Since leaks can occur throughout the circuit, the respirometer would not measure the volume as accurately downstream from the ventilator outlet. (Application)

Maximum score: 100
Incorrect answers: _____
Correct answers: _____
Minimum passing score: 70

INDEX

Note: Page numbers in *italics* refer to illustrations.